J. Freyschmidt · G. Freyschmidt

SKIBO-Diseases – Disorders Affecting the Skin and Bones

Springer

Berlin
Heidelberg
New York
Barcelona
Budapest
Hongkong
London
Mailand
Paris
Singapur
Tokio

J. Freyschmidt · G. Freyschmidt

SKIBO-Diseases
Disorders Affecting the Skin and Bones

A Clinical, Dermatologic, and Radiologic Synopsis

With 57 Figures in 236 Separate Illustrations, Some in Color
and 10 Tables

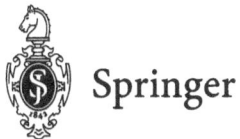 Springer

Prof. Dr. med. Jürgen Freyschmidt
Radiologische Klinik, Zentralkrankenhaus
St. Jürgen-Strasse, 28205 Bremen, Germany

Dr. med. Gisela Freyschmidt
Oberneulander Landstrasse 58, 28355 Bremen, Germany

Translator: Terry C. Telger, 6112 Waco Way, Forth Worth TX 76133, USA

Title of the original German edition:
Haut-, Schleimhaut- und Skeletterkrankungen – SKIBO-Diseases
© Springer-Verlag Berlin Heidelberg 1996. ISBN-13: 978-3-642-64159-6

ISBN-13: 978-3-642-64159-6   e-ISBN-13: 978-3-642-59867-8
DOI: 10.1007/978-3-642-59867-8

Library of Congress Cataloging-in-Publication Data
Freyschmidt, J. (Jürgen) [Haut-, Schleimhaut- und Skeletterkrankungen. English] SKIBO
diseases: disorders affecting the skin and bones: a clinical, dermatologic, and radiologic
synopsis / J. Freyschmidt, G. Freyschmidt. p. cm. Includes bibliographical references and
index.

1. Cutaneous manifestations of general diseases. 2. Musculoskeletal system - Diseases -
Diagnosis. 3. Skin - Radiography. 4. Diagnosis, Radioscopic. I. Freyschmidt, G. (Gisela)
II. Freyschmidt, J. (Jürgen) Haut-, Schleimhaut- und Skeletterkrankungen. English.
III. Title. [DNML: 1. Skin Manifestations. 2. Skin Diseases - diagnosis. 3. Bone Diseases - diag-
nosis. 4. Diagnosis, Differential. WR 143 F894h 1998a]   RL100.F74   1998   616.5-dc21
DNML/DLC 98-10617

© Springer-Verlag Berlin Heidelberg 1999
Softcover reprint of the hardcover 1st edition 1999

Cover Design: E. Kirchner, Heidelberg
Typesetting: K. Triltsch, Würzburg

SPIN: 10655970   21/3135-5 4 3 2 1 0 - Printed on acid free paper

For Carla

Preface

With the growing, necessary trend toward specialization in medicine, there is an increased likelihood that multisystem diseases with "interdisciplinary" features will be misclassified and misdiagnosed. Given the generally low prevalence of these diseases, at least for the present, even "generalists" cannot be expected to have the expertise to include such rare disorders in their primary differential diagnosis. But it is equally true that all patients have a right to an accurate diagnosis established by scientific and empirical means, regardless of whether a correct diagnosis will have different therapeutic implications than an incorrect one. Moreover, there are many rare congenital syndromes that, once recognized, should prompt a referral for genetic counseling.

Many of the diseases described in this monograph were correctly classified only because the authors, a long-married couple, were able to compare notes on unidentified, multisymptomatic disorders they saw in the hospital and office settings and pool the knowledge from their respective fields (dermatology and diagnostic radiology). The result of this collaborative effort is a practice-oriented monograph that will motivate diagnosing physicians to think of multisystem illnesses involving the skin, mucous membranes, and bones ("SKIBO" diseases) and render a specific diagnosis by interpreting the protean features of these diseases from a synoptic perspective. The critical step in making a correct diagnosis is to look specifically for symptoms that belong to another discipline (dermatology, orthopedics, internal medicine, radiology). Rather than try to interpret these changes "single handed," we hope that, with the help of this book, physicians will be able to suspect a SKIBO disease and recognize the need to seek proper specialist consultation in order to establish a diagnosis.

We thank Dr. Zimmermann-Schröder for her great help in procuring the dermatologic illustrations, many of which are from the collection of the Department of Dermatology (Director: Friedrich A. Bahmer, M. D., Ph. D.) of the Zentralkrankenhaus St. Juergen Strasse in Bremen.

Bremen, spring, 1998   The Authors

Contents

---

[1] Strictly speaking, the congenital disorders include some diseases and syndromes (e.g., pachydermoperiostosis and angiodysplasias) that are classified differently because of their dominant clinical and radiologic features.

Introduction

The etiology and pathogenesis of diseases that show synchronous or metachronous involvement of the skin, mucous membranes, and bones are well known in the case of some entities but are poorly understood in others. For example, in patients with mucosal inflammations due to immunvasculitis, symptoms will appear concomitantly or sequentially in anatomic regions with mucosal structures, involving for example the eyes, mouth, gastrointestinal tract, pleura, or the large and small joints of the axial and appendicular skeleton. While we know that the symptoms (e.g., conjunctivitis, diarrhea, joint swelling with limited motion) are based on the location of the inflamed mucosae, we do not yet know the principles that govern the timing of involvement of different organ systems in certain diseases.

A pattern of errors or defects simultaneously involving various known genes or gene locations gives rise to even more complex disorders with diverse symptoms that are not referable to a particular anatomic structure. An example is Gardner's syndrome.

Less is known about genetic syndromes that have not been adequately researched and are associated, perhaps randomly, with a combination of cutaneous and skeletal manifestations such as café-au-lait spots and nonossifying fibromas of bone or fibrous dysplasia.

Today for many disorders it is only speculated that they are caused by previously unknown genetic alterations that induce specific biochemical abnormalities in common basic structures of the skin and bone (i.e. collagen). Meanwhile there is hard scientific evidence that the proteoglycan loss is a common pathogenic principle for psoriatic arthritis and psoriatic spondylarthritis as well as for the mucocutaneous manifestations of psoriasis-associated musculoskeletal disorders that are genetically transmitted among others via the HLA-B27 locus. It would be fascinating to devote a whole chapter to similar disorders, but the authors of this book do not have the requisite expertise. Moreover, discoveries in molecular biology and other fields are progressing so swiftly that any information and hypotheses offered today may be outdated by the time the book is published. Instead, this monograph will focus on established clinical and radiologic features that can lead to a diagnosis and, in the case of the foregoing group of syndromes, should be learned even if their pathogenesis is not fully understood.

This book employs conventional nosologic and pathogenic classifications. The introductory tables list the dermatologic, clinical, and radiologic features that are essential in making an accurate differential diagnosis.

When is it worthwhile to consult this book?
In cases where skeletal radiographs reveal predominantly localized or generalized changes that have a discernible pathoanatomic pattern (e.g., destructive changes vs. sclerosis or new bone formation) but defy nosologic classification, the physician should first inspect the *disrobed* patient externally and look for any mucocutaneous lesions that would suggest a *preliminary* classification. Then, aided by this monograph, the examiner should try to relate the lesions to a specific disorder, provided the patient actually has a bi-, oligo- or multisymptomatic process involving the skin, mucous membranes, and bones. Of course, the preliminary dermatologic diagnosis will require confirmation by a specialist in dermatology.

Conversely, when predominantly cutaneous lesions are seen in a patient who *additionally* complains of general musculoskeletal or rheumatoid symptoms, the physician should consider whether an association may exist with the presenting skin lesions. A good example of this is Fabry's disease, in which diffuse angiokeratomatous skin lesions are frequently associated, especially in younger patients, with rheumatologic complaints based on occlusive vascular disease causing bone marrow infarction, arthropathies, etc. It is not enough in these cases to diagnose the diffuse angiokeratosis without also trying to recognize the underlying disease as a whole. A more common example, which we have studied intensively in recent years, is palmoplantar pustulosis (PPP), in which more than 10% of patients may exhibit unusual skeletal changes that, when considered in isolation, are usually misdiagnosed. Many of these patients have a long odyssey of fruitless doctor visits in which specialists have ignored symptoms voiced by the patient that fall within the domain of a different specialty. The conscientious physician should ask specifically about musculoskeletal complaints that are not volunteered by the patient. There are some dermatologic changes (e.g., skin lesions typical of sarcoidosis or Langerhans cell-histiocytosis) that warrant a specific radiologic workup in order to disclose, for example, a significant risk of spontaneous fracture or to establish a baseline for subsequent skeletal changes that would be difficult to interpret if cutaneous manifestations subside.

A secondary goal of this monograph is to help sharpen the physician's eye for rare, complex disorders that are likely to be missed if one is not prepared to recognize them.

Tables of Differential Diagnoses

The introductory tables list the entities that should be considered in the differential diagnostic interpretation of key dermatologic or radiologic features. Many diseases, of course, are notably pleomorphic and can have a variety of presentations. If suitable software is available, the data could be stored in a desktop computer to enable the physician to piece together the diagnostic "jigsaw puzzle" in any given case. This could make an effective supplement to the main clinical and radiologic features that are listed in a blue box at the start of each section in the text.

Main dermatologic features	Consider in differential diagnosis
▶ **Urticarial reactions**	
Urticaria	Rheumatic fever, plasmacytoma, Schnitzler's syndrome relapsing polychondritis
Wheals (induced by rubbing)	Mastocytosis
▶ **Erythematous, erythemosquamous, and papular skin lesions**	
Erythematous lesions	
– Centrifugal pattern of spread	Erythema chronicum migrans
– Lilac- or wine-colored	Dermatomyositis, Sharp's syndrome
– Periungual with telangiectases	Dermatomyositis
– Mottled	Rothmund-Thomson syndrome
– Diffuse	SLE, Sharp's syndrome
– Butterfly rash (face)	SLE
– Pale red	Leprosy (indeterminate type)
– Papules	Rheumatic fever
– Annular (Erythema annulare rheumaticum)	Rheumatic fever
Multiform and nodose erythemas	
– Erythema nodosum	Crohn's disease, ulcerative colitis, relapsing polychondritis, sarcoidosis, Reiter's syndrome, yersinia arthritis, enterospondylarthritis, rheumatic fever, Behçet's disease
– Erythema nodosum leprosum	Lepra reaction during therapy
– Erythema exudativum	Relapsing polychondritis, rheumatic fever
Erythemosquamous lesions	SLE, undifferentiated spondyloarthropathy, psoriasis vulgaris, Reiter's syndrome, tuberculoid leprosy, borderline leprosy, Rothmund-Thomson syndrome, mycosis fungoides, relapsing polychondritis
Erythroderma	Psoriasis vulgaris, mycosis fungoides
▶ **Vesicular and bullous lesions**	Epidermolysis bullosa dystrophica with acro-osteolysis
▶ **Pustular lesions**	
Sterile pustules	Pustular psoriasis, palmoplantar pustulosis, Reiter's syndrome, Behçet's disease, acne conglobata (in some cases)
▶ **Keratoses**	
Diffuse keratoses	
– Ichthyosis vulgaris	Refsum's syndrome
– Ichthyosiform erythroderma	Congenital ichthyosiform erythroderma with acro-osteolysis

Main dermatologic features	Consider in differential diagnosis
– Follicular keratoses	Scurvy
– Whorled keratoses	Ichthyosis with chondrodysplasia punctata
– Sporadic keratoses	Fabry's disease
– Circumscribed keratoses	SLE, dermatomyositis
– Palmoplantar keratoses	Psoriasis vulgaris, osteopoikilosis with dermatofibrosis lenticularis, Bureau-Barrière-Thomas syndrome, mutilating palmoplantar keratoderma, acro-osteolysis in guitar players and violinists, Werner's syndrome, Ainhum's syndrome
– Hyperkeratotic nailfold	Dermatomyositis
▶ Atrophic conditions	
▷ *Congenital atrophic skin disorders*	
– Diffuse	Goltz-Gorlin syndrome, Rothmund-Thomson syndrome, Werner's syndrome, epidermolysis bullosa dystrophica with acro-osteolysis, melorheostosis
– Sporadic	Proteus syndrome
– Follicular atrophy	Conradi-Hünermann disease
– Poikiloderma	Rothmund-Thomson syndrome
▷ *Acquired secondary atrophy of the skin*	
in collagen diseases:	
– Porcelain-white atrophy	Dermatomyositis
– Circumscribed atrophy	SLE
– Poikiloderma	Progressive systemic sclerosis, dermatomyositis
in granulomatous diseases:	
– Central atrophy	Sarcoidosis
in infectious diseases:	Acrodermatitis chronica atrophicans (borreliosis)
▶ Scleroderma-like skin lesions	
Cutaneous sclerosis	Progressive systemic sclerosis, Jo-1 syndrome, plasmacytoma, POEMS syndrome
Linear circumscribed scleroderma	Morphea, melorheostosis
Pseudosclerosis	Werner's syndrome
▶ Fistulation of the skin	Actinomycosis, mycetoma
▶ Fatty tissue lesions	
Fat hernia	Goltz-Gorlin syndrome
Fat atrophy	Lipoatrophic diabetes mellitus
Panniculitis	Relapsing polychondritis

Main dermatologic features	Consider in differential diagnosis
▶ **Vascular abnormalities**	
▷ *General*	
Telangiectases	Goltz-Gorlin syndrome, Rothmund-Thomson syndrome, sarcoidosis, collagen diseases (progressive systemic sclerosis, SLE, dermatomyositis)
Raynaud's phenomenon	Undifferentiated inflammatory systemic connective tissue disorders, collagen diseases (progressive systemic sclerosis, SLE, Sharp's syndrome, Jo-1 syndrome), plasmacytoma, fibroblastic rheumatism
Inflammatory angiopathies	
– Leukoclastic vasculitis	Relapsing polychondritis
– Vasculitis racemosa (livedo racemosa)	Rothmund-Thomson syndrome, relapsing polychondritis
– Marble skin (livedo reticularis)	Plasmacytoma
– Pyoderma gangrenosum	Plasmacytoma, enterospondylarthritis (Crohn's disease, ulcerative colitis)
▷ *Venous abnormalities*	
Varicosity	Periosteal ossification in varicose symptom complex
Varicose venectasia	Klippel-Trenaunay syndrome
Crural ulcer	Periosteal ossification in varicose symptom complex
Pseudo-Kaposi due to chronic venous insufficiency	Stewart-Bluefarb syndrome
Thrombosis and thrombophlebitis	Relapsing polychondritis, Behçet's disease
Venous angiomas	Angiodysplastic cutaneous and skeletal lesions (Servelle-Martorell type)
Venectasis	Angiodysplastic cutaneous and skeletal lesions (Servelle-Martorell type)
▶ **Hemorrhagic tendency**	
Purpura	Rheumatic fever, plasmacytoma (cold purpura), scurvy
Punctate hemorrhages in cuticle	Progressive systemic sclerosis, SLE
▶ **Edematous skin lesions**	POEMS plasmacytoma, early stage of progressive systemic sclerosis, early stage of Sudeck's disease, dermatomyositis, Jo-1 syndrome
Pretibial myxedema	EMO syndrome
Lymphedema	Fabry's disease, melorheostosis

Main dermatologic features	Consider in differential diagnosis
▶ **Pigmentation abnormalities**	
Hyper- and hypopigmentation	POEMS plasmacytoma
Hyperpigmentation	Fibrous dysplasia, Cronkhite-Canada syndrome, Goltz-Gorlin syndrome, Rothmund-Thomson syndrome, hemochromatosis, melorheostosis, collagen diseases (progressive systemic sclerosis, dermatomyositis)
– Melasma-like, stringy, streaky	Gaucher's disease
– Grayish-brown	Whipple's disease
Depigmentation (of the skin or hair)	Proteus syndrome, sarcoidosis, healing tertiary syphilis, leprosy, Rothmund-Thomson syndrome, congenital copper deficiency
Hypopigmentation	
– Café-au-lait pattern	Tuberous sclerosis
– Steely gray	Congenital copper deficiency
Lentigines	Neurofibromatosis
Axillary freckling	Neurofibromatosis
▶ **Diseases of the sweat glands**	
Hyperhidrosis	Buschke-Ollendorf syndrome, Bureau-Barrière-Thomas syndrome, mutilating palmoplantar keratoderma, Sudeck's syndrome, Pachydermoperiostosis
Hypohidrosis	Congenital ichthyosiform erythroderma with acro-osteolysis
Hypoplastic sweat glands and sebaceous glands	Rothmund-Thomson syndrome
▶ **Diseases of the sebaceous glands**	
Acne conglobata	Chronic recurrent multifocal osteomyelitis, pustulotic arthroosteitis-like lesions
▶ **Hair diseases**	
Alopecias	
– Diffuse	SLE, hemochromatosis
– Scarring	Progressive systemic sclerosis, Goltz-Gorlin syndrome, SLE
– Other	Cronkhite-Canada syndrome, Conradi-Hünermann disease, epidermolysis bullosa dystrophica with acro-osteolysis, Werner's syndrome, Satoyoshi's syndrome, syphilis
Hypotrichia	Rothmund-Thomson syndrome

Main dermatologic features	Consider in differential diagnosis
Atrichia	Rothmund-Thomson syndrome, metaphyseal chondrodysplasia with complete alopecia
Hirsutism	Lipoatrophic diabetes mellitus
Premature graying of hair	Rothmund-Thomson syndrome, Werner's syndrome
Hair shaft abnormalities (congenital trichorrhexis nodosa)	Congenital copper deficiency
▶ **Calcinoses**	
Interstitial calcinoses (with ulceration of calcific masses)	Progressive systemic sclerosis (CRESTA syndrome), dermatomyositis
Hard white papules, plaquelike lesions and perforations	Tumoral calcinosis
▶ **Nevi**	
▷ *Pigment cell nevi*	
Epidermal melanocytic nevi	
– Café-au-lait spots	Fibrous metaphyseal defects, fibrous dysplasia, neurofibromatosis, Maffucci's syndrome
– Nevus spilus	Proteus syndrome
– Lentigo simplex	Solomon's syndrome
▷ *Nevus cell nevi*	Neurofibromatosis
▶ **Tumors of the skin**	
Dermatofibromas	Buschke-Ollendorf syndrome (osteopoikilosis with dermatofibrosis lenticularis)
Neurofibromas	Neurofibromatosis
Cutaneous and subcutaneous lipomas	Neurofibromatosis
Epidermal cysts	Gardner's syndrome
Papillomas	Goltz-Gorlin syndrome
Sebaceous adenoma (angiofibroma)	Bourneville-Pringle disease (= tuberous sclerosis)
Lenticular fibromas	Goltz-Gorlin syndrome
Palmoplantar tumors	Proteus syndrome
Basal cell carcinomas	Goltz-Gorlin syndrome (= basal cell nevus syndrome)
Squamous cell carcinomas (frequent)	Rothmund-Thomson syndrome
Fungiform skin tumors	Mycosis fungoides
Neurogenic tumors	Glomus tumor
▶ **Tumors of blood vessels**	
Hemangiomas (cutaneous and subcutaneous)	Maffucci's syndrome, neurofibromatosis, Solomon's syndrome
Nevus flammeus	Klippel-Trenaunay syndrome
Angiokeratomas	Proteus syndrome, Fabry's disease

Main dermatologic features	Consider in differential diagnosis
Lymphangiomas	Neurofibromatosis
Angiomatous papule	Bacillary angiomatosis
▶ **Ulcerative skin lesions**	
Traumatic ulcers	Acroosteolysis in guitar players and violinists
Trophic ulcers	Mutilating palmoplantar keratoderma, Werner's syndrome, leprosy, Bureau-Barrière syndrome
Vasogenic ulcers	Stewart-Bluefarb syndrome
▶ **Papular skin lesions**	
Reddish brown or bluish	Sarcoidosis
▶ **Papulonodular skin lesions**	Multicentric reticulohistiocytosis, plasmacytoma, rheumatoid arthritis (chronic polyarthritis), leprosy (lepromatous type), rheumatic fever (rheumatic nodule)
– Juxta-articular	Fibroblastic rheumatism, borreliosis (late stage = juxta-articular nodules)
▶ **Papular and/or papulopustulovesicular skin lesions with petechial hemorrhages**	
Yellowish-brown	Abt-Letterer-Siwe disease, Hand-Schüller-Christian disease, eosinophilic granuloma
▶ **Maculopapular skin lesions**	Congenital syphilis
▶ **Papulonecrotic skin lesions**	Behçet's disease
▶ **Subcutaneous nodules**	
– Skin-colored	Sarcoidosis
– Yellowish-white	Gouty arthritis (tophi)
– Soft, erythematous	Pancreatic skin and skeletal diseases (subcutaneous fat necrosis)
▶ **Plaquelike infiltration of the skin**	
– Bluish-red	Sarcoidosis
– Red	Mycosis fungoides
– Indurated (woody)	Actinomycosis
▶ **Domelike skin lesions**	Tertiary syphilis
▶ **Necrosis of the skin**	
On the fingertips	Progressive systemic sclerosis

Main dermatologic features	Consider in differential diagnosis
▶ Contractures and clawhand	Epidermolysis bullosa dystrophica with acro-osteolysis, progressive systemic sclerosis
▶ Scars	Goltz-Gorlin syndrome, multilating palmoplantar keratoderma, epidermolysis bullosa dystrophica with acro-osteolysis
Molluscoid scars	Ehlers-Danlos syndrome
Cigarette-paper-like keloids	Ehlers-Danlos syndrome, Buschke-Ollendorf syndrome
▶ Annular constrictions of digital skin	Mutilating palmoplantar keratoderma, Ainhum
▶ Hyperelasticity of skin	Ehlers-Danlos syndrome
▶ Thickening of skin	
– Arms and legs	Pachydermoperiostosis
– With furrowing (= cutis verticis gyrata of the scalp)	Pachydermoperiostosis
– Palmoplantar gyriform hypertrophy	Proteus syndrome
▶ Lesions of oral mucosa	
Polypous	Plasmacytoma
Plaquelike	Late congenital syphilis
– Yellowish	Sarcoidosis
Aphthous (ulcerative)	SLE, Behçet's disease, undifferentiated spondyloarthropathy, enterospondylarthritis, Reiter's syndrome, ulcerative miliary syphilis, Langerhans cell histiocytosis
Nodules and plaques	Eosinophilic granuloma (Langerhans cell histiocytosis), Hand-Schüller-Christian syndrome
– Glassy nodules	Sarcoidosis
Papular	Reiter's syndrome, multisystemic Langerhans cell histiocytosis
Papillomatous	Goltz-Gorlin syndrome
Erythema and hemorrhages	Reiter's syndrome
Atrophic changes	Progressive systemic sclerosis
Macrocheilia	Tertiary syphilis
▶ Lesions of genital mucosa	
Circinate balanitis	Reiter's syndrome, undifferentiated spondyloarthropathy
Psoriatic balanitis	Psoriasis vulgaris
Ulcers	Behçet's disease
▶ Ocular changes	
Iridocyclitis	Oligoarticular juvenile rheumatoid arthritis, Reiter's syndrome, undifferentiated spondyloarthropathy

Main dermatologic features	Consider in differential diagnosis
Conjunctivitis	Reiter's syndrome, undifferentiated spondyloarthropathy, Behçet's disease
Keratitis	Behçet's disease
Uveitis	Sarcoidosis, intestinal arthropathies, undifferentiated spondyloarthropathy, Behçet's disease
Iritis	Behçet's disease, relapsing polychondritis
Retinitis	Behçet's disease
Scleritis	Relapsing polychondritis
▶ Nail changes	
– Aplasia	Nail patella syndrome
– Dysplasia	Nail patella syndrome
– Onychodystrophy	Osteopathia striata with focal atrophy of skin (Goltz-Gorlin syndrome), Cronkhite-Canada syndrome, Werner's syndrome, progressive systemic sclerosis, psoriasis, Reiter's syndrome, undifferentiated spondyloarthropathy
– Cross-ridges and mounds	Progressive systemic sclerosis, psoriasis
– Punctate bleeding sites in the cuticle	Progressive systemic sclerosis
– Pitting of nails	Psoriasis
– Yellow-brown discoloration (oil spots)	Psoriasis
– Crumbling nails	Psoriasis
– Spoonlike nail deformities	Osteopathia striata with focal hypoplasia of skin (Goltz-Gorlin syndrome)
– Leukonychia	Psoriasis
– Onycholysis	Rothmund-Thomson syndrome, undifferentiated spondyloarthropathy, psoriasis
– Hypertrophic nails	Rothmund-Thomson syndrome
– Nail loss	Epidermolysis bullosa dystrophica
– Watchglass nails	Congenital ichthyosiform erythroderma with acro-osteolysis, hereditary palmoplantar keratosis (Bureau-Barrière-Thomas syndrome), Crohn's disease, ulcerative colitis, pachydermoperiostosis, angiodysplasias

Main radiologic features	Consider in differential diagnosis
► **Predominantly sclerosing skeletal changes**	
Unifocal	POEMS syndrome (rare)
Oligofocal	
– "Dripping candle" pattern	Melorheostosis
– Irregular	Psoriatic arthritis and psoriatic spondylarthritis
– Patchy	Pustulotic arthro-osteitis, acne-associated, POEMS syndrome, sarcoidosis
Multiple	
– Round	Osteopoikilosis, Gardner's syndrome
– Linear	Osteopathia striata
– Irregular	Psoriatic arthritis and psoriatic spondylarthritis
– Patchy	Pustulotic arthro-osteitis, acne-associated, POEMS syndrome, sarcoidosis, mastocytosis
Disseminated	
– Uniform	POEMS syndrome (rare), mastocytosis, pyknodysostosis, lipoatrophic diabetes mellitus
– Irregular	Gaucher's disease (Erlenmeier flask deformities), lipoatrophic diabetes mellitus
► **Localized skeletal hypertrophy**	
Unilateral	Proteus syndrome, Klippel-Trenaunay-type angiodysplasia, Weber-type angiodysplasia
► **Osteoporosis**	
Generalized	Werner's syndrome, congenital copper deficiency, mastocytosis
Localized (hands, feet)	Progressive systemic sclerosis, SLE, Jo-1 syndrome, Sharp's syndrome, Sudeck's disease
► **Bone marrow infarction**	Gaucher's disease, Fabry's disease, pancreatogenic
► **Bone necrosis**	
Classic (hip, knee)	Gaucher's disease, Fabry's disease
Osteomyelitis-like	Pancreatogenic
► **"Cystic" bone lesions** [a]	
Unifocal, mono-osseous	Neurofibromatosis in a child with tibial bowing or nonunion
Multiple, multifocal	Tuberous sclerosis, basal cell nevus syndrome, progressive systemic sclerosis (wrist), SLE (hand), hemochromatosis (subarticular), sarcoidosis, pancreatogenic

Main radiologic features	Consider in differential diagnosis
► Acroosteolysis	See Table 8.1, p. 191
► Periosteal disorders	See Tables 7.1 and 7.2, p. 179
► Joint destruction	
Hands, feet	Sharp's syndrome, rheumatoid arthritis, gout
Polyarticular	Sharp's syndrome, rheumatoid arthritis, fibroblastic rheumatism, gout, relapsing polychondritis, multicentric reticulohistiocytosis, Cronkhite-Canada syndrome
► Osteoarthritic symptoms (mainly affecting the hands)	Fabry's disease, protracted gout, hemochromatosis
► Sacroiliitis, "variegated" type	Ankylosing spondylitis, relapsing polychondritis (in some cases), psoriatic arthritis and psoriatic spondylarthritis, Reiter's syndrome and other reactive arthritides, acne-associated
► Enthesopathy	Ankylosing spondylitis, psoriatic arthritis and psoriatic spondylarthritis, Reiter's syndrome and other reactive arthritides, acne-associated
► Interstitial calcinoses	
Localized (fingers)	Idiopathic in elderly women
Disseminated	Thiebièrge-Weissenbach syndrome in progressive systemic sclerosis, CRESTA syndrome, dermatomyositis, Sharp's syndrome
Coarse, packet-like, usually unifocal	Tumoral calcinosis

[a] "Cystic" as used here refers to all round or oval lucencies with sharp borders, regardless of whether they are caused by a necrotic process, foreign body deposition, or similar processes. It does not refer to a true cyst, defined as a fluid-filled cavity with a cystic sac.

1 Congenital Disorders and Developmental Anomalies

1.1 Nail-Patella Syndrome

Synonyms: onycho-osteodysplasia, osteo-ony-chodysplasia, osteo-onychodysostosis

> Dysplastic nails, especially on the thumb and index finger.
> **Roentgen signs:** hypoplastic patellae, posterior iliac horns. Dysplasia of the distal, radial, articular portion of the humerus with dislocation of the radial head.

Definition

Nail-patella syndrome is an autosomal dominant disorder marked by a combination of nail dystrophy, absence or hypoplasia of the patellae, posterior dislocation of the radial heads, and "iliac horns." Nephropathy may also be present.

General Clinical Features

The defective gene has been mapped to chromosome 9. The incidence of the syndrome in Central Europe is approximately 22 per 1 million population. Nail changes occur in about 98% of cases. Patellar hypoplasia is present in about 92%, and a smaller percentage have patellar aplasia with absence of the anterior cruciate ligament. Elbow mobility is limited in about 90% of cases, and bilateral iliac horns, palpable through the abdominal wall, are present in about 81% (Vogel and Wiegers 1980).

While the patellar and knee abnormalities lead to corresponding mechanical symptoms (frequent falls in childhood and delayed walking with eventual secondary osteoarthritis), and the radial head dislocation is either asymptomatic or causes limitation of extension, pronation, and supination, almost 60% of cases are complicated by a nephropathy that may progress to end-stage renal failure (Bennet et al. 1973). Electron microscopy confirms the nephropathic changes, which may produce no clinical or histologic abnormalities.

There are reports of associations with other anomalies such as clinodactyly of the fifth finger, abnormal pigmentation of the iris (Lester's sign), renal dysplasia, and occasional clubfoot, coxa valga, congenital hip dislocation, spinal deformities, etc.

Dermatology

The nail changes are highly variable and can range from mild dysplasia to complete anonychia. Typically, one-half to one-third of the nail plate is missing. The hands – especially the thumb and index finger – are more commonly affected than the feet (Fig. 1.1 a).

Radiology

The patellae are hypoplastic and occasionally absent. Radiographs also show general dysplasia of the knee joints eventually leading to secondary degenerative arthritis.

The "iliac horns" appear as symmetric, palpable, horn-like bony prominences, sometimes pyramid-shaped, that project up to 4 cm from the posterior surface of the ilium 2–3 fingerwidths lateral to the sacroiliac joints (Fig. 1.1 b).

Hypoplasia and deformity of the radial side of the elbow joint are associated with lateral and posterior dislocation of the radial head (Fig. 1.1 c).

Other possible abnormalities were noted above.

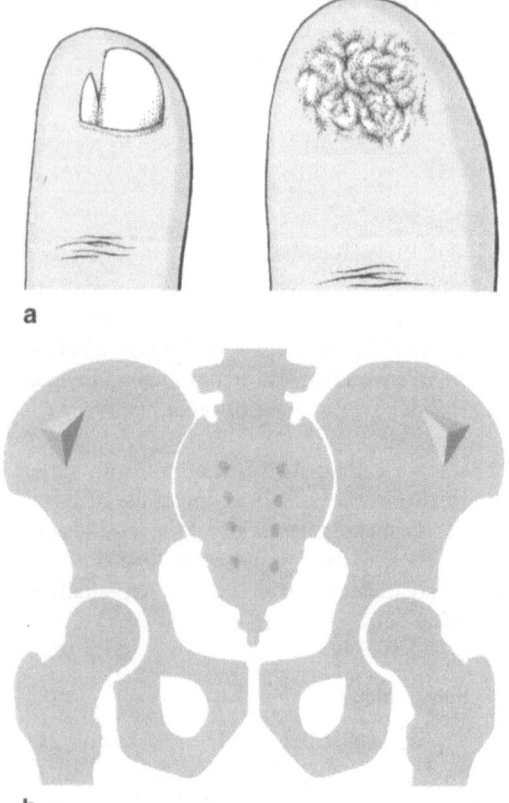

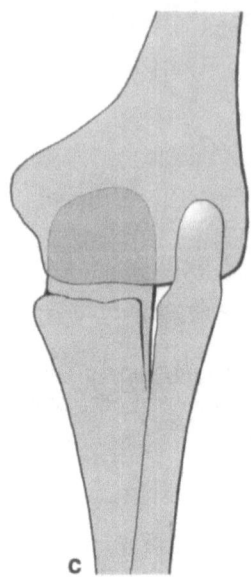

Fig. 1.1. a Raised scarlike lesions replace the normal thumbnail (*right*), and the ulnar half of the nail of the index finger is dystrophic (*left*). **b** Each of the iliac wings bears a horn-like triangular or pyramid-shaped bony prominence called an "iliac horn." **c** Hypoplasia of the radial head and distal articular humerus on the radial side. The head of the radius is dislocated

References

Bennet WM, Musgrave JE, Campbell RA et al. (1973) The nephropathy of the nail-patella syndrome. Am J Med 54: 304

Ferguson-Smith MA, Aitken DA, Turleau C et al. (1976) Localisation of the human AB0: Np-1: AK-1 linkage group by regional assignment of AK-1 to 9q34. Hum Genet 34: 35

Korting GW, Gebhardt R (1967) Weitere Befunde zum Nagel-Patella-Syndrom. Arch Klin Exp Dermatol 229: 372

Pilling DW, Levick RK (1978) Radiological abnormalities associated with anomalies of the ninth chromosome. Pediatr Radiol 6: 215

Renwick JH, Lawler SD (1955) Genetical linkage between AB0 and nail patella loci. Ann Hum Genet 19: 312

Spichtin H, Mihatsch MJ (1979) Diagnostic progress in familial nephropathy. Alport's syndrome, nail-patella syndrome and benign familial hematuria. Pathol Res Pract 164: 80

Vogel H, Wiegers U (1980) Das Nail-Patella-Syndrom. Röfo 133: 555

1.2 Enchondromatosis with Cavernous Hemangiomas (e.g., Maffucci's Syndrome)

Cavernous hemangiomas of variable size appearing anywhere on the skin.
Roentgen signs: multiple or generalized enchondromas of the tubular bones and flat bones, with or without vertebral body dysplasia and cranial deformity. "Fan-like" septation, esp. in the metaphyses of the long bones. Calcified phleboliths appear on radiographs of the hemangiomas. Rarely: interstitial calcinosis.

Definition

Enchondromatoses of various forms and etiologies may be associated with the presence of cutaneous and subcutaneous cavernous hemangiomas. Maffucci's syndrome in the strict sense is characterized by multiple enchondromas of the long and flat bones showing an irregular distribution, sparing the calvarium and spine, and accompanied by multiple, predominantly cutaneous hemangiomas.

General Clinical Features

The eponymous syndrome described by A. Maffucci in 1881 is generally understood to be a combination of enchondromas (more "dysplastic" cartilage than true tumor) and multiple hemangiomas. But as various forms of enchondromatosis have been discovered, each showing distinctive etiologic, clinical, and radiologic features and some associated with cutaneous hemangiomas, Maffucci's syndrome is now considered but *one* of the entities that manifest a combination of enchondromatous skeletal changes and hemangiomatous skin lesions. For example, Creveld et al. (1971) and Spranger et al. (1978) described cases that conformed to group VI (generalized enchondromatosis) in Table 1.2 and also featured cutaneous hemangiomas. Kaibara et al. (1982) followed one case of generalized enchondromatosis for 12 years in a patient who, at 4 years of age, developed multiple hemangiomas ranging from a few millimeters to 1.5 cm in size. Some of these lesions involved the nose and mouth. The patient also had diffuse interstitial calcifications in the subcutaneous tissues of the right thigh, detected radiographically at age 4

Table 1.2. Classification of enchondromatoses. (According to Spranger et al. 1978)

Disease	Key radiographic signs	Etiology	Assessment of the classification
I. Ollier's disease	Multiple enchondromas of the tubular and flat bones, unevenly distributed, variable in degree and sparing the calvarium and vertebral column	Sporadic	Definitive
II. Maffucci's syndrome	Same features as Ollier's disease, but with multiple cutaneous hemangiomas	Sporadic	Definitive
III. Metachondromatosis	Multiple enchondromas with prominent marginal or solid calcification, exostoses, rapid progression and regression; tends to involve small tubular bones	Autosomal dominant	Definitive
IV. Spondylo-enchondrodysplasia	Irregularly distributed, usually subtle enchondromas of long tubular bones; severe generalized platyspondylia	Autosomal recessive?	Probably permanent
V. Enchondromatosis with irregular vertebral lesions	Multiple enchondromas of long tubular bones and flat bones, generalized, irregular dysplasia of vertebral bodies	No hereditary factor is known	Tentative
VI. Generalized enchondromatosis	Generalized, uniformly distributed enchondromas with massive involvement of hands and feet, mild platyspondylia and cranial deformity	No hereditary factor is known	Tentative

months. Interestingly, these radiographic changes were accompanied by multiple café-au-lait spots of varying size on the trunk and extremities, sparse scalp hair, and closed fontanelles. The general clinical presentation of patients with enchondromatosis depends entirely on the location of the enchondromas, the type of the disease (see Table 1.2), and the onset of manifestations. Type VI cases are the easiest to diagnose in small children owing to the external deformities caused by the mass effect of the enchondromas. Other signs in this subgroup are limb length discrepancies and delays in learning to walk and sit upright. Some enchondromas can reach grotesque proportions, eroding through the cortical bone and projecting into the soft tissues. Carriers of enchondromatosis are at high risk for the malignant transformation of indi-

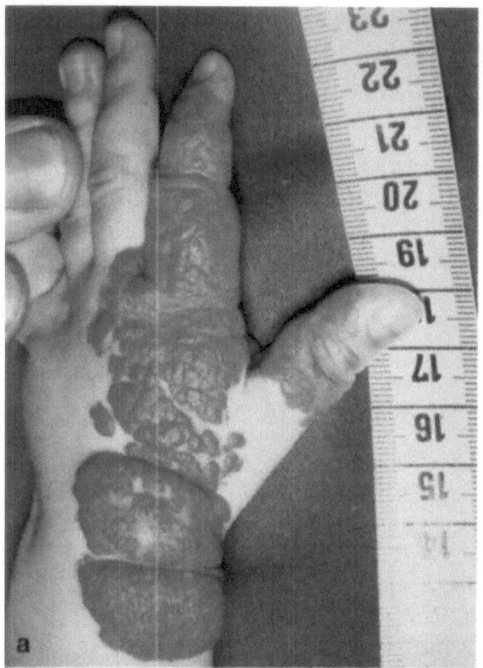
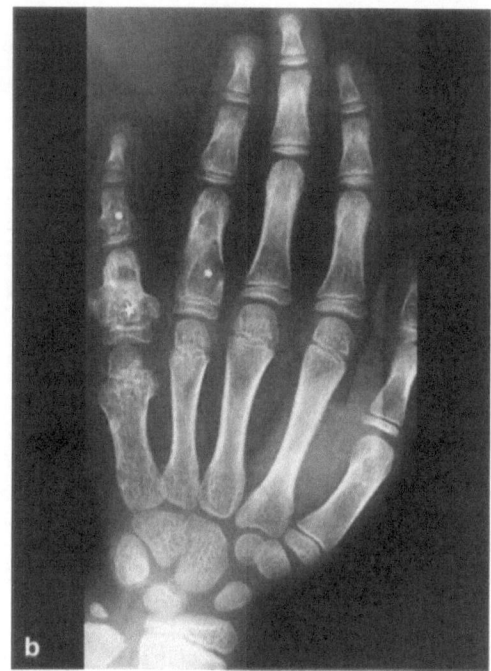
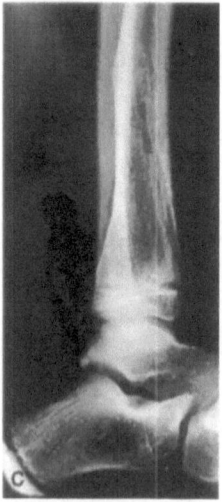
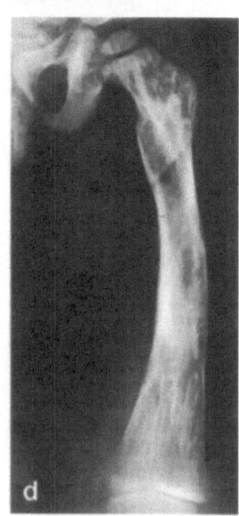

Fig. 1.2 a–g. Typical cases of Maffucci's syndrome. **a–c** 9-year-old girl presenting with cutaneous and subcutaneous hemangiomas on the trunk, the left distal forearm, and the radial side of the hand (**a**). The chondromatous lesions mainly involve the left hand and left leg. Note the predominantly endosteal chondromas of the fourth and fifth digits, causing marked expansion of the proximal phalanges (**b**, *asterisks*). Osteochondromatous lesions also involve the metaphysis of the fifth metacarpal. Note the "fan-like" septations in the distal tibial diametaphysis (**c**). **d–g** Grotesque enchondromatosis in a 12-year-old boy. Involvement of all tubular bones. "Fan-like" septations in the distal femur metaphysis and mixed enchondromas (islands of cartilage) and "fan-like" septation in all metatarsal bones. CT-scans of the distal metaphyses of the femur (**f**) and tibia (**g**) demonstrate the columns of cartilage. In plain film (**d, e**) they appear as "fan-like" septations. **e–g** see p.17

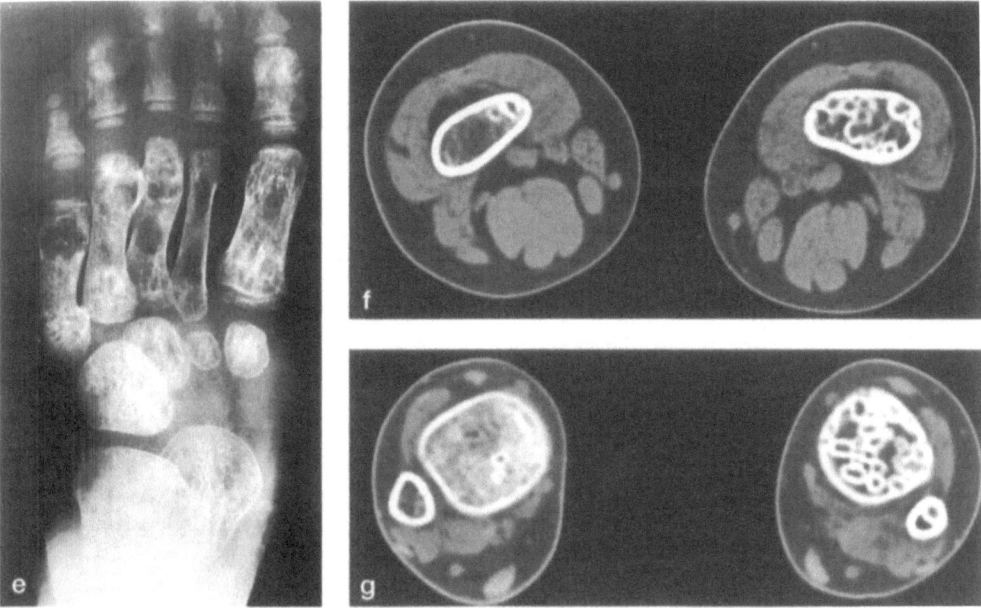

Fig. 1.2 (*continued*). See legend on p. 16

vidual lesions; the incidence of malignant transformation is approximately 30–35%. There is controversy as to whether these cases actually involve the malignant transformation of a primarily benign lesion or the eventual activation of an indolent chondrosarcoma. Clinically, malignant transformation is marked by a sudden or gradual increase of pain in the affected skeletal area, usually associated with a palpable mass lesion. We personally observed a case of true Maffucci's syndrome that was associated with a chondrosarcoma of the scapula (Freyschmidt 1997).

Dermatology

Hemangiomas of the skin and subcutaneous tissue are cavernous in nature. The cutaneous type presents as surface raised lesions that are engorged with blood, giving them a deep red color (Fig. 1.2 a). Subcutaneous hemangiomas form a soft subcutaneous mass that often can be expressed like a sponge and may elevate the skin level. Sometimes it is visible as a bluish mass beneath the skin. Hemangiomas can occur anywhere on the skin and mucosal surfaces, ranging from a few millimeters to several centimeters in diameter. Larger angiomas, like enchondromas,

may undergo malignant change (to angiosarcoma).

Radiology

The typical enchondroma appears radiographically as an osteolytic lesion that may erode through the original cortex while forming a new bony shell ("neocortex"). The cartilaginous matrix undergoes popcorn-like calcification. In typical cases of enchondromatosis the "dysplastic" cartilage forms columns in the metaphyses of enchondrally formed bones, giving the X-ray appearance of "fanlike septation" (Brien et al. 1997). The "dysplastic" cartilage emanates from the physeal plate (dyschondroplasia). Columns of cartilage usually coexist with enchondromas or "islands" of cartilage in various bones of the same patient. Lesions in small tubular bones quickly cause significant bone deformity with expansion and, in early cases, bowing and longitudinal growth disturbance (Fig. 1.2 b). Involvement of the radius and ulna lead to pseudo-Madelung deformity. The cartilage-forming lesions in enchondromatosis (Fig. 1.2 b–g) do not necessarily arise from inside the bone; they may develop subperiosteally or in the form of exostoses. Type VI cases of enchondromatosis are associated with slight flattening of the vertebral bodies (platyspondylia) and cranial deformity.

Larger enchondromas can perforate the cortex and expand into the soft tissues. This may cause bowing of adjacent tubular bones (e.g., the tibia and fibula). The matrix calcifications often extend far into the shafts of the tubular bones. Malignant transformation is usually marked by rapid enlargement of the lesion with increasing cortical bone destruction and the development of a large paraosseous mass. The previously ordered matrix calcifications are partially destroyed and may be replaced by new, irregular amorphous or stippled calcifications.

References

Brien EW, Mirra JM, Keir R (1997) Benign and malignant cartilage tumors of bone and joint: their anatomical and theoretical basis with an emphasis on radiology, pathology and clinical biology. Skeletal Radiol 26: 325

Creveld S van, Kozlowski K, Pietron K et al. (1971) Metaphyseal chondrodysplasia calcificans. A report of two cases. Br J Radiol 44: 773

Freyschmidt J (1997) Skeletterkrankungen. Klinisch-radiologische Diagnose und Differentialdiagnose, 2. Aufl. Springer, Berlin Heidelberg New York, S 506

Holzmann H, Wessmann D, Schlieter A (1994) Chondrodysplasie-Hämangiom-Syndrom (Maffucci-Syndrom). Aktuelle Dermatol 20: 292

Kaibara N, Mitsuyasu M, Katsuki I et al. (1982) Generalized enchondromatosis with unusual complications of soft tissue calcifications and hemangiomas. Skeletal Radiol 8: 43

Maffucci A (1881) Di un caso enchondroma ed angioma multiplo. Mov Med-Chir 3: 399

Spranger J, Langer LO, Wiedemann HR (1974) Bone dysplasias: an atlas of constitutional disorders of skeletal development. Saunders, Philadelphia, p 199

Spranger J, Kemperdieck H, Bakowski H et al. (1978) Two peculiar types of enchondromatosis. Pediatr Radiol 7: 215

1.3 Fibroosseous Lesions with Café-au-lait Spots

1.3.1 Fibrous Metaphyseal Defects with Café-au-lait Spots (Jaffé-Campanacci Syndrome)

Synonyms for fibrous metaphyseal defect: nonossifying fibroma, fibrous cortical defect

> Café-au-lait spots.
> **Roentgen signs:** fibrous metaphyseal defects predominantly involving the femur and tibia.

Definition

Fibrous metaphyseal defect (FMD) is a spontaneously resolving, tumorlike bone defect with fibrous replacement involving the metaphyses of growing tubular bones. Multiple defects are almost invariably associated with the presence of café-au-lait spots.

General Clinical Features

As the definition states, FMD is an innocuous, tumorlike lesion of the metaphyses that primarily affects the bones about the knee. It most likely represents a simple growth disturbance. Clinically asymptomatic, FMD is detected incidentally on X-ray films obtained for some other indication (e.g., trauma). Spontaneous fractures from larger lesions are very rare. In Germany, FMD has been noted in almost 2–3% of all knee radiographs taken in patients from 1 to 20 years of age (Freyschmidt et al. 1981). Approximately 96% of all FMDs occur on the lower extremity with only 4% involving the upper extremity. The site of predilection is the distal femoral metaphysis, where 62% of lesions occur. Most FMDs are detected between 10 and 15 years of age. No associated changes are seen in patients with FMDs, and laboratory findings are normal.

Children with neurofibromatosis, who invariably have café-au-lait spots, have a very strong tendency to develop FMDs. Usually these lesions are relatively large and may lead to spontaneous fractures. Solitary FMDs are rarely associated with café-au-lait spots, but this combination is not unusual in patients with multiple defects (Freyschmidt et al. 1998; Mirra et al. 1982).

Dermatology

The café-au-lait spot is a type of pigment cell nevus belonging to the subgroup of epidermal melanocytic nevi. It appears as a round to oval macule, 1–10 cm in diameter, of a light brown ("coffee with milk") or grayish brown color (Fig. 1.3 a). The spots may have an irregular shape. The presence of more than five spots should raise suspicion of neurofibromatosis, especially if there is concomitant axillary freckling. The combination of multiple FMDs and café-au-lait spots may represent a forme fruste of neurofibromatosis (see p. 20 and Fig. 1.3 a).

Café-au-lait spots are considered to be benign.

Radiology

Long-term observations have identified various stages in the natural history of FMD. Radiographs in early cases show a sometimes multifocal, elliptical cortical lucency 2–30 mm in diameter whose long axis parallels that of the affect-ed bone. The lesion is very sharply demarcated and sometimes causes an hourglass-shaped protrusion of the overlying ossified periosteum into the soft tissues. Larger specimens have a sclerotic rim, and there may be thickening of adjacent cortical bone. Occasionally there is complete external erosion of the cortex, causing its boundary with the calcified periosteum to appear frayed and irregular. This stage is called a *fibrous cortical defect*.

If the fibrous cortical defect is not "modeled away" by metadiaphyseal tapering during a growth spurt, it will develop into a true *nonossifying* fibroma, which typically appears as a cluster-of-grapes lucency beneath the residual, slightly bulging compact bone (Fig. 1.3 b). The cluster-of-grapes pattern is caused by reeflike projections on the inner surface of the lesion. Usually the lesions are surrounded by a dense, scalloped, sclerotic border, and most lesions show extension into the cancellous bone. Lesions may become up to 70 mm long and 30 mm wide and may "travel" for some distance along the diaphysis during longitudinal growth.

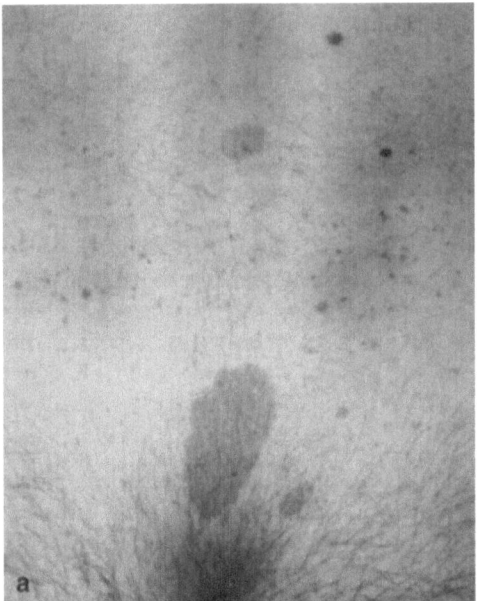
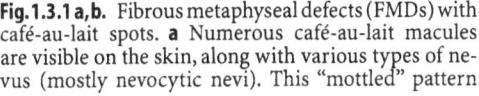

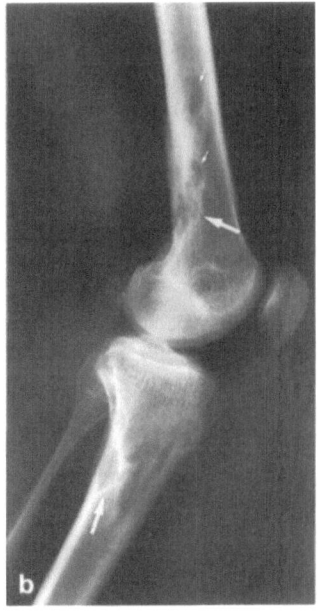

Fig. 1.3.1 a,b. Fibrous metaphyseal defects (FMDs) with café-au-lait spots. **a** Numerous café-au-lait macules are visible on the skin, along with various types of nevus (mostly nevocytic nevi). This "mottled" pattern may represent a forme fruste of neurofibromatosis. **b** Radiograph shows multiple FMDs (nonossifying fibromas) in the distal femur and proximal tibia. The lesions are bilaterally symmetric

The close relationship of FMD to the cortical bone is useful for differentiating these defects from other osteolytic lesions. Most FMDs involve the posteromedial portion of the distal femoral metaphysis. Another differentiating criterion is patient age, since FMD invariably develops during the first two decades of life. Lesions that appear at a later age and resemble nonossifying fibroma should be viewed with great suspicion. A radionuclide bone scan should be obtained in these cases, as a true FMD generally will not show radiotracer uptake. As a rule, typical FMDs (including nonossifying fibromas) do not require further investigation by other imaging modalities such as CT or MRI.

1.3.2 Fibrous Dysplasia

Fibrous dysplasia is a not uncommon bone disease with specific radiographic features, that usually do not challenge interdisciplinary (dermatologic – radiologic) considerations. Therefore it will not be discussed in detail here. In 50% of the polyostotic form of the disease patients have café-au-lait spots.

In *McCune-Albright-syndrome* (association of fibrous dysplasia with various endocrine disorders) patients usually have hyperpigmentations of the skin at the buttock, thigh, neck and back, that follow the so-called Blaschko-Lines. These hyperpigmentations present in a whirl-like or storiform pattern.

References

Freyschmidt J, Ostertag H, Jundt G (1998) Knochentumoren. Klinik, Radiologie, Pathologie, 2. Aufl. Springer, Berlin Heidelberg New York

Freyschmidt J, Saure D, Dammenhain S (1981) Der fibröse metaphysäre Defekt. I. Untersuchungen zur Häufigkeit. Röfo 134: 169

Mirra JM, Gold RH, Rand F (1982) Disseminated nonossifying fibromas in association with café-au-lait spots (Jaffé-Campanacci syndrome). Clin Orthop 168: 192

1.4 Neurofibromatosis Type 1

Various forms of pigment cell nevi, neurofibromas, optic glioma, Lisch nodules (pigmented iris hamartomas).

Roentgen signs: angular scoliosis, sphenoid dysplasia, thinning of long bones with pseudarthrosis, notching of ribs, nonossifying fibromas of bone.

Definition

Neurofibromatosis is an autosomal dominant disorder that is classified among the neurocutaneous syndromes, or phacomatoses. The variable penetrance of the disease leads to a diversity of clinical presentations.

General Clinical Features

The incidence of neurofibromatosis is approximately 1 case per 3000 births. Eight different forms of neurofibromatosis are recognized. Neurofibromatosis type 1 accounts for most cases that present with a combination of cutaneous and skeletal changes.

The diagnostic criteria for neurofibromatosis type 1 are as follows:

– six or more café-au-lait spots;
– two or more neurofibromas of any kind or one plexiform neurofibroma;
– axillary and inguinal freckling;
– optic glioma;
– two or more Lisch nodules (iris hamartomas);
– distinctive skeletal changes such as sphenoid dysplasia or cortical thinning of long bones that may be complicated by pseudarthrosis;
– a first-degree relative (parent, twin, or offspring) with neurofibromatosis type 1 by the above criteria.

Identical to classic von Recklinghausen's disease, neurofibromatosis type 1 represents a mixture of hereditary disorders involving neuroectodermal and mesodermal tissues. The spectrum of clinical changes is broad. The diagnosis relies on demonstrating involvement of the peripheral nerves and cranial nerves by neurofibromas. These tumors may cause clinical symptoms at a relatively late stage, but the skeletal malformations usually become symptomatic in childhood. A notable example is angular kyphoscoliosis (see Fig. 1.4 b), whose more severe forms may lead to paraplegia. Severe neurologic deficits can also result from myelomeningoceles, particularly those occurring in the thoracic region. Extreme hypertrophy may affect individual fingers or whole limbs, especially in patients who also have plexiform neurofibromas. Skeletal bowing, usually of the tibia, is an obvious sign in small children and may be associated with congenital pseudarthrosis (see Fig. 1.4 d). Endocrine disorders involving the thyroid gland, adrenals, and pituitary are occasionally observed. The effects of tumors of the cranial nerve roots (e.g., optic nerve, statoacoustic nerve) and the potential for malignant transformation in neurofibromatous tumors are beyond our present scope.

Dermatology

The spectrum of dermatologic changes in neurofibromatosis type 1 is extremely broad. The neural tumors may be relatively inconspicuous, and occasionally the examiner must hunt for them. Sometimes, minute brownish "spots" are the only lesions that are found on initial inspection. Other patients may have very large neurofibromas, usually on the trunk. The tumors generally have a broad base but may be pedunculated; they are soft and may be bluish or skin-colored (Fig. 1.4 a). Many tumors that penetrate the skin from the subcutaneous tissue can be pushed down into the panniculus by digital pressure and spring back when released ("bell-push phenomenon"). Palpation of the skin reveals more deeply seated nodules that may be tender to pressure and often are distributed along nerve pathways in the extremities. The skin may form circumscribed lobular folds like those seen in dermatochalasis; larger folds may appear as flabby, pendulous masses. Other types of pigment cell nevi are found in addition to the distinctive café-au-lait spots (see above and Fig. 1.3 a). They include:

- Nevus spilus, appearing as a large, tan pigmented area speckled with smaller, darker macules 1–2 mm in size.
- Lentigo simplex, a small, flat, sharply circumscribed, tan to dark-brown macular lesion.

Lentigines are often visible at birth and may become more numerous as the child grows. Multiple disseminated lesions are referred to as lentiginosis.

- Nevus cell (nevocytic) nevi (see Fig. 1.3 a), which include nevus pigmentosus, molluscoid nevus cell nevus, nevus pigmentosus et pilosus, and nevus pigmentosus et papillomatosus. A separate description of these lesions is beyond the scope of this book.
- Freckle-like pigmentation of the axillae, often giving the skin an overall "mottled" appearance (Fig. 1.4 a). Other dermatologic changes may take the form of hemangiomas and lymphangiomas, and skin changes may be combined with sebaceous adenoma and tuberous sclerosis of the brain (see p. 24ff.). Cutaneous and subcutaneous lipomas are also observed.

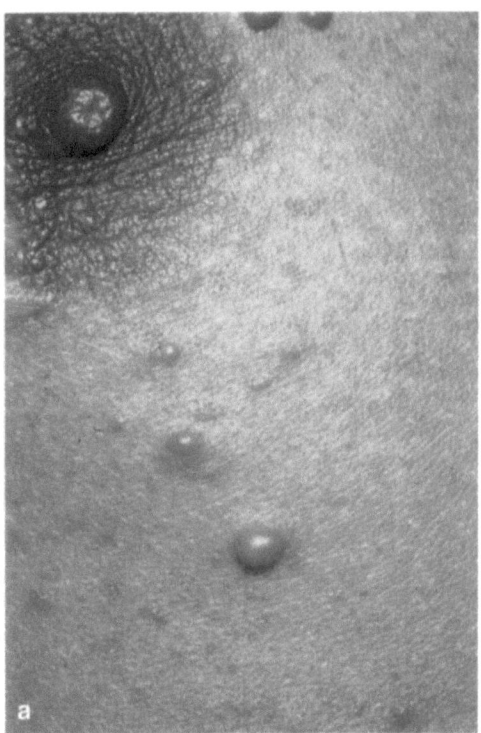

Fig. 1.4 a–d. Neurofibromatosis. **a** Mottled skin bearing innumerable small nevi, some very faint, along with typical, prominent neurofibromas. Note also the finer lesions that are barely raised above skin level, representing incipient neurofibromas. The patient had conspicuous café-au-lait spots on the back, similar to those in Fig. 1.3 a, and freckle-like axillary pigmentation. **b–d** see p. 22

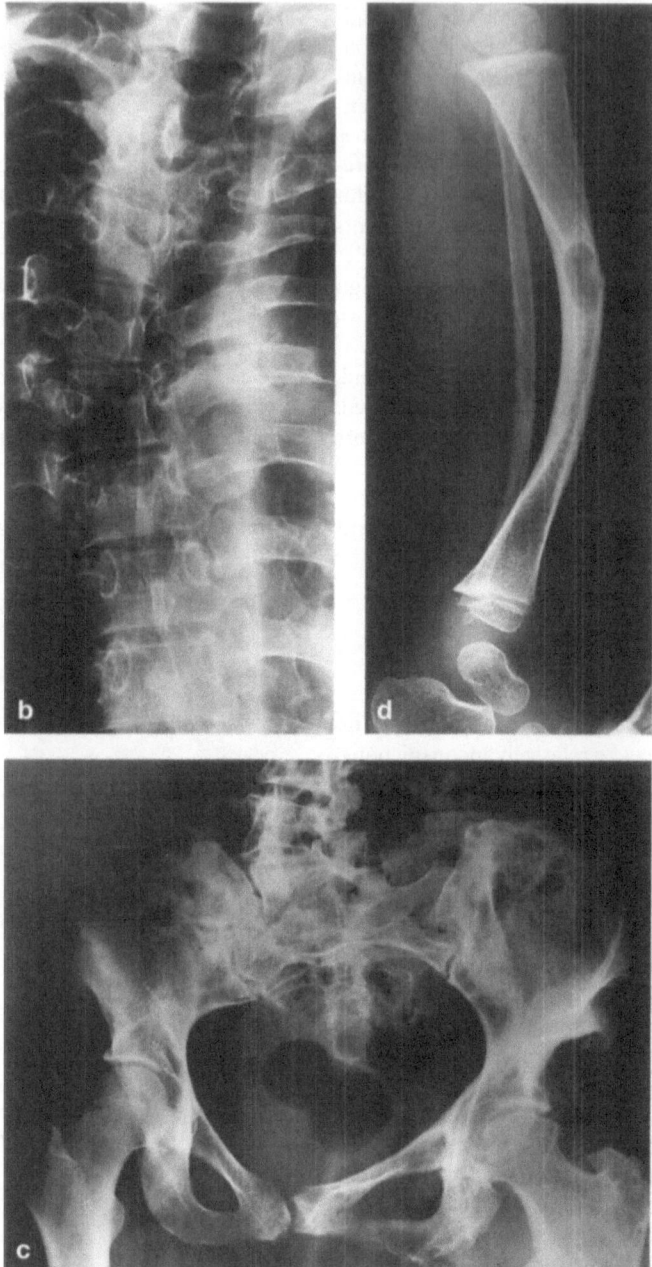

Fig. 1.4 (*continued*). **b, c** Skeletal changes commonly seen in neurofibromatosis. **b** Coarse scoliosis of the upper and mid-thoracic spine in a 28-year-old man with neurofibromatosis, found to have typical left-sided sphenoid dysplasia in addition to other changes (e.g., rib notching by neurofibromas, FMDs, etc.). **c** Woman 33 years of age with gross kyphoscoliosis of the lower lumbar spine due to wedging of the vertebrae. The sacrum and left bony pelvis also show severe dysplastic changes. Note the tubercle-like sites of new bone formation on the left anterior inferior iliac spine and left ischium, the dysplastic left hip, and the broadened intertrochanteric area. **d** Significant bowing and thinning of the tibia and, to a lesser degree, of the fibula in a 2-year-old boy. In the midshaft tibial lucency there is a spontaneous fracture. The cystlike lucency contained fluid and connective tissue but was devoid of neurofibromatous tissue. A more distal spontaneous fracture occurred 9 months later and progressed to pseudarthrosis. Clinically, years passed before the café-au-lait spots and neurofibromas appeared

Radiology

Skeletal abnormalities may result from a primary bone dysplasia or may be caused by erosions from adjacent soft-tissue tumors.

The dysplastic changes predominantly affect the spine, with nearly half of all patients showing an angular kyphoscoliosis that usually involves the thoracic region (Fig. 1.4 b). Other vertebral malformations consist of wedged vertebrae, neural arch defects, etc. (Fig. 1.4 c). Almost half of the cases show scalloping of one or more vertebral bodies, usually posteriorly, caused by dural ectasia or local neurofibromas. There may be concomitant anterior scalloping due to dysplasia. There is a high association with myelomeningoceles, especially at the thoracic level, which appear on X-ray films as gross paravertebral opacities that resemble neurofibromatous masses.

In the skull, it is common to find a defect in the posterosuperior orbital wall caused by defective development of the sphenoid wings and the orbital part of the frontal bone. The temporal lobe may protrude into the orbit through this defect, resulting in pulsating exophthalmos. The clinoid processes may be absent or malformed, and the calvarium may contain defects of variable size. Macrocranium is commonly seen in children.

Neurofibromas of the intercostal nerves can cause varying degrees of rib erosion at various levels. The tubular bones may be markedly thinned (e.g., fibula), or they may appear hypertrophic when plexiform neurofibromas are present (e.g., individual fingers). A common feature is bowing of the distal tibia, sometimes combined with a congenital pseudarthrosis (Fig. 1.4 d). Interestingly, the pseudarthrosis itself is devoid of neurofibromatous tissue.

Intraosseous neurofibromas are rare. They appear radiographically as subperiosteal or cortical lucencies surrounded by a thin bony shell. Nonossifying fibromas tend to occur in large numbers (see Fig. 1.3). Sporadic cases of osteomalacia have been described in neurofibromatosis. They are probably due to neurofibroma-induced stenotic changes in the renal arteries, leading gradually to renal failure. It has also been postulated that neurofibromas may secrete substances that prevent the hydroxylation of vitamin D into its active form ("tumor-induced hypophosphatemic osteomalacia").

References

Braun-Falco O, Plewig G, Wolff HH, Winkelmann RK (1991) Dermatology, 3rd edn. Springer, Berlin Heidelberg New York

Freyschmidt J (1997) Skeletterkrankungen. Klinisch-radiologische Diagnose und Differentialdiagnose, 2. Aufl. Springer, Berlin Heidelberg New York

1.5 Tuberous Sclerosis

Synonyms: adenoma sebaceum (Pringle type), Bourneville-Pringle disease, Pringle's disease

Facial angiofibromas, "white spots," epileptic seizures.
Roentgen signs: predominantly subependymal calcifications on cranial CT, cerebral cortical lesions on MRI; sclerotic foci in the cancellous bone of the vertebrae and pelvis; fine "cystic" lucencies in the bones of the hands and feet; interstitial pulmonary changes; renal angiomyolipomas.

Definition

Tuberous sclerosis is an autosomal dominant disorder with high penetrance and diverse clinical manifestations, but whose dominant features are facial angiofibromas and other hamartomas that may affect virtually any organ including the brain, leading to convulsive seizures.

General Clinical Features

Tuberous sclerosis belongs to the group of phakomatoses. Rott and Fahsold (1993) state that its pathogenesis is based on "multiple, localized areas of incomplete or abnormal tissue differentiation" (hamartial defects). If benign proliferation occurs in these areas, hamartomas develop; if malignant differentiation occurs, the lesions are called hamartoblastomas. "Hamartial defects" are considered intermediate between malformations and benign neoplasms. The hamartomas that occur in tuberous sclerosis include angiofibromas, angiomyolipomas, glial vegetations, and rhabdomyomas. Rott and Fahsold (1993) may be consulted for a detailed discussion on the etiology of the faulty tissue differentiation.

The incidence of tuberous sclerosis in Germany is approximately 1 in 10,000 births. It is known to have an autosomal dominant mode of inheritance, but 60–80% of all cases are based on a new mutation. The genetic aberration has been localized to chromosome 9.

The epileptic seizures begin in infancy (in about 80% of cases), and some 50% of patients who

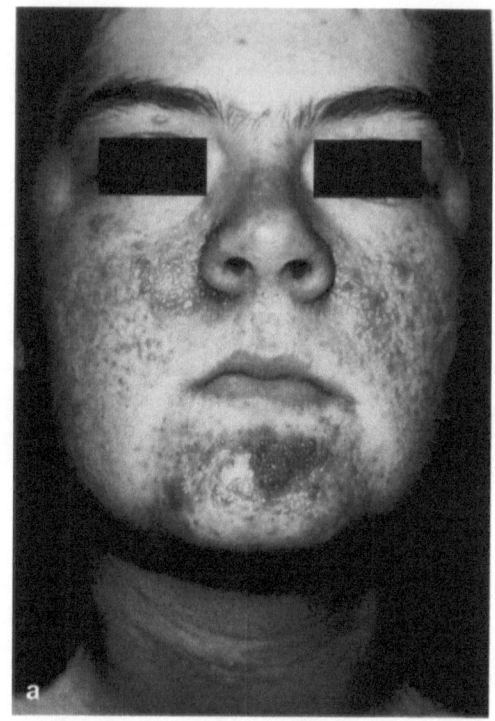

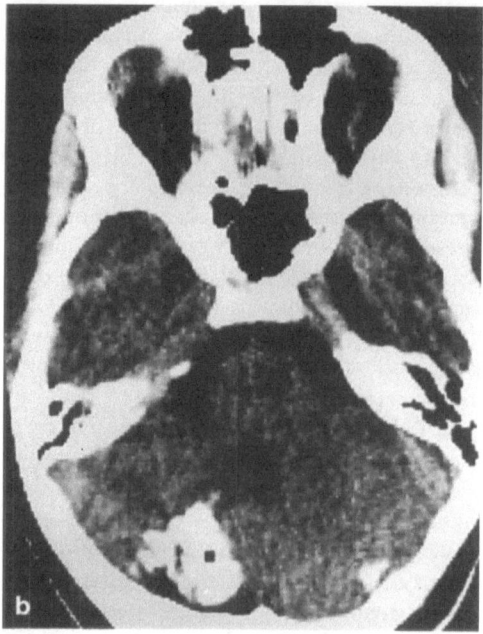

Fig. 1.5 a–g. Tuberous sclerosis. **a** Conspicuous angiofibromas on the chin and a butterfly lesional pattern on the cheeks. **b** Unusual calcifications in both hemispheres of the cerebellum. **c–g** see p. 25

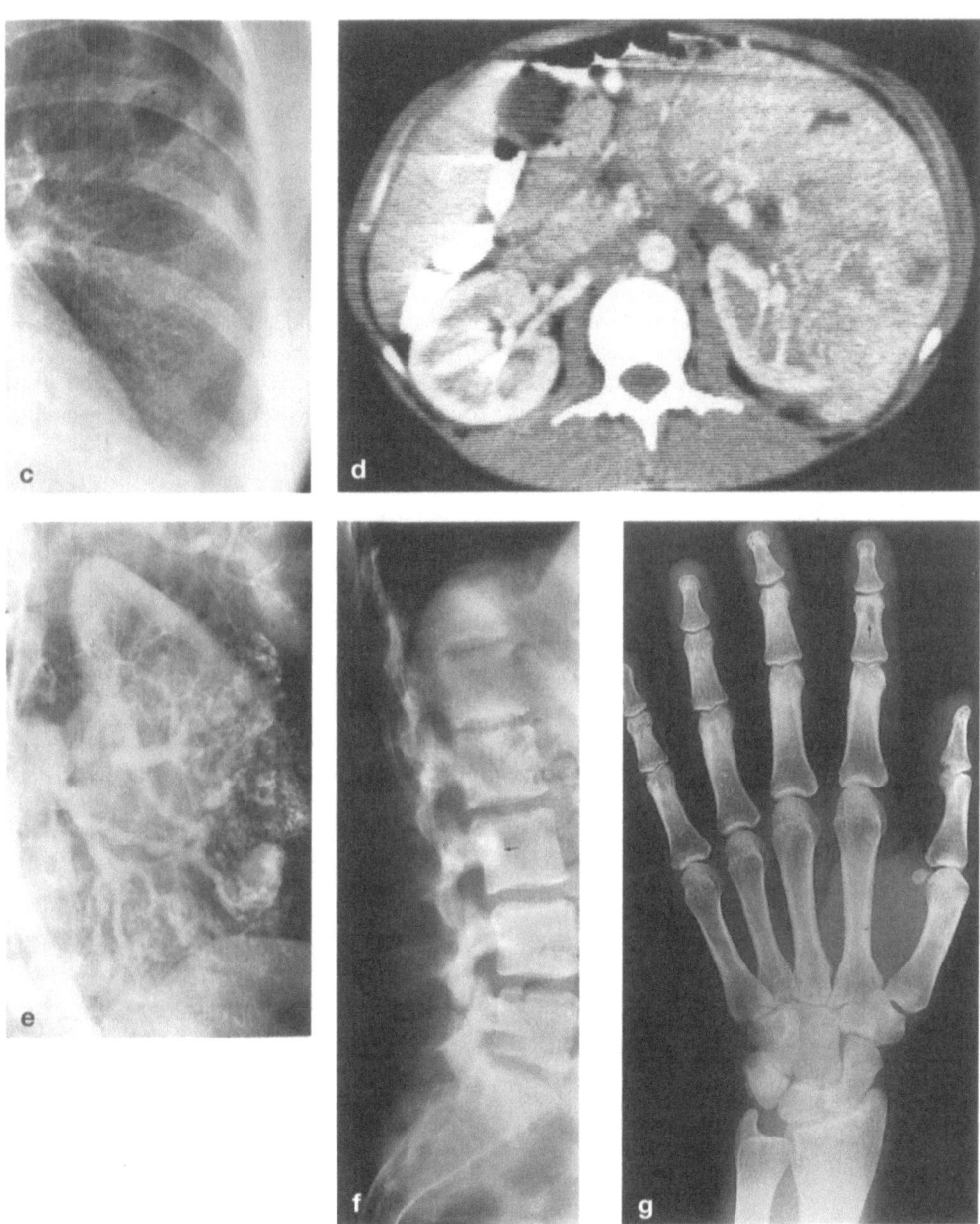

Fig. 1.5 (*continued*). **c** Diffuse lymphangiomyomatous interstitial lung disease with development of a left spontaneous pneumothorax. Note the cystlike areas in the left middle and upper zones. Similar changes were found on the opposite side. **d, e** Gross hamartoma of the left kidney with extension to the lateral and anterior abdominal wall. Angiography (**e**) defines the angiomatous component of the angiomyolipoma in the form of a large hypervascular mass and disordered vascular pattern. **f** Sclerotic foci in the cancellous bone of the lumbar spine. Note in particular the focus in the posterior part of the third lumbar vertebra. **g** "Cystic" changes in the metacarpophalangeal bones of the hand. The lesion in the distal part of the second middle phalanx is particularly striking (*arrow*). Similar changes were found in the opposite hand and in the bones of the feet

have seizures are mentally retarded. The lesions consist of pinhead- to thumbnail-size subependymal glial nodules that develop in the walls of the lateral ventricles. Usually the lesions calcify, making them visible on CT scans. The CT visualization of these calcified nodules, which may project into the ventricular cavities, is a fairly strong indicator of tuberous sclerosis in infants and small children. It is less common to find calcified foci in the cerebellum or other sites (Fig. 1.5 b). T2-weighted MR images, but not CT, can demonstrate whitish areas of firm consistency in the cerebral cortex and on the cortical surface. These are the "tubers" that give the disease its name, and they are responsible for the convulsive seizures.

Renal angiomyolipomas are very typical of tuberous sclerosis, occurring in up to 80% of cases, and are frequently combined with cysts (Fig. 1.5 d, e). Similar changes may occur in the liver and pancreas, and polypous lesions may develop in the gastrointestinal tract. Less common but still typical of tuberous sclerosis are interstitial lung changes (Fig. 1.5 c), which may lead to pulmonary fibrosis. Spontaneous pneumothorax is a common presenting sign in many patients. Lymphangiomyomatosis is the pathologic process that underlies these changes. Rhabdomyomas may be detectable in the heart at a very early stage (as early as 19 weeks' gestation), but they rarely produce clinical symptoms.

Examination of the retina in about 50% of patients reveals multiple, mulberry-like astrocytic hamartomas accompanied by small, nonpigmented areas that have a "punched-out" appearance. If the macula is unaffected, the ocular changes do not produce clinical symptoms.

Point defects in the dental enamel can already be recognized in the deciduous teeth.

Dermatology

The typical cutaneous lesions (seen in about 90% of cases) are angiofibromas, which appear after 2 years of age and, by puberty, spread over the chin and form a butterfly pattern across the cheeks (Fig. 1.5 a). The lesions appear as pinhead-sized, hemispheric nodules of a reddish or yellowish color. Originally they were misclassified as benign sebaceous gland tumors, giving rise to the term "adenoma sebaceum."

Up to 50% of adults with tuberous sclerosis develop angiofibromas in the area of the nailfold ("Koenen tumors"). They may reach 1 cm in diameter and occur mainly in women, most commonly on the toes.

"White spots" are considered typical of tuberous sclerosis when combined with the symptoms described above. They appear as areas of *hypopigmentation* having the same configuration as café-au-lait spots. Another dermatologic lesion consists of leathery skin areas up to several centimeters in diameter ("chagrin patches"), which occur mainly in the pelvic region. They are caused by a dense, cobblestone arrangement of connective tissue nevi.

Radiology

Radiographs in up to 80% of cases show circumscribed sclerotic foci of pea to half-dollar size that have rounded, ellipsoid, or irregular margins and predominantly involve the pelvis and lumbar spine (Fig. 1.5 f). Similar lesions may be found in the cranial vault. Bony lesions in the hands and feet appear as fine, cystlike lucencies that are occasionally combined with sites of periosteal ossification (Fig. 1.5 g). These skeletal abnormalities do not produce clinical symptoms.

References

Hatlinghus S, Sager M (1982) Tuberous sclerosis: bone and lung changes mimicking metastatic malignancy. Eur J Radiol 2: 90

Holland B, Kubale R, Freyschmidt J, Lucka D (1985) Radiologische Befunde beim Bourneville-Pringle-Syndrom. Z Hautkr 61: 1524

Rott HD, Fahsold R (1993) Klinik und Genetik der tuberösen Sklerose. Dtsch Ärztebl 90: C-274

1.6 Osteopoikilosis with Dermatofibrosis Lenticularis Disseminata and Other Cutaneous Lesions

Synonyms for osteopoikilosis: osteopathia condensans disseminata, osteopathia condensans generalisata, "spotted bones"
Synonyms for the disease when combined with dermatofibrosis lenticularis: Buschke-Ollendorf syndrome, osteodermatopoikilosis, McKusick's syndrome

> **Roentgen signs:** rounded cancellous bone densities, 2–5 mm in size and usually located near joints.
> **Cutaneous signs:** dermatofibrosis lenticularis disseminata, keratoma hereditarium dissipatum (palmar and plantar), tendency for keloid formation.

Definition

Osteopoikilosis is a rare hereditary bone disease, usually detectable only on X-rays, that is associated with well-circumscribed round or oval areas of increased density in cancellous bone. The foci range in size from 2–5 mm and primarily involve the epiphyses and metaphyses of the appendicular bones. They may be one feature of a syndrome that often is completed by dermatofibrosis lenticularis disseminata (Buschke-Ollendorf syndrome or osteodermatopoikilosis).

General Clinical Features

The incidence of osteopoikilosis in Central Europe is approximately 20 cases per 100,000 population. It chiefly affects males and has a dominant mode of inheritance.
The disease is clinically asymptomatic. Osteopoikilotic lesions are apparent only on roentgen examination and assume pathologic significance only when associated with dermatofibrosis lenticularis disseminata. Laboratory tests are normal. Coexistence with other skeletal anomalies has been described.

Dermatology

The combination of osteopoikilosis and dermatofibrosis lenticularis disseminata is a familial mesenchymal dysplasia often referred to as *Buschke-Ollendorf syndrome*. The upper trunk and thighs are affected with multiple lentil-sized dermatofibromas showing varying grades of differentiation (Fig. 1.6 b). Usually the lesions do not appear until adulthood.
Cases have been described that combine osteopoikilosis with abnormalities of palmoplantar keratinization (keratoma or keratosis). Classic palmoplantar keratoma hereditarium dissipatum is an autosomal dominant disease that has its onset in childhood or adolescence. Thick, yellowish, waxy-looking horny plaques appear in a symmetric distribution on the palms and soles and may be subdivided by fissures. They are separated from normal skin by a pale red border up to 1 cm wide. Frequently there is concomitant hyperhidrosis. The *differential diagnostic spectrum* is broad and ranges from palmoplantar psoriasis and hyperkeratotic rhagadiform hand and foot eczema to hyperkeratotic tinea manus and pedis, Darier's disease, and many other conditions.
Another rare association with osteopoikilosis is a tendency for keloid formation, which appears to have genetic roots.

Radiology

Three forms of osteopoikilosis are recognized:

1. a patchy or lenticular form
2. a linear or striate form
3. a mixed form.

Most common is the lenticular form, characterized by rounded, well-circumscribed, usually multifocal areas of increased cancellous bone density ("spotted bones") varying from 2 to 5 mm in size and chiefly involving the epiphyses and metaphyses of the appendicular bones as described above (Fig. 1.6 a). The linear or striate form may represent a transitional form to osteopathia striata, and indeed osteopoikilosis and osteopathia striata may be different manifestations of the same disease. Mixed forms that feature other hyperostotic skeletal changes are described in the section on osteopathia striata

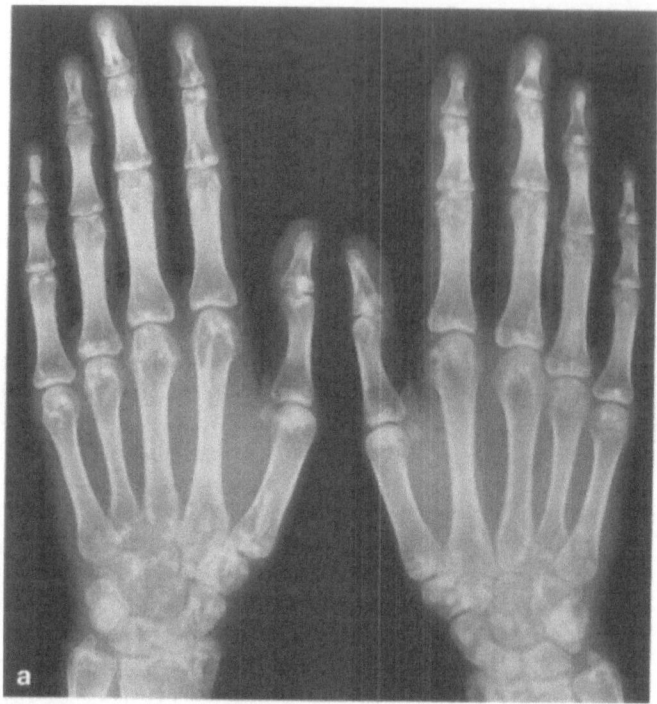

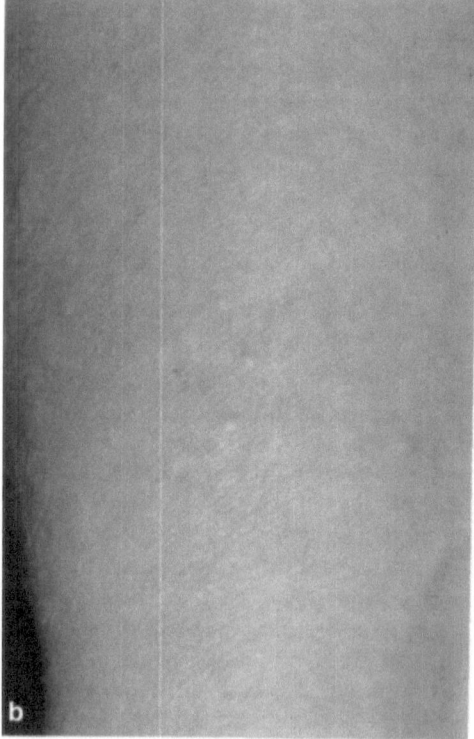

Fig. 1.6. a Typical "spotted bones" pattern in osteopoikilosis, with innumerable well-defined sclerotic foci, some very dense, involving the cancellous bone. Note the more linear densities in the distal part of the left second metacarpal, at the base of the second middle phalanx, and in the third distal phalanx of the left hand. These represent the striated form of osteopoikilosis that is transitional to osteopathia striata. Cutaneous manifestations consisted of dermatofibrosis lenticularis disseminata on the trunk and thighs (**b**)

(1.7). Osteopoikilotic foci may enlarge during skeletal growth and may become smaller after skeletal maturity is attained (Lagier et al. 1984).

Problems in the differential diagnosis of osteosclerotic metastases may occur only, if the sclerotic foci are asymmetric, especially in the pelvic region. Radiographs of the hands or knees are sufficient to confirm osteopoikilosis by demonstrating the symmetric distribution of the lesions. Radionuclide bone scans are rarely necessary but will differentiate metastases from osteopoikilosis by showing an absence of increased radiotracer uptake in osteopoikilotic foci. The differential diagnosis may be facilitated, if one takes a look to the skin and finds Buschke-Ollendorf's syndrome.

References

Atherton DJ, Wells RS (1982) Juvenile elastoma and osteopoikilosis (the Buschke-Ollendorf syndrome). Clin Exp Dermatol 7: 109

Freyschmidt J (1997) Skeletterkrankungen. Klinisch-radiologische Diagnose und Differentialdiagnose, 2. Aufl. Springer, Berlin Heidelberg New York

Lagier R, Mbakop A, Bigler A (1984) Osteopoikilosis: a radiological and pathological study. Skeletal Radiol 11: 161

McKusick VA (1972) Heritable disorders of connective tissue. Mosby, St. Louis

Uitto J, Santa Cruz DJ, Starcher BC et al. (1981) Biochemical and ultrastructural demonstration of elastin accumulation in the skin lesions of the Buschke-Ollendorf syndrome. J Invest Dermatol 76: 284

Verbov J (1977) Buschke-Ollendorf syndrome (disseminated dermatofibrosis with osteopoikilosis). Br J Dermatol 96: 87

1.7 Osteopathia Striata and Other Skeletal Malformations with Focal Cutaneous Hypoplasia or Cutaneous Atrophy (e.g., Goltz-Gorlin Syndrome)

Synonyms for Goltz-Gorlin syndrome: ectomesodermal dysplasia, osteo-oculodermal dysplasia

Roentgen signs: linear or patchy densities primarily involving the epiphyses of the long tubular bones as well as the pelvis, hands, and feet; flaring of the iliac wings.

Cutaneous signs: congenital, scarlike skin changes, widely distributed but asymmetric, marked by linear hyperpigmentation, cutaneous atrophy, and telangiectases. Hernia-like protrusions of subcutaneous fat in the atrophic areas, visible at birth or developing later and occurring primarily at the level of the iliac crest, in the inguinal area, and on the backs of the thighs. Multiple mucosal and perioral papillomas, scarring alopecia, nail abnormalities.

Other signs: mental retardation; chorioretinal and iris colobomas.

Definition

Hereditary osteopathia striata may occur as an isolated skeletal abnormality that is clinically asymptomatic and detectable only on radiographs. The striations may be combined with other hyperostotic changes, various skeletal malformations, and cutaneous lesions. The combination of osteopathia striata with focal dermal hypoplasia (atrophy), with various skeletal malformations, and with dental and ocular changes is referred to as Goltz-Gorlin syndrome, ectomesodermal dysplasia, or osteo-oculodermal dysplasia.

General Clinical Features

Osteopathia striata is, in itself, an innocuous condition that probably is inherited as a dominant trait and is detected incidentally on radiographs. Laboratory findings are unremarkable. Larregue et al. (1973) note that osteopathia striata may be associated with other skeletal changes such as osteopoikilotic foci, partial osteopetrosis, melorheostosis, and progressive diaphyseal dysplasia (Engelmann's disease). There is an occasional association with skin changes in the form of lenticular fibromas.

As part of an interdisciplinary syndrome, osteopathia striata is of interest when recognized in patients who suffer from Goltz-Gorlin syndrome. This condition is defined as consisting of cutaneous atrophy and linear hyperpigmentation, secondary herniations of subcutaneous fat visible on the skin surface, multiple mucosal and perioral papillomas, nail changes, and a variety of skeletal abnormalities chiefly affecting the extremities. Ginsburg et al. (1970) published an excellent description of the Goltz-Gorlin syndrome, noting that it occurs almost exclusively in Caucasian women. It probably has an X-linked dominant mode of inheritance. Interestingly, Goltz-Gorlin syndrome in women has a high association with complicated pregnancies and stillbirths. General developmental retardation is common, and mental retardation is quite frequent. Chorioretinal and iris colobomas are among the most common ocular abnormalities, and other changes such as strabismus, nystagmus, and microphthalmia have been described. A variety of auricular malformations, including hypoplasia of the auricular cartilage, have been cited. It is unclear whether the many other malformations at other sites described by Ginsburg et al. (1970) bear any causal relationship to true focal dermal hypoplasia. This also applies to skeletal changes such as microcephaly and dyscephaly, scoliosis and spinal segmentation anomalies, and countless asymmetric malformations of the appendicular bones, particularly in the hands and feet. At the same time, syndactyly and dental malformations with hypo- or oligodontia, microdontia, dental deformities, and malposed teeth appear to be associated with Goltz-Gorlin syndrome with some regularity.

Dermatology

The newborn presents with initially erythematous, then circumscribed atrophic skin changes that show a reticular, linear, or systematic arrangement. The lesions are reddish-brown in color and are slightly indrawn like scars; the skin is thin, delicate, and wrinkled like cigarette paper (Fig. 1.7 a, b). In some cases the atrophic areas contain hernia-like protrusions of subcutaneous fat, pigmentary changes, and telangiectases, the latter showing a predilection for the head and the back of the neck. The herniated fat is yellowish or pinkish yellow and usually occurs at the level of the iliac crests, the inguinal area, and the backs of the thighs. This is the most characteristic feature of focal dermal hypoplasia. Ginsburg et al. (1970) note that the theory of fat herniation in hypoplastic skin areas is somewhat controversial. They cite histologic studies by Hobel (1965) showing that fat accumulations in the skin may represent linear hamartomas (e.g., nevoid neoplasms), whereas circumscribed areas of skin atrophy, linear hyperpigmentation, and telangiectases belong to a different group of skin lesions. The authors speculate whether the early lesions they described as scar-like changes (e.g., linear areas of hyperpigmentation, atrophy, telangiectasis) may be the result of vesicle-like changes that were already present in utero and at birth.

Other characteristic skin changes are papillomas involving the lips, genital mucosa, and anal mucosa, scars secondary to deeper tissue defects, scarring alopecia, onychodystrophies, and occasional spoon-shaped deformities of the nails. It is unknown whether other skin changes such as photosensitivity, hypo- and hyperhidrosis, palmar hyperkeratosis, skin hyperelasticity, and acrocyanosis – like the various skeletal malformations – are only incidentally associated with the cardinal features of Goltz-Gorlin syndrome.

Radiology

Radiographs of simple osteopathia striata typically demonstrate fine, dense longitudinal striations in tubular bones representing lines of increased cancellous bone density (Fig. 1.7 c). The striations are most pronounced in the epiphyses and metaphyses, becoming narrower and less distinct toward the shaft. They primarily involve the area about the knee, showing a symmetric distribution. Striations are also described in the pelvis and in the tarsal and carpal bones. Except for the flaring of the iliac wings, all other bones that harbor these lesions show a normal configuration.

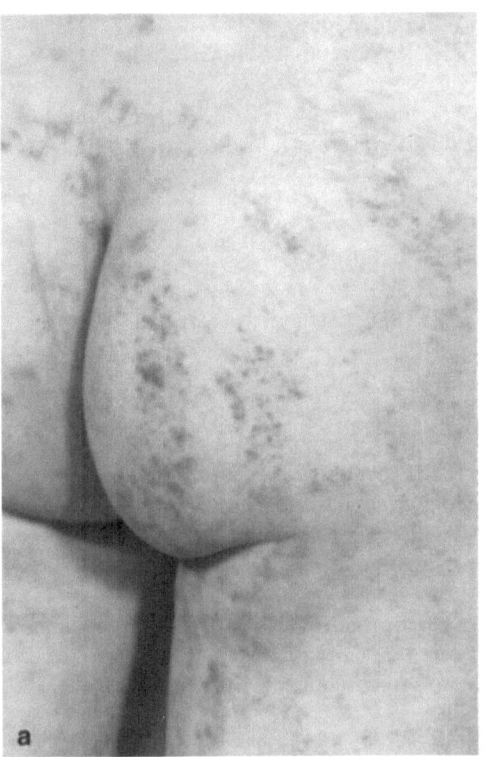

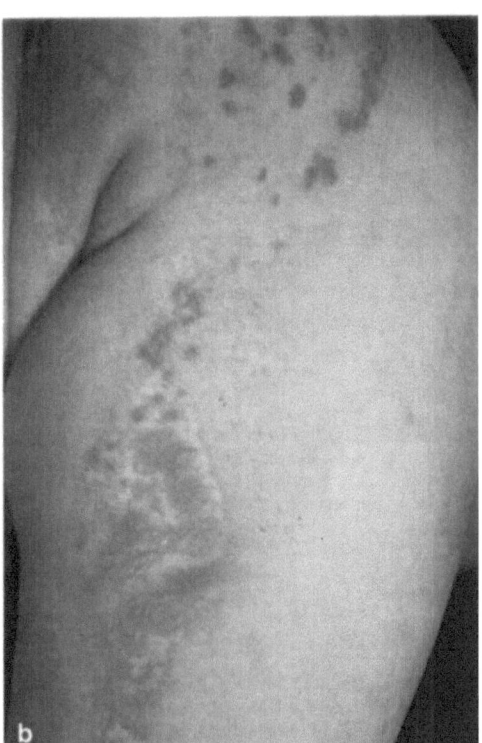

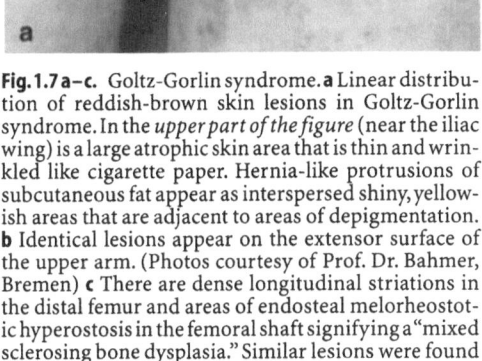

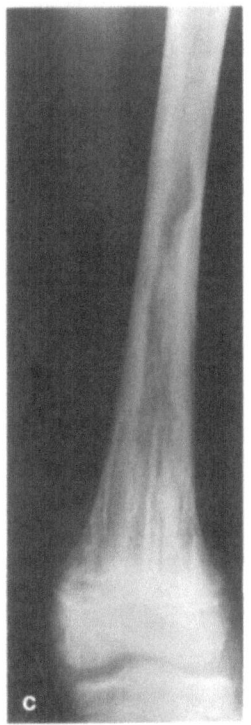

Fig.1.7a–c. Goltz-Gorlin syndrome. **a** Linear distribution of reddish-brown skin lesions in Goltz-Gorlin syndrome. In the *upper part of the figure* (near the iliac wing) is a large atrophic skin area that is thin and wrinkled like cigarette paper. Hernia-like protrusions of subcutaneous fat appear as interspersed shiny, yellowish areas that are adjacent to areas of depigmentation. **b** Identical lesions appear on the extensor surface of the upper arm. (Photos courtesy of Prof. Dr. Bahmer, Bremen) **c** There are dense longitudinal striations in the distal femur and areas of endosteal melorheostotic hyperostosis in the femoral shaft signifying a "mixed sclerosing bone dysplasia." Similar lesions were found in the other extremities

As noted earlier, osteopathic striations have been found to coexist with osteopoikilosis, partial osteopetrosis, melorheostosis, and progressive diaphyseal dysplasia (Engelmann's disease). Beighton and Cremin (1980) described an association of osteopathia striata with cranial sclerosis and classified this syndrome as having an autosomal dominant mode of inheritance. These authors observed sclerosis of the skull base accompanied by slight expansion and increased density of the calvarium, sometimes limited to its anterior or posterior portion. Clinically, these sclerotic changes are often associated with increased cranial circumference, frontal bossing, and deafness.

The long-bone striations in this syndrome may be accompanied by patchy sclerotic areas in the ribs and pelvis and near vertebral end plates, the latter sometimes associated with scoliosis or other spinal deformities.

The combination of osteopathia striata with other sclerosing skeletal changes is also referred to as *mixed sclerosing bone dysplasia or dystrophy* (e.g., Whyte et al. 1981).

References

Beighton P, Cremin BJ (1980) Sclerosing bone dysplasias. Springer, Berlin Heidelberg New York

Ginsburg LD, Sedano HO, Gorlin RJ (1970) Focal dermal hypoplasia syndrome. Am J Roentgenol 110: 561

Holden JD, Akers WA (1967) Goltz's syndrome: focal dermal hypoplasia; combined mesoectodermal dysplasia. AMA Am J Dis Child 114: 292

Howell JB (1965) Nevus angiolipomatosus vs. focal dermal hypoplasia. AMA Arch Dermatol Syph 92: 238

Larregue M, Michel Y, Maroteaux J et al. (1973) L'ostéopathie striée et dysmorphies squelettiques associées dans l'hypoplasie dermique en aires. Rev Rhum Mal Osteoartic 6: 415

Whyte MP, Murphy WA, Fallon MD et al. (1981) Mixed-sclerosing-bone-dystrophy: report of a case and review of the literature. Skeletal Radiol 6: 95

1.8 Melorheostosis with Circumscribed Scleroderma

Synonyms for circumscribed scleroderma: localized scleroderma, morphea

Roentgen signs: tracks of hyperostotic bone resembling wax flowing down a burning candle, segmental distribution.
Cutaneous signs: circumscribed linear and band-like areas of scleroderma.

Definition

Melorheostosis is a rare disease of unknown etiology characterized by wavy tracks of periosteal and endosteal new bone formation that appear to flow along the cortex of the affected bone. Affected areas present clinically with swelling and induration, and various cutaneous manifestations (e.g., circumscribed scleroderma) occur with some frequency.

General Clinical Features

The term "melorheostosis" is derived from the Greek *melos* ("limb") and *rheos* ("flow"). It describes the radiographic appearance of melorheostosis, in which periosteal and endosteal hyperostosis "flows down" the surface of the affected bone like wax flowing down the side of a burning candle (see Fig. 1.8 b, c). Approximately 200 to 300 cases have been published to date, and we have personally diagnosed 11 cases.

The etiology of this congenital condition is unclear, and genetic factors apparently do not play a role. Because the segmental distribution pattern of the lesions follows the distribution of the sclerotomes (zones of the skeleton supplied by individual spinal sensory nerves), Murray and McCredie (1979) suggested a pathogenesis analogous to that of herpes zoster, i.e., an early infection of the sensory nerves causing nerve scarring that leads secondarily to the segmental sclerotic bone changes. The frequent association of subcutaneous fibrosis and soft-tissue ossification with muscle contractures could perhaps be analogous to the involvement of dermatomes and myotomes of the same sensory nerve roots. Interestingly, it has been suggested that both peripheral and central nerve lesions are involved in the pathogenesis of linear and band-like morphea as a special, localized form of scleroderma (Korting 1979).

Patients with melorheostosis usually become symptomatic no later than the second or third decade of life, presenting with chronic pain, soft-tissue swelling, and limited motion in the affected skeletal segment. Laboratory findings are normal. Contractures and even ankylosis may develop in the affected limb as bony deposits form across articular surfaces. Circumscribed scleroderma and particularly childhood morphea are associated with muscular abnormalities (myosclerosis, myositis, muscular atrophy). Lengthening or shortening of the affected extremity may be observed.

Approximately 17% of patients with melorheostosis exhibit skin changes in the form of patchy hyperpigmented areas, especially over affected bone, in addition to blood and lymphatic vascular malformations and circumscribed scleroderma (see below). Occasionally the skin lesions may antedate the skeletal changes. Raby and Vivian (1988) and Garver et al. (1982) described melorheostosis combined with spinal lipomas in rare cases of spinal involvement and with calcified fibrolipomatous tissue in the retroperitoneal region in front of a sacrum affected by melorheostosis.

While no sex predilection is known for melorheostosis, circumscribed scleroderma reportedly shows a 2:1 to 3:1 female preponderance.

Dermatology

The major cutaneous manifestation of melorheostosis is circumscribed scleroderma, whose predominant form consists of linear or band-like lesions in children. Circumscribed scleroderma, known also as localized scleroderma or morphea, is a chronic disease of unknown etiology in which circumscribed skin areas undergo sclerosis following an initial inflammatory phase (Fig. 1.8 a). A variety of patterns have been described, including focal circumscribed scleroderma, mottled circumscribed scleroderma, erythematous circumscribed scleroderma, disseminated circumscribed scleroderma, and linear or band-like circumscribed scleroderma (Braun-Falco et al. 1991). The skin lesion of circumscribed scleroderma starts as a large, round or oval, moderately inflamed erythematous macule that may spread. Later the periphery of the lesion becomes more heavily pigmented while its center remains hypopigmented or depigmented. Next a yellowish-white, indurated plaque appears, surrounded by a distinctive violaceous border of variable width called the "lilac ring" (Fig. 1.8 a). Finally the lesion may become atrophic, losing its hair and sebaceous glands and showing internal pigmentary changes. In the linear or band-like form of localized scleroderma, which is the form most closely associated with melorheostosis, the extremities bear linear band-like lesions, sometimes widespread, that follow the longitudinal axis of the affected limb. Indurated sclerotic foci that cross joints can cause significant limitation of motion. As mentioned, patients may have coexistent muscular disorders such as myosclerosis, muscular atrophy, and myositis.

Goldschlag (1929, quoted in Morris et al. 1963) described an association of melorheostosis with a Meige type of primary lymphedema. This hereditary lymphedema differs from Nonne-Milroy trophedema in that it does not appear until puberty and is almost twice as common in females as in males. Examination reveals firm, painless swellings on the lower legs and feet caused by a fibrotic reaction to previous edema. Other associated changes that have been described include mental retardation, hypogenitalism, short stature, hip and thigh obesity, drooping eyelids, and recurrent intrahepatic cholestases. Hall (1961) described an association of melorheostosis with cutaneous hemangioma and "lymphatic bullae." Höffken et al. (1951) described areas of hyperpigmentation, particularly over the skeletal segments affected by melorheostosis.

In their review of the literature, Morris et al. (1963) found associations with hemangiomas, glomus tumors, enlarged femoral veins and capillaries, arteriovenous malformations, and vascular nevi. Concomitant melorheostosis and neurofibromatosis was also described.

Radiology

The "limb and flow" etymology of the disease describes its basic radiographic features. The are-

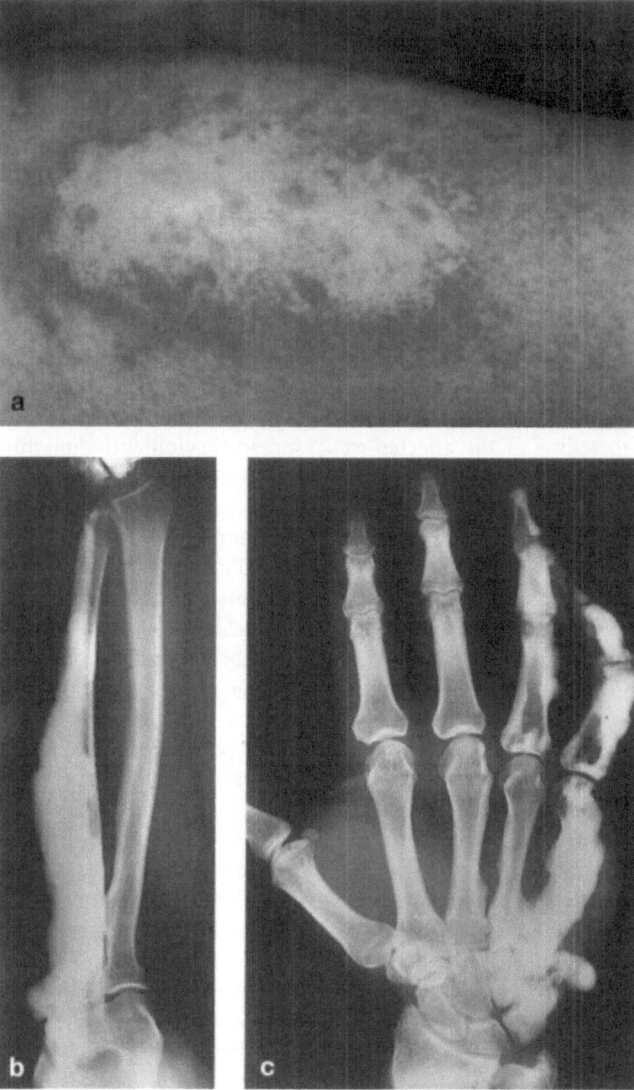

Fig. 1.8 a–c. Melorheostosis with circumscribed scleroderma. **a** Indurated plaquelike lesion with central depigmentation surrounded by a violaceous border ("lilac ring"). This lesion was preceded by an area of inflammatory erythema. Eventually the change progresses to atrophy with hyper- and depigmentation and local hair loss. **b,c** "Dripping candle" pattern of hyperostosis on the ulna and on the fourth and fifth digits, showing a predominantly eccentric distribution. Note the flexion contracture of the small finger. The changes were localized to the right side of the extremity (ulnar nerve region). Axillary examination revealed sites of soft-tissue ossification with firm subcutaneous fibrosis. Clinically, the ulnar and hand lesions were associated with significant pain and fibrosis that rendered the right arm useless. The patient, now 36 years of age, did not become symptomatic until puberty

as of new bone formation typically show a segmental distribution (e.g., a hemipelvis plus the ipsilateral thigh and lower leg). They form wavy tracks along the cortical surface of the bone, resembling wax flowing down a candle (Fig. 1.8 b, c). Endosteal new bone formation also occurs, primarily affecting and sometimes filling flat and irregular bones. The most common sites of involvement are the long tubular bones of the lower extremity, but the small bones of the foot may also be affected. The hyperostotic changes are usually eccentric, i.e., confined to one side of the bone. Garver et al. (1982) and Raby and Vivian (1988) described unusual sites of occurrence on the ribs, pelvis, and spine.

The characteristic roentgen appearance of melorheostosis usually allows a simple *differential diagnosis*. Juxtacortical osteosarcoma should be considered when monostotic involvement is seen. Generally, however, osteosarcoma is not as dense, solid, or wavy as melorheostosis. Also, juxtacortical osteosarcoma is usually associated with a broader area of ossification, often with destruction of the underlying cortex. CT and MR scans of sarcoma usually demonstrate a nonossified tumor component that is not seen with melorheostosis. The differential diagnosis may also include cortical osteoid osteoma, which usually has a shorter history than monostotic melorheostosis and whose pain symptoms are easily controlled with aspirin. Cortical osteomas are indistinguishable from melorheostosis and may in fact be a "miniature version" of the more extensive lesions of melorheostosis.

The histologic features of melorheostosis are so nonspecific that tissue examination cannot confirm the diagnosis.

References

Braun-Falco O, Plewig G, Wolff HH, Winkelmann RK (1991) Dermatology, 3rd edn. Springer, Berlin Heidelberg New York

Garver P, Resnick D, Haghighi P et al. (1982) Melorheostosis of the axial skeleton with associated fibrolipomatous lesions. Skeletal Radiol 9: 41

Hall R (1961) A case of Melorheostosis with cutaneous haemangioma and lymphatic vesicles. J Bone Joint Surg Br 43: 335

Höffken W, Heim G (1951) Melorheostose mit Sklerosierung der Knochen im rechten oberen Körperquadranten, Schädelbeteiligung und Hautveränderungen. Röfo 74: 289

Korting GW (1979) Dermatologie in Klinik und Praxis, Bd III 34. Thieme, Stuttgart

Morris JM, Samilson RL, Corley CL (1963) Melorheostosis. Review of the literature and report of an interesting case with a nineteen-year follow-up. J Bone Joint Surg Am 45: 1191

Murray RO, McCredie J (1979) Melorheostosis and the sclerotomes: a radiological correlation. Skeletal Radiol 4: 57

Raby N, Vivian G (1988) Case report 478 (Melorheostosis of the axial skeleton with associated intrathecal lipoma). Skeletal Radiol 17: 216

1.9 Gardner's Syndrome

Roentgen signs: multiple osteomas, most commonly affecting the mandible, the tubular bones, and occasionally the pelvis; dental abnormalities.
Mucocutaneous signs: epidermoid cysts, intestinal polyposis.

Definition

Gardner's syndrome is a variant of familial adenomatous polyposis with an autosomal dominant mode of inheritance. It is associated with multisystem abnormalities, and skeletal changes with multiple osteomas are a characteristic feature.

General Clinical Features

Gardner's syndrome in the strict sense (colonic polyposis, multiple osteomas, epidermoid cysts) and familial adenomatous polyposis are probably based on various mutations of the same gene on the long arm of chromosome 5. The penetrance of the dominant gene is 95%, with 40% of cases occurring sporadically, i.e., based essentially on new mutations.

Because Gardner's syndrome is a variant of familial adenomatous polyposis, it may present with any or all features of that disorder. Briefly, hundreds of tubular and tubulovillous adenomas ("polyps") appear throughout the colon during the first and second decades of life and no later than the third decade, the polyps becoming more numerous from the ascending colon toward the rectum (Fig. 1.9 a). Patients present clinically with blood and mucus in the stool. Without treatment, it is virtually certain that some of the polyps will undergo malignant transformation. Up to 50% of patients have benign polyps in the gastric fundus, and a similar percentage develop adenomas, which are especially common in Japanese patients. Duodenal adenomas have a very high risk of malignant transformation. Approximately 4% of patients have benign desmoid tumors in the form of an aggressive mesenteric fibromatosis, especially after colectomy. High-dose tamoxifen therapy can inhibit the growth of these lesions.

Congenital hypertrophy of the retinal pigmented epithelium occurs in some 85% of cases but does not affect vision. The incidence of epidermoid cysts in familial polyposis is approximately 50–65%. Patients with familial polyposis frequently have endocrine abnormalities and endocrine tumors (of the thyroid, ovaries, adrenals, etc.).

Dermatology

The cutaneous manifestations of Gardner's syndrome appear shortly after birth or in early childhood and predominantly involve the face, head, and neck. Two types of lesions may be seen:

1. Slow-growing *epidermal cysts*. These are round, raised subcutaneous lesions ranging from about 1 to 5 cm in diameter. The contents of the cysts have a soft, semiliquid consistency and a fetid odor.
2. *Sebaceous cysts*. These are epithelial cysts that exhibit small nests of sebocytes in the cyst wall. Multiple sebaceous cysts occur in Gardner's syndrome and chiefly involve the neck and scrotal regions.

Radiology

The radiologic features of the colonic polyps are beyond the scope of this text. The main skeletal abnormalities are osteomas of the jaws and long tubular bones. They occur in more than 50% of patients with familial polyposis and are considered pathognomonic for Gardner's syndrome. Osteomas are especially common in the mandible (mandibular angle, Fig. 1.9 b), the frontal sinus, and the outer table of the skull. The mandibular changes are frequently accompanied by dental abnormalities (hypercementomas, odontogenic cysts, extra teeth, numerous caries). Osteomas of the pelvis appear as punctate densities, while osteomas on the long bones look like cortical hyperostoses and primarily affect the diaphyses. Melorheostosis-like hyperostosis can also occur (see p. 32). The skeletal changes in Gardner's syndrome may antedate the intestinal lesions.

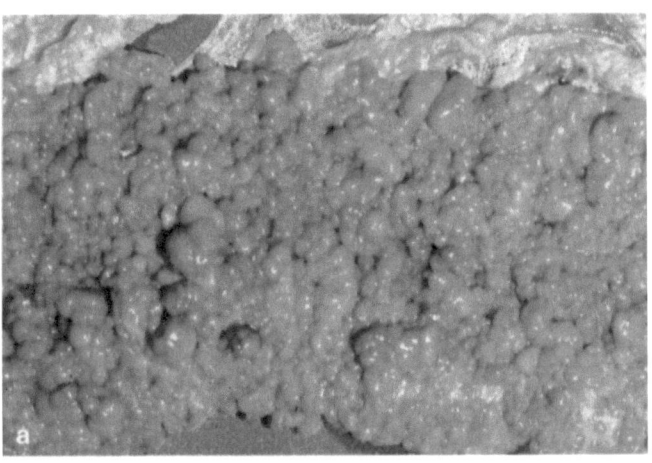

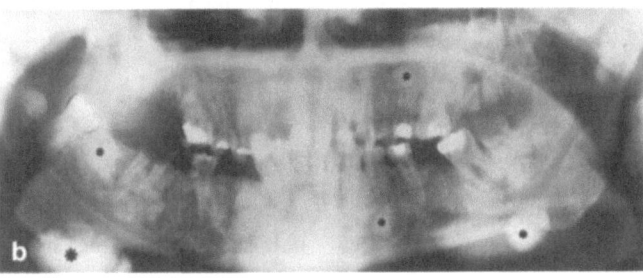

Fig.1.9a,b. Gardner's syndrome in a 27-year-old woman with multiple maxillary and mandibular osteomas (*asterisks*, **b**). The conspicuous, lobulated tumor on the right mandibular angle prompted referral of the patient to our oral surgery clinic. The panoramic film also shows marked dental abnormalities and advanced caries. Skeletal radiographs showed additional hyperostotic lesions: osteomas of the calvarium and periosteal and cortical osteomas of the long tubular bones. Myriad polyps line the colectomy specimen in **a**. The patient's mother had generalized polyposis and died from colon carcinoma, thus identifying the disorder as a familial polyposis with skeletal abnormalities. The patient had other abnormalities including thyroid and ovarian endocrine dysfunction and an epidermal oil cyst above the anal fissure (full radiographic documentation of this case may be found in Freyschmidt, 1997)

References

Freyschmidt J (1997) Skeletterkrankungen. Klinisch-radiologische Diagnose und Differentialdiagnose, 2. Aufl. Springer, Berlin Heidelberg New York

Harned RK, Buck JL, Olmsted WW et al. (1991) Extracolonic manifestations of the familial adenomatous polyposi syndromes. Am J Roentgenol 156: 481

1.10 Cronkhite-Canada Syndrome

Synonym: Ménétrier's syndrome

Because this condition is mainly of interest in gastroenterology, it will be discussed only briefly here. Cronkhite-Canada syndrome is a rare systemic disorder in which multiple hamartomatous gastrointestinal polyps are associated with ectodermal changes such as alopecia, onychodystrophy, and hyperpigmentation of the skin. Only about 60 cases have been described to date.

The etiology of this syndrome is unclear. The disease takes a remitting and relapsing course marked clinically by diarrhea and weight loss. Sanders et al. (1985) described the case of a 72-year-old woman with severe clinical symptoms and extensive polyposis involving all portions of the gastrointestinal tract (demonstrated radiographically and endoscopically). The diarrhea was associated with progressive alopecia and loss of the eyebrows and nails. The alopecia and other symptoms regressed in response to massive alimentary replacement. One year later the patient relapsed, developing joint symptoms in the shoulder and distal interphalangeal joints. Radiographs showed erosive changes with marginal and central destruction of the distal interphalangeal joints, similar to the pattern in multicentric reticulohistiocytosis. Synovial biopsy from a bursa showed only nonspecific synovitis with focal hyperemia. The joint effusion was blood-tinged and bacteriologically sterile. Maurer and Beck (1980) described a similar case with joint manifestations in a 62-year-old woman.

The erosive arthritis seen in association with psoriasis, Reiter's disease, and multicentric reticulohistiocytosis is readily distinguished clinically and radiologically from that in Cronkhite-Canada syndrome.

References

Cronkhite LW, Canada WJ (1955) Generalized gastrointestinal polyposis: an unusual syndrome of polyposis, pigmentation, alopecia and onychotrophia. N Engl J Med 252: 1011

Maurer H-J, Berek L (1980) Knochen- und Gelenkveränderungen bei Ménétrier- bzw. Cronkhite-Syndrom. Röfo 132: 728

Sanders KM, Resnik CS, Owen DS (1985) Erosive arthritis in Cronkhite-Canada-Syndrome. Radiology 156: 309

1.11 Proteus Syndrome

Unilateral hypertrophy affecting one body half or extremity, macrodactyly; nodular gyriform thickenings on the palms and soles; epidermal nevi in the form of multiple small verrucous papules; subcutaneous lipomas, hamartomas; cartilaginous exostoses; scoliosis due to vertebral hypertrophy.

Definition

Proteus syndrome is a genetically determined disorder that is associated with more or less circumscribed areas of hypertrophy and with hamartomatous lesions of the skin, subcutaneous tissues, and bones.

General Clinical, Dermatologic, and Radiologic Features

Fewer than 100 cases of the syndrome have been published to date. Its etiology is poorly understood but presumably involves a spontaneous mutation of autosomal dominant genes, possibly the genes responsible for the local production and regulation of tissue growth factors. Apparently all three germ layers are affected. The clinical hallmark is complete or incomplete unilateral hypertrophy limited to one body half or one extremity. Other features are macrodactyly, subcutaneous mesodermal tumors, palmoplantar tumors, exostoses, epidermal nevi, and scoliosis. Less common cutaneous manifestations are depigmented areas, café-au-lait spots, subcutaneous atrophy, superficial varicosities, and angiokeratomas.

The *cardinal features* will be described in somewhat greater detail. The palmoplantar lesions usually appear as nodular thickenings with a symmetric, gyriform distribution. There may be yellowish discoloration of the overlying skin. Sometimes the lesions appear only as palpable cutaneous thickenings on the palms and soles. Epidermal nevi are another striking feature of proteus syndrome. They occur primarily on the neck, trunk, axillae, groin, and extremities. They may be hyperpigmented and often are described as multiple, small, verrucous papules with indistinct borders.

The hemihypertrophy affecting isolated musculoskeletal regions or an entire body half is obvious on visual inspection and involves both the skeleton and the soft tissues. This can result in significant arm- or leg-length discrepancies. Clinical and radiographic abnormalities consist of facial asymmetries and calvarial bulging (bony protuberances), macrodactyly of one or more fingers or toes, cartilaginous exostoses on the metaphyses and apophyses of long tubular bones, and scoliotic deformity secondary to more or less localized vertebral hypertrophy (megalospondylodysplasia).

From a dermatologic standpoint, proteus syndrome mainly requires differentiation from *Solomon's syndrome* (epidermal nevus syndrome), which may feature epidermal nevi, spinal abnormalities, and hemangiomas. Solomon's syndrome may actually be a variant of proteus syndrome. Neurofibromatosis should also be considered in the differential diagnosis (see p. 20). The hemihypertrophy and macrodactyly serve to differentiate proteus syndrome from *Klippel-Trenaunay syndrome* and *Parkes-Weber syndrome*.

Since proteus syndrome is a hamartomatous disease with a potential for malignant transformation, it is imperative that regular follow-ups be maintained.

References

Baykal C, Gögüs A, Gürsoy EÖ et al. (1994) Proteus-Syndrom. Hautarzt 45: 237

Costa T, Fitch N, Azouz EM (1985) Proteus syndrome: report of two cases with pelvic lipomatosis. Pediatrics 76: 984

Maassen D, Voigtlaender V (1991) Proteus-Syndrom. Hautarzt 42: 186

Samlaska CP, Levin SW, James WD et al. (1989) Proteus-Syndrome. Arch Dermatol 125: 1009

Solomon LM, Fretzin DF, Dewald RL (1968) The epidermal nevus syndrome. Arch Dermatol 97: 273

Wiedemann HR, Burgio GR, Aldenhoff P et al. (1983) The proteus syndrome. Eur J Pediatr 140: 5

1.12 Basal Cell Nevus Syndrome (Gorlin-Goltz Syndrome)

Synonyms: Syndrome of jaw cysts, hereditary cutaneomandibular polyoncosis

Multiple broad-based, brownish or skin-colored tumors that become true basal cell cancers on the face, neck, trunk, and proximal extremities.

Roentgen signs: large maxillary and mandibular cysts; cysts in tubular bones; frontoparietal bossing, calcification of the falx cerebri, shallow sella; rib deformities; scoliosis.

Definition

Basal cell nevus syndrome is an autosomal dominant hereditary disorder associated with multiple nevoid, pigmented or keratinizing basal cell epitheliomas, multiple jaw cysts, solitary or multiple rib deformities, and other skeletal abnormalities.

General Clinical Features

Since basal cell nevus syndrome was first described by Gorlin and Goltz (1960), more than 150 cases have been reported in the literature. There is disagreement as to whether the disease can be classified as a fifth phakomatosis based on its ocular and central nervous system manifestations. The skin lesions may appear in childhood but usually are first noticed between 20 and 30 years of age. In most cases the fully developed presentation of the syndrome is delayed until age 30 or after. Not infrequently, the mandibular cysts are the first presenting symptom and lead the patient to consult a dentist or oral surgeon (see Fig. 1.12 b).

Besides the cutaneous and osseous abnormalities described below, patients may have ocular manifestations consisting of hypertelorism, canthal dystopia, congenital blindness, or internal strabismus. Neurologic manifestations are rare and may consist of mental retardation, congenital hydrocephalus, medulloblastomas, dural calcifications, and agenesis of the corpus callosum.

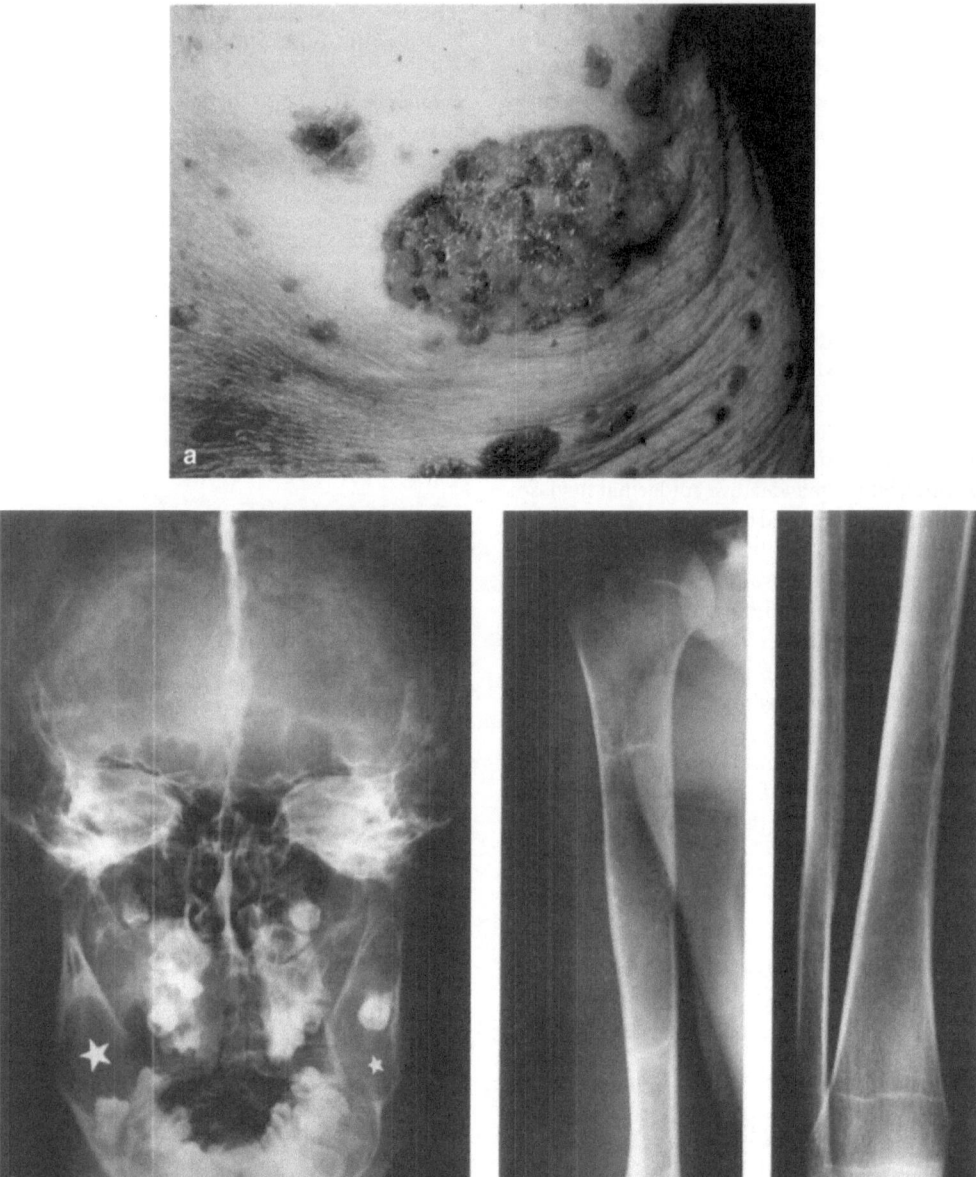

Fig. 1.12 a–d. Basal cell nevus syndrome (Gorlin-Goltz syndrome). **a** Disseminated basal cell carcinomas. The large tumor at the center of the photo shows small ulcerations and areas of crusting. **b–d** This 20-year-old man sought medical attention for multiple prominent cysts of the mandible (**b**) accompanied by extensive dental abnormalities. Other cysts were found in the right humerus (**c**), coalescing in the midshaft region to form one large cyst. Multiple cysts up to 2 cm in diameter were also found in other tubular bones (**d**) including the bones of the hand. Skull radiograph (**b**) shows marked frontal and parietal bossing and significant calcification of the falx. CT scan (not shown) revealed internal hydrocephalus and meningeal calcifications

Less common manifestations are hypogonadism in males and ovarian tumors in females.

Dermatology

The cutaneous manifestations of this syndrome are a form of nevoid systemic disease that may present in a nevoid or oncogenic stage. The nevoid stage is characterized by multiple broad-based brownish or skin-colored tumors that appear during childhood or puberty and may ulcerate and form crusts. These tumors occur on the face, the back of the neck, the trunk, and the proximal parts of the extremities. Progression to the oncogenic stage occurs at about age 20, when the lesions are clearly identifiable, both clinically and histologically, as basal cell carcinomas (Fig. 1.12 a). Lesions on the palms and soles are called "pits."

Radiology

Rib deformities and mandibular cysts are classic features and an integral component of the Goltz-Gorlin syndrome. The rib deformities (seen in about 45% of cases) are diverse, ranging from rudimentary ribs, synostoses, shortened ribs, and bifid ribs to widening or thinning of the ribs. As Novak and Bloss (1976) showed in 4 of their own cases and 105 cases from the literature, these rib deformities are not incidental findings, as their incidence in the population as a whole is only 2–5%.

The most common bony lesions in basal cell nevus syndrome are mandibular cysts (Fig. 1.12 b). Histologically, these lesions are benign follicular or odontogenic keratocysts. As noted earlier, they may antedate the appearance of skin lesions. The cysts are multiple and show a tendency to recur. Maxillary cysts are found in approximately 35% of cases. Radiographs may also demonstrate frontal and/or parietal bossing (see Fig. 1.12 b). Another possible cranial abnormality is prognathia. Calcification of the falx is noted in almost 50% of cases (Fig. 1.12 b) versus about 7% in the population at large. Other potential sites of calcification are the tentorium and the dura. The sella may be markedly small and shallow, and sellar bridges with petrosellar calcification may be observed.

Approximately 32% of patients have scoliosis. Many other spinal deformities may occur, including block vertebrae and spina bifida.

Cystic changes in the tubular bones can be highly characteristic (Fig. 1.12 c, d). Novak and Bloss (1976) described cystlike lucencies 2–3 mm in diameter in the radius, ulna, and the bones of the hand. Blinder et al. (1984) published the case of three family members with pronounced cystic lesions in all the tubular bones combined with spotty osteopoikilotic lesions. The cystic lesions were sharply demarcated without sclerotic margins or soft-tissue changes, and some had a distinctive flame shape.

In our case we observed a large confluent cyst in the right humerus (Fig. 1.12 d) along with smaller cystic lesions, also flame-shaped, in the forearms, tibiae, and the bones of the hand. There is about a 50% incidence of cystic changes in the bones of the hand.

References

Blinder G, Barki Y, Pezt M et al. (1984) Widespread osteolytic lesions of the long bones in basal cell nevus syndrome. Skeletal Radiol 12: 196

Camisa C, Rossana C, Little L (1985) Naevoid basal-cell carcinoma syndrome with unilateral neoplasms and pits. Br J Dermatol 113: 365

Gorlin RJ, Goltz RW (1960) Multiple nevoid basal cell epithelium jaw cysts and bifid rib syndrome. N Engl J Med 262: 908

Lile HA, Rogers JF, Gerald B (1968) The basal cell nevus syndrome. Radiology 103: 214

Novak D, Bloss W (1976) Röntgenologische Aspekte des Basalzell-Naevus-Syndroms (Gorlin-Goltz-Syndrom). Röfo 124: 11

Potaznik D, Steinherz P (1984) Multiple nevoid basal cell carcinoma syndrome and Hodgkin's disease. Cancer 53: 2713

Ramström G, Anniko M (1985) Clinical and histopathologic findings in a patient with Gorlin's Syndrome. Arch Otorhinolaryngol 241: 157

1.13 Ichthyosis with Chondrodysplasia Punctata (Conradi-Hünermann Syndrome, Happle's Syndrome)

Synonyms for chondrodysplasia punctata: chondrodystrophia calcificans congenita punctata, stippled epiphyses, Conradi-Hünermann disease

Whorled or gyrate pattern of hyperkeratosis, follicular cutaneous atrophy of the distal extremities, foci of scarring alopecia.
Roentgen signs: stippled epiphyses and other skeletal abnormalities.

This syndrome is known in the radiological literature mainly for its distinctive stippled pattern of epiphyseal calcifications. It constitutes a rare type of epiphyseal dysplasia marked by the appearance of small punctate calcifications in the epiphyses during the first year of life before the ossification centers appear (Fig. 1.13). The sites most commonly involved are the hips, knees, shoulders, wrists, and tarsi. The underlying pathoanatomy involves hypervascularization of the epiphyseal cartilages with patchy mucoid degeneration and fragmentation. The fragments form niduses for pathologic calcification. The densities may disappear by 3 years of age or may coalesce to form a normal-appearing ossification center. There may be asymmetric shortening of the tubular bones, and accelerated growth has been observed. The stippling of the epiphyses is finer than the epiphyseal fragmentation that occurs in cretinism or multiple epiphyseal dysplasia. Clubfoot, dislocation of the hip, and various spinal deformities have also been observed. Other possible abnormalities include saddle nose, microcephaly, flexion contractures, cataracts, cardiac anomalies, and calcifications of the synovial membrane.

Mental retardation is a common associated finding.

Chondrodysplasia punctata is known to be associated with ichthyosis. Happle et al. (1977, 1979) described X-linked dominant chondrodysplasia punctata that only occurs in female newborns while the underlying (X-linked) gene defects is lethal in (hemizygous) males. Cutaneous anomalies of this syndrome are congenital ichthyosiform erythroderma with linear patterns of whorled or gyrate hyperkeratoses that regress during the first months of live and are subsequently leaving atrophic skin lesions and alopecia with the same pattern.

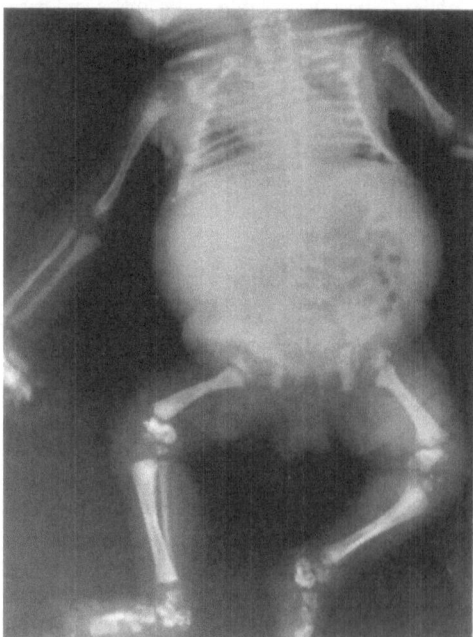

Fig. 1.13. Newborn with classic chondrodysplasia punctata. Stippled calcifications of irregular density, some confluent, involve all the epiphyses of the upper and lower extremities. Whorls of ichthyosiform hyperkeratosis were noted clinically

References

Brogdon BG, Grow NE (1958) Chondrodysplasia calcificans congenita. Am J Roentgenol 80: 443
Happle R, Mathiass HH, Macher E (1977) Sex-linked chondrodysplasia punctata? Clin Genet 11: 73
Happle R, Kästner H (1979) X-gekoppelt dominante Chondrodysplasia punctata. Hautarzt 30: 590
Korting GW et al. (Hrsg) (1980) Dermatologie in Praxis und Klinik. Band 2, 21.11. Thieme, Stuttgart
Mason RC, Kozlowski K (1973) Chondrodysplasia punctata. Radiology 109: 145

1.14 Congenital Ichthyosiform Erythroderma with Acro-osteolysis

Fishscale-like keratinization disorders involving the neck, the periumbilical and peri-areolar skin, and the flexor surfaces of the extremities; watchglass nails, clubbing of the fingers.
Roentgen signs: acro-osteolysis.

Ichthyosiform erythroderma is a rare, probably autosomal recessive skin disease with variable expression that is classified as a relatively mild form of congenital ichthyosis. Fishscale-like keratinization disorders are present at birth. The skin is slack, dry, and creases easily and is covered with small, plate-like horny scales. In some cases the lesions predominantly involve the back and sides of the neck, the periumbilical and peri-areolar areas, and flexor surfaces. The case with acro-osteolysis described by Vidal et al. (1979) displayed mild generalized erythema at birth that was most pronounced on flexor surfaces of the extremities. The syndrome is associated with parchment-like facial skin and the development of ectropion at an early age. Braun-Falco et al. (1991) also observed hypotrichosis, mental deficiency, general growth retardation, and cardiac abnormalities. The case of ichthyosiform erythroderma described by Vidal et al. (1979) was associated with watchglass nails and clubbed fingers (drumstick fingers). Examination of the patient at 16 years of age disclosed resorption of the distal portions of the distal phalanges of the hands and feet with thickening of the surrounding soft tissues.

The acro-osteolytic changes (a typical example is shown in Fig. 7.1 f) may well be a result of vascular insufficiency caused by the pronounced ichthyosis on the hands and feet.

References

Braun-Falco O, Plewig G, Wolff HH, Winkelmann RK (1991) Dermatology, 3rd edn. Springer, Berlin Heidelberg New York
Vidal JJ, Ruiz, Santiago T et al. (1979) Case report 106: Ichthyosiform erythroderma associated with osteolysis of the terminal tufts of the hands (and feet). Skeletal Radiol 4: 251

1.15 Refsum's Syndrome

Synonyms: Refsum's disease; phytanic acid thesaurismosis

Night blindness, peripheral neuropathy, cerebellar ataxia, ichthyosis of the trunk and extremities.
Roentgen signs: epiphyseal flattening and sclerosis of the femoral condyles, shortening and broadening of small tubular bones in the hands and feet, irregularities of the vertebral end plates.

Refsum's syndrome is based on an autosomal recessive defect of phytanic acid metabolism. The body lacks the essential oxidative enzyme that breaks down phytanic acid as an initial step in the metabolic pathway. Since phytanic acid is a fatty acid, its persistence leads to widespread lipid deposition in red blood cells, the liver, kidneys, heart, peripheral nerves, and other organs. Phytanic acid is absorbed by foods that contain chlorophyll. Initial symptoms usually appear between ages 20 and 40 with an atypical form of retinitis pigmentosa that causes night blindness. This is followed later by chronic progressive peripheral neuropathy, cerebellar ataxia, and occasional cutaneous manifestations: mild *ichthyosis* of the trunk and extremities and an ichthyosiform erythroderma. The ichthyosis closely resembles the dominant ichthyosis vulgaris in its clinical and histologic features. Laboratory tests show elevated levels of phytanic acid in the serum and cerebrospinal fluid.

Radiographs show distinctive epiphyseal abnormalities that consist mainly of flattening and subchondral sclerosis of the femoral condyles, similar to ischemic necrosis. Additionally there is marked symmetric shortening and broadening of individual small tubular bones in the hands and/or feet. Vertebral end-plate irregularities are seen most commonly in the thoracic and lumbar regions of the spine (Lovelock and Griffiths 1981).

References

Lovelock J, Griffiths H (1981) Case report 175. Skeletal Radiol 7: 214
Wall WJH, Worthington BS (1979) Skeletal changes in Refsum's disease. Clin Radiol 30: 657

1.16 Hereditary Palmoplantar Keratosis with Drumstick Fingers and Bony Hypertrophy

Synonym: Bureau-Barrière-Thomas syndrome

Diffuse, symmetric keratoses on the palms and soles; clubbing of the fingers and toes, watchglass nails, palmoplantar hyperhidrosis.

Roentgen signs: periosteal new bone formation, mainly involving the hands and feet, with a gradual increase in thickness, acro-osteolysis.

▨ Definition

Bureau-Barrière-Thomas syndrome, inherited as an autosomal recessive trait, is characterized by typical hyperkeratotic changes on the hands and feet with hyperhidrosis, digital clubbing, watchglass nails, and periosteal new bone formation on the tubular bones.

▨ General Clinical Features

Bureau-Barrière-Thomas syndrome should first be distinguished from *Bureau-Barrière syndrome*, an ulcerative, mutilating acropathy first described by Bureau and Barrière (1955). Whether this represents a separate entity or only a description of the dermatologic complications of various metabolic disorders (see below) is open to discussion.
The hallmark of Bureau-Barrière syndrome is the development of painless (trophic) ulcers (mala perforantia) on weight-bearing areas of the sole of the foot. These lesions are preceded by callus-like hyperkeratoses with fissuring, vesiculation, and secondary infection. Usually there are associated peripheral sensory disturbances and subsequent bone destruction, creating an overall picture similar to trophic osteoarthropathy. In most cases there is an underlying latent or overt diabetes mellitus with diabetic neuropathy and primary or secondary (alcoholic) disturbances of fat metabolism combined with polyneuropathy. Of the 17 patients with Bureau-Barrière syndrome studied by Thoma

et al. (1993), 8 had diabetes mellitus, and almost all had some disturbance of fat metabolism (14 were alcoholics!).
Bureau-Barrière-Thomas syndrome is inherited as an autosomal recessive trait. Symptoms begin in childhood with the characteristic palmoplantar keratoses described below and with a generalized hyperhidrosis, as stated in the definition. The hyperostotic changes in the tubular bones can occasionally cause rheumatoid aches and pains. Digital clubbing and watchglass nails develop at a very early stage. Laboratory findings are normal.

▨ Dermatology

The diffuse hyperkeratosis (by thickening of the stratium corneum) on the palms and soles is sharply demarcated from surrounding healthy skin. The dorsal surfaces of the hands and feet are always spared. The hyperkeratosis itself is diffusely distributed and consists of a thick, waxy, yellowish, fissured horny layer (Fig. 1.16 a, b). Usually it is separated from healthy skin by a well-defined pink rim several millimeters wide. These changes are often associated with hyperhidrosis. The digital clubbing and watchglass nails mentioned earlier are probably due to impaired vagal regulation of acral blood flow.

▨ Radiology

Sites of periosteal new bone formation appear on the tubular bones of the hands and feet, most commonly involving the metacarpals and metatarsals but also affecting the long bones of the forearm and lower leg (Fig. 1.16 c–g). The proliferative periosteal ossifications gradually lead to thickening of the cortical bone. The distal phalangeal tufts may acquire coarse spiculations or undergo increasing resorption. The overall picture mimics pachydermoperiostosis (see p. 181) including acro-osteolysis (Fig. 1.16 d). Differentiation from hypertrophic osteoarthropathy (see p. 185) is also required.

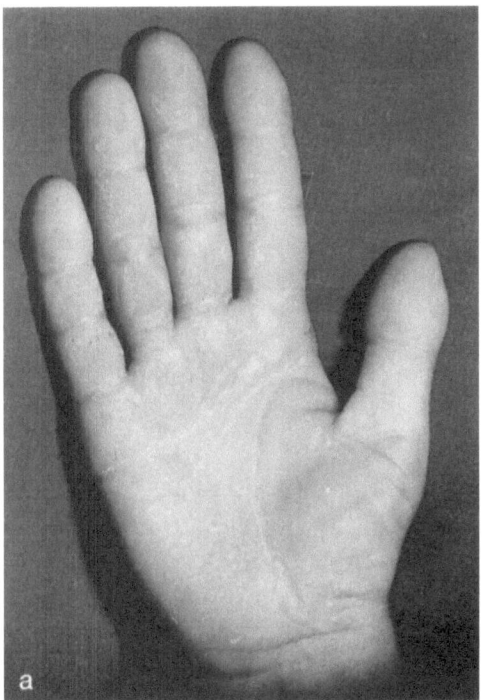

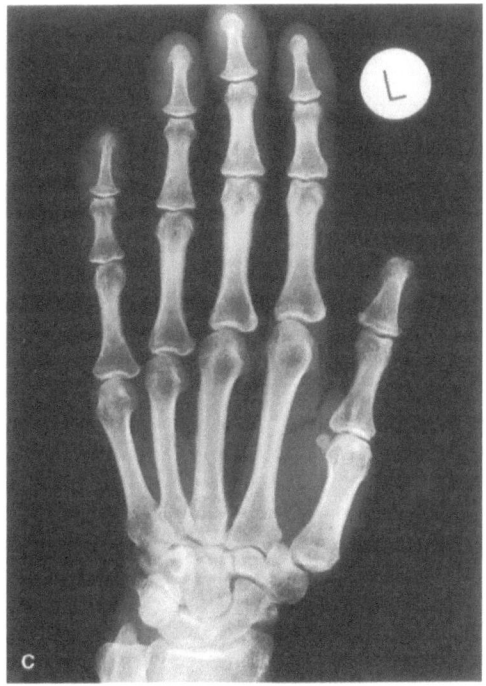

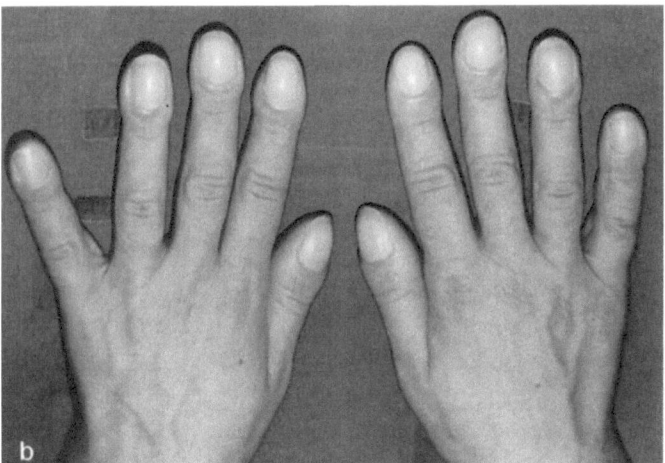

Fig. 1.16 a–g. Hereditary palmoplantar keratosis with drumstick fingers and bone hypertrophy (27-year-old female). **a** Diffuse hyperkeratosis with thick, waxy, yellowish fissured horny layers. **b** Digital clubbing and watchglass nails. Same changes in the feet. **c, d** X-rays from the left hand and right foot. Note the clubbing phenomenon in the distal phalanges with broadening of the soft-tissue shadow and spiculation of the terminal tufts. Acro-osteolysis in the distal phalanges of the foot with pencil-like configuration, same changes on the opposite side (not shown here). **e** Bone scan demonstrates increased tracer uptake in the distal radius and ulna. Same changes in the opposite side and in the distal tibiae and fibulae, caused by periosteal new bone formation. These are well demonstrated in the X-rays of the distal leg (**f**) and the forearm (**g**). The patient suffered from rheumatoid aches and pains since childhood. Numerous operations under the diagnosis of osteomyelitis had been performed in the past. **d–g** see p. 46

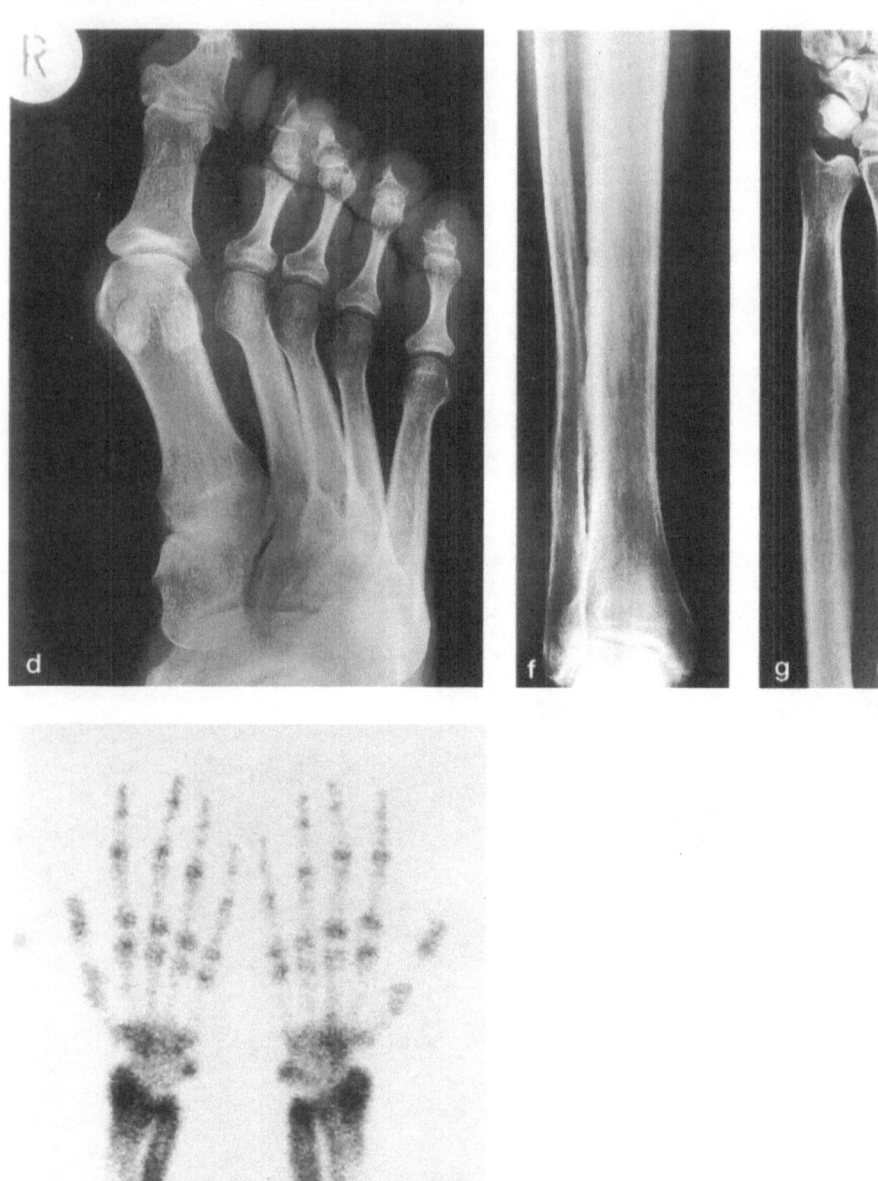

Fig. 1.16 (*continued*). See legend on p. 45

References

Bureau Y, Barrière H, Thomas M (1959) Hippocratisme digital congénital avec hyperkératose palmoplantaire et troubles osseux. Ann Dermatol Syph 86: 611

Freyschmidt J (1997) Skeletterkrankungen. Klinischradiologische Diagnose und Differentialdiagnose, 2. Aufl. Springer, Berlin Heidelberg New York

Rauch HJ, Neumayer K (1981) Bureau-Barrière-Thomas-Syndrom. Eine seltene hereditäre Palmoplantarkeratose mit assoziierten Symptomen. Z Hautkr 56: 102

Thoma E, Ruzicka T, Dornhauser G (1993) Bureau-Barrière-Syndrom. Hautarzt 44: 5

1.17 Mutilating Palmoplantar Keratoderma

Synonyms: Brauer's syndrome, keratosis palmoplantaris mutilans, Vohwinkel's syndrome

Massive palmoplantar keratosis, beginning in early childhood, characterized by annular keratotic constriction and mutilation of the affected digits and disabling contractures.

Definition

Mutilating palmoplantar keratoderma is an autosomal dominant disorder in which extreme hyperkeratosis leads to deep strictures with subsequent mutilation, contractures, and severe trophic disturbances principally involving the adjacent bone.

General Clinical Features

The disease generally has its onset in the third or fourth month of life and never appears after 6 months. The most striking feature is the appearance of massive hyperkeratotic lesions on the hands and feet, which soon lead to significant disability. Patients develop contractures of the fingers or toes, and trophic ulcerations appear. Spontaneous digital amputations occur at a relatively early stage (pseudoainhum disease). The disease takes a relentless course and has a poor prognosis. It is likely that surgical amputations in the hands and feet will eventually prove necessary, especially if infection supervenes.

Dermatology

The cutaneous lesions of palmoplantar keratosis are surrounded by a livid margin, and hyperhidrosis is present. The padlike, verruciform, hyperkeratotic lesions coalesce and spread to the dorsal side, soon leading to maceration, ainhumlike annular constrictions, and infection, especially of trophic ulcerations (Fig. 1.17 a). Verruciform keratoses may also occur on the malleoli, Achilles tendons, elbows, and knees. As mentioned, the deep scarring leads to contractures and vascular occlusions that culminate in autoamputations. Nguyen et al. (1986) reported oth-

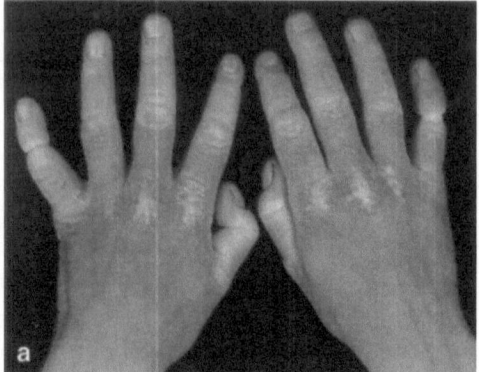

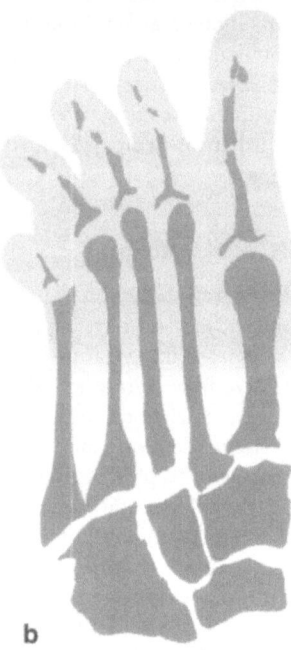

b

Fig. 1.17 a, b. Mutilating palmoplantar keratoderma. **a** Typical clinical presentation with conspicuous annular constrictions on the small fingers, an incipient constriction on the left ring finger, and flexion contractures of the thumbs. It is easy to see how these very severe cicatricial changes could strangulate the blood supply, leading gradually to necrosis of the bone. For clarity, it should be noted that the palmoplantar hyperkeratosis develops on the palmar side of the hand before gradually spreading to the dorsal aspect. This photo was selected because of the deep constrictions visible from the dorsal side. **b** Drawing of the severe mutilating changes, illustrated here for the foot (ainhum-like changes)

er ectodermal dysplasias with abnormalities of the hair, teeth, nails, and mucous membranes. The differential diagnosis should include *Olmstedt's syndrome*, which additionally features circumscribed hyperkeratotic plaques (perioral, perinasal, and perianal) that are at high risk for malignant transformation. The differential diagnosis to the hereditary palmoplantar keratosis (see p. 44) must consider the age of onset and the pattern of distribution of the hyperkeratotic changes.

Radiology

The affected tubular bones of the hands and feet are atrophic, show pathologic fractures, and finally undergo mutilative changes, with affected phalanges showing a tapered and dissolved appearance ("candy stick" configuration; Fig. 1.17 b). The metacarpals and metatarsals may also become atrophic, showing marked overconstriction of the shafts and mutilation of the epiphyses. Differentiation is required from other diseases associated with trophic disturbances such as leprosy and frostbite. Only the clinical presentation can differentiate mutilating palmoplantar keratoderma from other rare mutilating disorders such as Werner's syndrome.

References

Haußer I, Frantzmann Y, Lamprecht IA et al. (1993) Olmstedt-Syndrom. Hautarzt 44: 394
Kaveggia L, Afshani E, Gole D et al. (1989) Mutilating palmoplantar keratoderma. Case Report 581. Skeletal Radiol 18: 610
Nguyen TQ, Greer KE, Fisher GB Jr. et al. (1986) Papillon-Lefevre Syndrome. Report of two patients treated successfully with isotretinoin. J Am Acad Dermatol 15: 46

1.18 Epidermolysis Bullosa Dystrophica with Acro-osteolysis

Thin, shiny, parchment-like skin that is extremely fragile; trauma causes vesicular lesions that heal with scarring, causing contractures of the fingers and toes; hyperpigmentation on the pressure sites of extremities; numerous postbullous milia; nail loss. **Roentgen signs:** acro-osteolysis.

Definition

Epidermolysis bullosa is an autosomal recessive disorder that is present at birth and marked by an extreme, etiologically obscure vulnerability of the epidermis and mucous membranes to the slightest trauma, which causes nonspecific vesiculation culminating in rupture, infection, and scarring. The pathogenesis of the epidermolytic vesiculation is based on a separation of the epidermis and dermis secondary to degenerative changes in the basal cells.

General Clinical, Dermatologic, and Radiologic Features

The disease primarily affects the hands and feet, where scarring can lead to grotesque *contractures of the fingers and toes* and dystrophy and *loss of the nails*. Lesions behind the hairline can leave patches of scarring alopecia, the skin becoming thin, shiny, and parchment-like with hyperpigmentation and postbullous milia. Vascular occlusions lead to foci of *acro-osteolysis* in the distal phalanges. Radiographs of a patient's hands published by Hoeffel et al. (1992) show acro-osteolytic lesions and grotesque deformities involving almost all the joints. Blistering of the esophageal mucosa in the same patient led to a progressive esophageal stricture starting at 10 years of age, and numerous bullae formed in the mouth, on the lips, and in the perianal region. In cases where the dystrophic or atrophic form of the disease begins shortly after birth, two-thirds of the patients die, usually from sepsis-related complications. Survivors later manifest bullae and scarring of the conjunctiva, oral mucosa, esophagus, anal canal, and external genitalia.

References

Hoeffel JC, Bigard MA, Merle M et al. (1992) Epidermolysis bullosa: radiological patterns in childhood. Röfo 157: 427

1.19 Rothmund-Thomson Syndrome

Synonym: congenital poikiloderma

> Short stature with small hands and feet; complex skeletal anomalies; juvenile cataract and hypogonadism; premature graying of the hair; livedo reticularis-like striae, starting on the face and spreading to the buttocks and extremities with gradual progression to poikiloderma.

Definition

Rothmund-Thomson syndrome is an autosomal recessive disease that is associated with short stature, complex skeletal anomalies, and general progerian manifestations and whose distinctive feature is poikiloderma. The syndrome is distinguished from Werner's syndrome by its early onset at about 6 months of age.

General Clinical Features

Slightly more than 100 cases of Rothmund-Thomson syndrome have been described to date. The syndrome is inherited as an autosomal recessive trait and affects males about twice as often as females. The cutaneous signs appear as early as 6 months of age, quite unlike Werner's syndrome, which it closely resembles by virtue of its progerian features. Patients present clinically with short stature, small hands and feet, and dystrophic nails. The hair turns prematurely gray. Bilateral cataracts occur in about 50% of cases, and hypogonadism is not uncommon. Gaetani et al. (1988) state that the absence of osteoporosis, growth retardation, leg ulcers, and atherosclerosis are among the features that distinguish Rothmund-Thomson from *Werner's syndrome.* The disease develops early in life and progresses no further, so patients can live a normal life, though they are at increased risk for developing malignant neoplasms. This tendency is attributed in part to absent or deficient DNA repair processes, especially in fibroblasts (Moss 1990; Paterson et al. 1984). Increased incidences of basal cell carcinomas, gastric carcinomas, squamous cell carcinomas, and osteosarcomas have been reported.

Dermatology

Striae similar to those seen in livedo reticularis first appear on the forehead, chin, cheeks, and ears and later involve the buttocks and extremities. The trunk is unaffected. The lesions typically appear around 6 months of age, giving way gradually to a poikiloderma with diffuse atrophy, mottled or reticular areas of hyper- and depigmentation, and irregular or reticular telangiectases (Fig. 1.19). Erythematous mottling and pityriasiform scaling are also described. The skin lesions take a waxing and waning course and usually cease to progress by 6 years of age. Other dermatologic abnormalities are hypo- or atrichia, hypoplasia or aplasia of the sebaceous and sweat glands, and nail dystrophy (hypertrophy, onycholysis, etc.).

Bloom's syndrome (parental consanguinity, short stature, skeletal anomalies, low birthweight, immunopathies with susceptibility to malignant neoplasms) is distinguished from Rothmund-Thomson syndrome mainly by its dermatologic

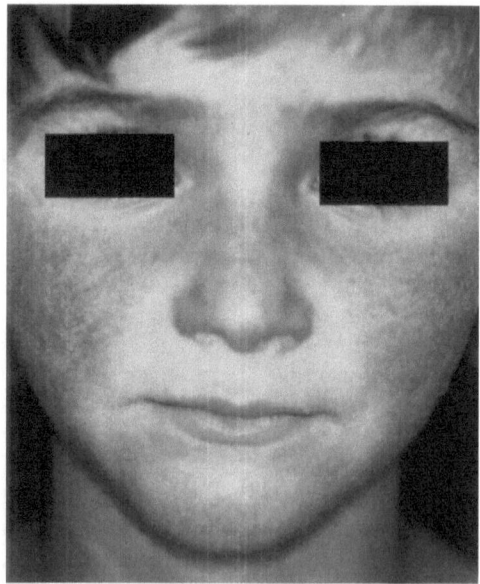

Fig.1.19. Congenital poikiloderma. Typical triangular facial shape with teleangiectases and erythema involving the nose, cheeks, and chin. Other typical poikilodermal lesions were present on the ears, buttocks, hands, and feet and exhibited the depigmentation component of the disease. (Photo courtesy of Prof. Dr. O. E. Hornstein, Director, Department of Dermatology, University of Erlangen)

features. Bloom's syndrome is marked by exzematoid skin lesions on the trunk and face, and increased photosensitivity has been described.

Radiology

In addition to various deformities involving the spine (kyphoscoliosis) and pelvis (hip dysplasia), radiographs mainly show hypoplasia of the ulna, radius, and thumbs and possible absence of the patella. Chondrodysplastic metaphyseal changes, broadening of the tubular bones ("undertubulation"), and osteopathia striatalike changes have also been described. Sim et al. (1992) published the unusual case of multicentric osteosarcoma occurring in a patient with Rothmund-Thomson syndrome.

References

Braun-Falco O, Plewig G, Wolff HH (1984) Dermatologie und Venerologie, 3. Aufl. Springer, Berlin Heidelberg New York, S. 510 f.
Gaetani SA, Ferraris AM, D'Agosta A (1988) Werner's syndrome. Skeletal Radiol 17: 298
Gerecht K, Fuhrmann U (1993) Rothmund-Thomson-Syndrom bei zwei Brüdern. HG Z Hautkrankh 68: 814
Hall JG, Pagon RA, Wilson KM (1980) Rothmund-Thomson syndrome with severe dwarfism. Am J Dis Child 134: 165
Katzenellenbogen J, Larun Z, Tiquva P (1960) A contribution to Bloom's syndrome. Arch Dermatol 82: 177
Moss C (1990) Rothmund-Thomson syndrome: a report of two patients and a review of the literature. Br J Dermatol 122: 821
Paterson MC, Bech-Hansen NT, Smith PJ et al. (1984) Radiogenic neoplasia, cellular radiosensitivity, and faulty DNA repair. Prog Cancer Res Ther 26: 319
Sim FH, DeVries EMG, Miser JS et al. (1992) Osteoblastic osteosarcoma (grade 4) with Rothmund-Thomson-syndrome. Case Report Nr. 760. Skeletal Radiol 21: 543

1.20 Werner's Syndrome

Synonym: progeria adultorum

Short stature, premature senility, cataract, cutaneous and subcutaneous atrophy with scleroderma-like dermal fibrosis, especially involving the lower extremities; muscular atrophy, trophic ulcerations in areas of cutaneous lesions; diabetes mellitus, generalized osteoporosis, trophic deformities and osteomyelitis-like lesions of the feet; soft-tissue atrophy, heterotopic calcifications at the insertions of tendons, ligaments, and the synovial membrane.

Definition

Werner's syndrome is a rare, familial, systemic mesenchymal disorder that probably is inherited as an autosomal recessive trait. Its essential features are short stature, premature senility, cataracts, sclerodermal and ulcerative skin lesions, and diabetes mellitus. The skeletal changes are basically complications due to trophic disturbances.

General Clinical Features

Werner's syndrome represents an adult form of progeria. Patients have short stature due to the premature cessation of skeletal growth. The symptoms appear no later than about 20 years of age and include progressive cutaneous and muscular atrophy and the development of a scleroderma-like cutaneous fibrosis that chiefly involves the lower extremities (especially the feet and ankle region). Patients also report premature graying of the hair and alopecia. Clinically, the cutaneous atrophy produces a birdlike facies with a pointed nose and loss of orbital fat, taut skin, and impaired mimetic function. A hoarse high falsetto voice results from thinning of the vocal cords. There is early onset of cataracts, diabetes mellitus, and endocrine abnormalities such as premature menopause in women and testicular atrophy in men. Early-onset atherosclerosis and its complications lead to death in the fourth or fifth decade of life. As in Rothmund-

Thomson syndrome, patients are predisposed to developing malignant neoplasms.

Dermatology

There is an increasing loss of subcutaneous fat in the feet and ankles and later in the lower leg, accompanied by muscular atrophy. Cutaneous atrophy leads to a fibrosis that is called "pseudo-scleroderma" after its resemblance to that disease. As the atrophic skin becomes "hidebound" due to the loss of subcutaneous fat, very poorly healing trophic ulcers form over distal pressure sites such as the malleoli and Achilles tendon insertion. Areas of hyperkeratosis appear on the soles of the feet. The nails become dystrophic.

Radiology

Patients exhibit a generalized osteoporosis that has a patchy appearance, especially on the hands, due to concomitant sclerotic changes. Trophic disturbances of the skin and subcutaneous tissue lead to spindling of the small tubular bones, particularly in the feet. Additionally there are typical acro-osteolytic lesions with pencil-like bone deformity. Gaetani et al. (1988) described osteomyelitis-like changes in the foot with soft-tissue swelling and extensive heterotopic calcifications at the insertions of tendons, ligaments, and joint capsules. Interstitial subcutaneous calcifications are also observed. On X-rays, the tubular bones show similarities to neuropathic osteoarthropathy like seen in diabetes mellitus.

References

Epstein CJ, Martin GM, Schultz AL et al. (1966) Werner's syndrome: A review of its symptomatology, natural history, pathologic features, genetics and relationship to the natural aging process. Medicine 45: 177
Gaetani SA, Ferraris AM, D'Agosta A (1988) Werner's syndrome. Case Report 485. Skeletal Radiol 17: 298
Jacobson HG, Rifkin H, Zucker-Franklin D (1960) Werner's syndrome: a clinical-roentgen entity. Radiology 74: 373

1.21 Ehlers-Danlos Syndrome

Fragile and hyperelastic skin; darkly pigmented "cigarette paper" scars; hypermobility of the joints; kyphoscoliosis; blue sclerae, epicanthus; prepubertal periodontitis and tooth loss; hemorrhages; hernias.
Roentgen signs: intestinal diverticula, aortic aneurysm, spondylolisthesis.

Definition

Ehlers-Danlos syndrome comprises a complex group of inherited disorders that are associated with congenital connective-tissue weakness and whose major features include hyperelastic skin, hypermobile joints, tissue fragility, ocular changes, and proneness to vascular hemorrhages.

General Clinical Features

The congenital defect in the connective tissues leads to clinical symptoms of varying form and severity. Today, 10 distinct variants of Ehlers-Danlos syndrome are distinguished according to the involvement of particular organs or organ systems, specific enzyme defects, and mode of inheritance. The autosomal dominant type I (gravis type) being the most common. Below we shall briefly review the essential features of the syndrome as a whole.

The most striking feature is hypermobility of the joints with a predisposition to instability, dislocation, and intra-articular hemorrhage. Musculoskeletal abnormalities consist of kyphoscoliosis and a high incidence of spondylolisthesis. Flat foot is also observed. Ocular changes consist of blue sclerae, frequent strabismus, and epicanthus. Dislocation of the lens is also common, as are retinal detachment and ocular tears in response to even minor trauma. Many patients are near-sighted. Prepubertal periodontitis may develop, leading to early tooth loss. Other manifestations of the connective-tissue weakness are inguinal and diaphragmatic hernias and scar disruption. Gastrointestinal abnormalities include small-bowel and colonic diverticula, which are susceptible to perforation. Systemic signs include rapid fatigability on physical exertion. Raynaud's phenomenon may also be present.

Hemorrhages at a variety of sites are a typical feature. Dental extractions provoke heavy bleeding, and even light pressure can cause punctate hemorrhaging ("Rumpel-Leede sign"). Dissecting aneurysm is a potentially grave complication of the syndrome. Pregnant patients may develop serious complications due to vascular ruptures, uterine tears, or severe postpartum hemorrhage.

Some symptoms may appear shortly after birth. The prognosis is generally guarded due to the potential complications listed above.

Dermatology

The most striking symptom is hyperelasticity of the skin, which can be stretched out like a rubber band and returns to its normal position when released (Fig. 1.21). The skin has also an increased vulnerability and tears easily, especially over the knees and elbows and on the face. Minor trauma produces gaping, jagged wounds that heal poorly and form thin "cigarette paper" scars. With repeated trauma, the scarred areas darken. Inspection may also reveal *molluscoid pseudotumors* over bony prominences and musculotendinous insertions. The ears are highly elastic and stretchable. Subcutaneous fat cysts as well as cutaneous and soft-tissue hemorrhages tend to form calcifications appearing as rice bodie-shaped opacities on X-ray films.

Radiology

The skeletal radiology of Ehlers-Danlos syndrome is nonspecific and usually demonstrates orthopedic problems such as subluxations and hemarthrosis (soft-tissue swelling). Other features are genu recurvatum and hyperabductibility of the thumbs. Spinal abnormalities may include kyphoscoliosis, spondylolisthesis, spina bifida, and many other changes. Dental X-rays show prepubertal resorption of the alveolar processes with premature tooth loss. The chest film shows relatively nonspecific pulmonary changes consisting of interstitial fibrosis and honeycomb lung. Similar changes are seen in Langerhans cell-histiocytosis and other disorders.

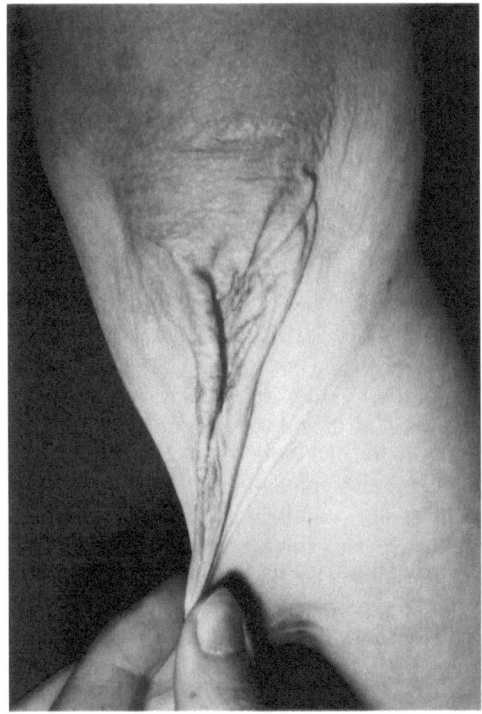

Fig. 1.21. Hyperextensible skin in Ehlers-Danlos syndrome

References

Fridrich KL, Fridrich HH, Kempf KK et al. (1990) Dental implications in Ehlers-Danlos syndrome. Oral Surg Oral Med Oral Pathol 69: 431

McKusick VA (1974) Multiple forms of the Ehlers-Danlos syndrome. Arch Surg 109: 475

Sartoris DJ, Luzzatti L et al. (1981) Type IX Ehlers-Danlos syndrome. Radiology 152: 665

1.22 Metaphyseal Chondrodysplasia with Complete Alopecia

Complete alopecia at birth; short stature. **Roentgen signs:** cone-shaped epiphyses, cupping of the metaphyses; various other skeletal anomalies.

This appears to be an extremely rare disorder, with only two cases (in Italy) having been reported to date (Bellini and Bardare 1966; Jequier and Bellini 1981). Both children were completely hairless at birth and were of short stature. One child (Bellini and Bardare 1966) also had hypospadias and cryptorchidism, while the second child (Jequier and Bellini 1981) was born with scoliosis, flexion contractures of both knees, ulnar deviation of the fingers with an arachnodactyly-like appearance, bilateral hip dysplasia, hyperextension of the distal interphalangeal joints, a high palatal arch, retrognathism, a small pointed nose, and bilateral epicanthus. Both sets of parents were normal.

Radiographs in both children showed cone-shaped epiphyses and metaphyseal cupping involving the long bones and the tubular bones of the hands and feet. The films also showed central indentations of the vertebral bodies and hypoplasia of the odontoid process. While bone growth in these patients was initially accelerated (with the premature appearance of epiphyseal ossification centers before 1 year of age), growth after 1 year of age was retarded.

This disorder is distinguished from *Ellis-van Creveld syndrome* and from *"hair-cartilage hypoplasia"* by the greatly accelerated closure of the epiphyseal growth plates.

References

Bellini F, Bardare M (1966) Su un caso di disotosi periferica. Minerva Pediatr 18: 105

Jequier S, Bellini F, Mackenzie DA (1981) Metaphyseal chondrodysplasia with ectodermal dysplasia. Skeletal Radiol 7: 107

1.23 Satoyoshi's Syndrome

Alopecia; diarrhea; progressive muscle spasms with secondary changes, particularly involving the growth regions. **Roentgen signs:** epiphyseal separations, metaphyseal irregularities, etc.

Satoyoshi's syndrome is a disease of unknown etiology that is associated with progressive muscle spasms, alopecia, diarrhea, and skeletal anomalies. The syndrome was first described by Satoyoshi and Yamada in Japan in 1967. There are no reports of occurrences outside Japan.

The disease begins in childhood with progressive, intermittent muscle spasms primarily involving the legs. Gradually these spasms increase in severity and intensity and additionally involve the arms, trunk, neck, and masseters. The spasms are paroxysmal, occurring in transient attacks that last for several minutes and recur over periods lasting from 30 min to 1 week. Reportedly, the spasms are so severe that the affected extremities become fixed and rigid. Alopecia and diarrhea are variable in degree. Laboratory findings are normal.

Ikegawa et al. (1993) state that the skeletal abnormalities are largely traumatic in nature and result from the spasms. They consist basically of widened, irregular epiphyseal plates, lucencies and sclerotic changes in the metaphyses, epiphyseal separations, cystic lesions (e.g., of the olecranon or fibular head), acro-osteolysis, bone fragmentation at tendon insertion sites, fatigue fractures, and early osteoarthritis.

References

Ikegawa S, Nagano A, Satoyoshi E (1993) Skeletal abnormalities in Satoyoshi's syndrome: a radiographic study of eight cases. Skeletal Radiol 22: 321

Satoyoshi E (1978) A syndrome of progressive muscle spasm, alopecia, and diarrhea. Neurology 28: 458

Satoyoshi E, Yamada K (1967) Recurrent muscle spasms of central origin. Arch Neurol 16: 254

1.24 Gaucher's Disease

Cutaneous manifestations: brownish hyperpigmented areas on exposed sites.
Roentgen signs: osteopenia, Erlenmeier-flask deformity of long tubular bones, irregular lucencies and sclerosis of cancellous bone with a coarsened trabecular pattern, periosteal new bone formation, aseptic necrosis, pseudo-osteomyelitis (crisis).
Clinical signs: hepatosplenomegaly, anemia, thrombocytopenic hemorrhages.

Definition

Gaucher's disease is a congenital, autosomal recessive metabolic disorder characterized by the accumulation of glucocerebrosides in the reticuloendothelial system and central nervous system with clinical manifestations involving the liver, spleen, bone, skin, and central nervous system.

General Clinical Features

Gaucher's disease is based on a congenital deficiency of glucocerebroside-β-glucosidase, the severity of the enzyme defect determining the severity and rate of progression of clinical disease. The diagnosis is established by the histopathologic demonstration of typical Gaucher cells in the reticuloendothelial system.
A distinction is drawn between the infantile form of the disease, which is swiftly fatal, and the visceral form, which appears between 6 months and puberty and whose dominant feature is hepatosplenomegaly. Early death may occur as a result of infection or hemorrhage.
Our primary interest is in the *skeletal form*, which may appear between 6 months and adulthood and whose major features are splenomegaly and skeletal changes. Patients may live to a normal age. Males and females are affected equally, but the disease is especially common in Ashkenasic Jews. Hepatosplenomegaly and slight enlargement of the lymph nodes are accompanied by general weakness, fatigue, weight loss, and nonspecific abdominal complaints. Rare involvement of the lungs presents as interstitial fibrosis with dyspnea and dry cough. Massive bone marrow infiltration can cause anemia and thrombocytopenic hemorrhaging in many tissues including bone.
The *cutaneous manifestations* consist of brownish, melasma-like areas of hyperpigmentation on the face and linear or patchy areas on the legs and exposed sites. Some of the hyperpigmented areas may acquire a bronze or dark leaden color and continue to darken with aging. External inspection may occasionally reveal thickening of the conjunctiva.
Skeletal abnormalities occur in 50–75% of patients with Gaucher's disease. The clinical and radiologic features of the skeletal changes are described below in greater detail.

Radiology

The massive infiltration of the bone marrow with Gaucher storage cells and reactive proliferative tissue disrupts the normal bony architecture, leading to osteopenia, bone destruction, osteosclerosis, pathologic fractures, ischemic necrosis, subperiosteal hemorrhages, and cortical abnormalities due to periosteal new bone formation (Fig. 1.24 a, b).
A specific radiographic sign is the *Erlenmeier-flask deformity* of the tubular bones caused by an expansive infiltration of the bone marrow by kerasin-laden cells with gradual thinning of the cortex from the inside and periosteal bone deposition on the outside. This leads to a typical underconstriction of the tubular bones. The resorption of cancellous bone may create a motheaten appearance. The original cortex is thin, irregular, and split, but there is a net overall thickening due to *periosteal new bone formation*. The general response to the resorptive changes is *sclerosis*, which may show a patchy, irregular pattern. Proliferative bone marrow changes that penetrate through the cortical shell can produce solid or lacelike periosteal new bone formation. In areas of ischemic necrosis, buttressing may occur due to subperiosteal hemorrhage or pathologic fracture. Since the bone loses stability, fractures are common. Fractures involving the vertebral bodies generally produce a typical *kyphoscoliosis*.
Larger regional accumulations of abnormal Gaucher cells and proliferative tissue lead to

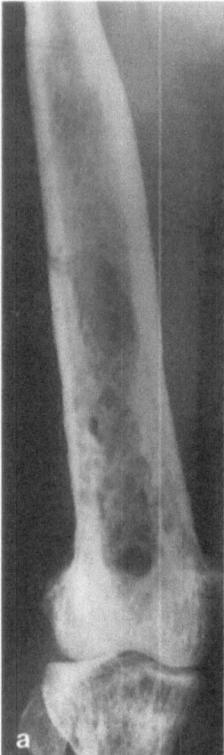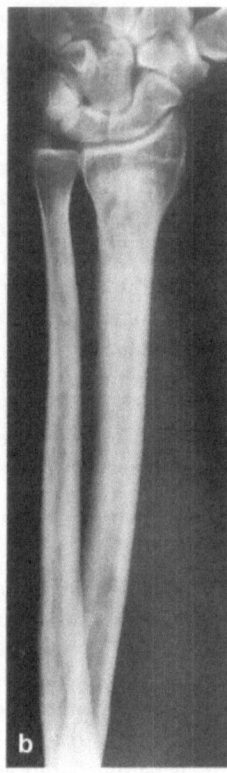

Fig. 1.24 a, b. Typical radiographic changes in Gaucher's disease. The patient, a 40-year-old man, presented clinically with brownish areas of hyperpigmentation on the face and the extensor surfaces of the thigh and lower leg. Physical examination revealed hepatosplenomegaly. Radiographs (**a**) showed marked Erlenmeier-flask deformity of both femurs with expansion of the medullary cavity and solid, mostly medial periosteal ossification, giving the cortex an almost normal thickness. The coarsened trabecular pattern is most pronounced in the epiphyses and metaphyses. In the distal shaft and metaphysis there is a plug-like formation containing mottled, irregular densities that are separated from the medullary cavity by a very thin sclerotic border. This plug-like structure represents an extensive bone infarction. The large osteolytic area proximal to the infarct is probably the result of profuse intraosseous hemorrhage with bone resorption, or it may represent an accumulation of abnormal Gaucher cells and proliferative tissue that have replaced the local bone. A spontaneous fracture has occurred in this area. Similar changes are seen in the upper extremity. Irregular sclerosis of the medullary cavity and cancellous bone and fine scattered lucencies were noted in the humerus, forearm bones (**b**), and tibiae

bubble-like *lytic lesions.* Hemorrhage in these lesions is possible. On the other hand, reperfusion following vascular occlusions and avascular necrosis can lead to profuse bleeding within the bone.

A typical radiographic sign of Gaucher's disease is *aseptic necrosis* caused by the compression of small veins with secondary edema formation due to the accumulation of Gaucher cells. Aseptic necrosis most commonly affects the femoral heads but may also involve the knee, the humeral head, the tali, and the diaphyses, especially of the femurs. Acute vascular occlusions affecting a long bone segment cause severe pain and swelling in the affected area, especially in children, that may be accompanied by high fever, leukocytosis, and an elevated ESR. This situation is termed a *crisis* or *pseudo-osteomyelitis.*

References

Goldblatt J, Sacks S, Beighton P (1978) The orthopedic aspects of Gaucher's disease. Clin Orthop 137: 208

Goldman AB, Jacobs B (1984) Femoral neck fractures complicating Gaucher disease in children. Skeletal Radiol 12: 162

Greenfield GB (1970) Bone changes in chronic adult Gaucher's disease. Am J Roentgenol 110: 800

Groen J (1964) Gaucher's disease: hereditary transmission and racial distribution. Arch Intern Med 113: 543

Hermann G, Pastores GM, Abdelwahab IF et al. (1997) Gaucher disease: assessment of skeletal involvement and therapeutic responses to enzyme replacement. Skeletal Radiol 26: 687

1.25 Fabry's Disease

Synonym: angiokeratoma corporis diffusum

Angiokeratomas developing on the buttock, scrotum, and periumbilical area, less commonly on the trunk and extremities, from dark red or black papules.

Clinical signs: rheumatoid features with febrile episodes and elevated ESR.

Roentgen signs: bone marrow infarction and necrosis, early interphalangeal osteoarthritis, acro-osteolysis.

Childhood onset.

Definition

Fabry's disease, a lipid storage disease with an X-linked recessive mode of inheritance, is characterized by the deposition of ceramides in vessels and tissues of the internal organs and skin. The clinical picture is dominated by vascular occlusions leading to foci of ischemic necrosis, mainly in the skeleton, osteoarthritic changes in the interphalangeal joints, and angiokeratomas.

General Clinical Features

The deposition of ceramides is caused by a deficiency of ceramide trihexoside-α-galactosidase, impairing the breakdown of certain glycosphingolipids and leading to the ubiquitous intracellular accumulation of ceramides. Preferential deposition in the vascular endothelium and smooth muscle leads to luminal narrowing and ischemic complications in the organs supplied by the vessels. The clinical symptoms are correspondingly diverse. Most patients are quite young, and many present with cerebral infarction. Deposition in the heart and kidneys can lead to cardiomyopathy and renal failure. Vascular occlusions in the synovial membrane give rise to painful rheumatoid symptoms with limitation of motion, especially extension. Bone marrow infarcts can produce nonspecific, gnawing pains in the tubular bones. Febrile attacks are less common. The ESR is always elevated. The appearance of these musculoskeletal signs and symptoms in childhood or adolescence may prompt an erroneous diagnosis of *rheumatoid arthritis* or *rheumatic fever.* The angiokeratomas described below are the key to the correct diagnosis.

Dermatology

The skin changes usually appear during the first decade of life and initially consist of dark red or black telangiectatic spots or papules up to 4 mm in diameter. The keratotic component is not always seen. The skin lesions are often inconspicuous and mainly involve the "bathing suit area" about the buttocks, scrotum, and umbilical region. More pronounced cases present with small angiokeratomas that spread like a rash over the trunk and extremities (Fig. 1.25). Only some of the lesions show keratotic changes.

Chevrant-Breton et al. (1981) described an association with lymphedema and an ulcerating, mutilating acropathy, apparently due to vascular occlusions.

Radiology

In the 20 to 30 cases published to date, only a few case reports describe the radiologic features of Fabry's disease in any detail. Lacroux (1960) and Wise et al. (1962) described foci of ischemic bone necrosis, "multiple densities in the femoral heads," and degenerative changes in the interphalangeal joints. Fone and King (1964) and Chevrant-Breton et al. (1981) noted extensive acro-osteolytic lesions involving several toes and metacarpophalangeal joints along with talar necrosis.

Fabry's disease should be considered in young males who present with nonspecific rheumatic symptoms (joint pain and mild swelling in the hand, febrile episodes, elevated ESR) combined with visible angiokeratomas (e.g., on the back), unusual degenerative changes in the interphalangeal joints, and bone marrow infarctions.

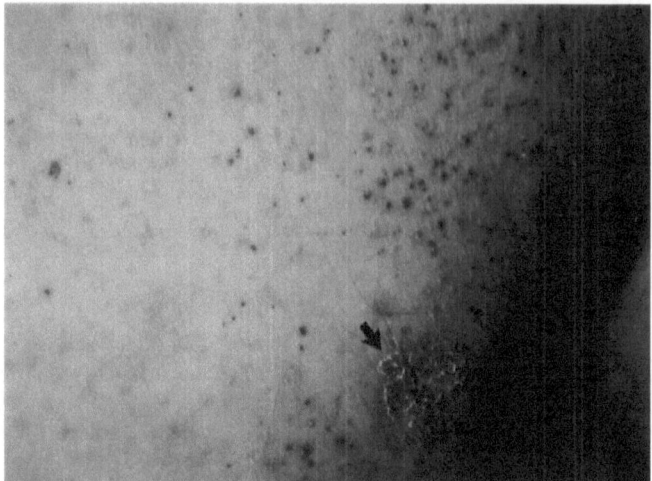

Fig.1.25. Fabry's disease with diffuse angiokeratomas in the inguinal region. The pattern of lesional spread is rash-like. The keratotic component in some angiokeratomas is manifested by scaling (*arrow*). The skin lesions had been present since childhood in this pa- tient, who presented with paroxysms of high fever and osteoarthritic changes in the interphalangeal joints with appreciable swelling. He also had a history of femoral head necrosis on the right side. The previous diagnosis had been "indeterminate rheumatic disease"

References

Chevrant-Breton J, Laudren A, Mazéas D et al. (1981) Maladie de Fabry. Lymphoédeme et acropathie ulcéro-mutilante – un cas. Ann Dermatol Venerol (Paris) 108: 366

Fone DJ, King WE (1964) Angiokeratoma corporis diffusum (Fabry's syndrome). Aust Ann Med 13: 339

Laroux R (1960) Angiokératome diffus (angiokeratoma corporis diffusum) de Fabry. Bull Soc Fr Dermatol Syph 67: 474

Sheth KJ, Bernhard GC (1979) The arthropathy of Fabry disease. Arthritis Rheum 2: 781

Wise D, Wallace HG, Jellinek EH (1962) Angiokeratoma corporis diffusum. A clinical study of eight affected families. Q J Med, N Ser 31: 177

1.26 Congenital Copper Deficiency

Depigmentation of skin and hair; generalized osteoporosis; cupped, sometimes frayed metaphyses of irregular density with beaks or spurs; metaphyseal fractures; periosteal ossification.

The manifestations of congenital copper deficiency may appear in newborns or as an hereditary disorder. While a healthy term infant has copper reserves in the liver sufficient for the first five months of life, enabling it to withstand a nutritional deficiency without harm, a premature or growth-retarded infant has copper reserves for only about 2 months. Consequently, a dietary or disease-related copper deficiency (prolonged parenteral nutrition, poor feeding, diarrhea, malabsorption, etc.) can cause true copper deficiency symptoms to appear between 6 and 9 months of age. These may consist of anemia, neutropenia, depigmentation of skin and hair, central nervous system abnormalities, generalized osteoporosis, and skeletal growth retardation with cupped, beaked, and sometimes frayed metaphyses of irregular density. This may be followed by metaphyseal surface fractures or impacted fractures and periosteal new bone formation. Periosteal ossification can cause expansion of the anterior rib ends. In the five cases described by Schmidt et al. (1991), the bone changes resolved completely in response to copper replacement therapy.

In contrast to nutritional copper deficiency, infants with an hereditary copper deficiency (X-linked recessive condition known as *Menke's syndrome*, also called kinky hair disease or trichopoliodystrophy) present in the first months of life with pronounced neurologic symptoms, growth retardation, hair changes (scalp hair is deficient in pigment, bristly, lusterless, feels like glass wool; a special form of pili torti), hypopigmentation (steely gray skin color), and skeletal abnormalities. These symptoms are the same as those of copper deficiency in premature infants. Menke's syndrome is not associated with anemia or neutropenia.

References

Schmidt H, Herwig J, Greinacher I (1991) Skelettveränderungen bei Frühgeborenen mit Kupfermangel. Röfo 155: 38

2 Collagen Diseases

Collagen diseases is a collective term for a group of diseases whose basic pathoanatomic feature is a fibrinoid degeneration (fibrinoid necrosis) of the connective tissues. The pathogenesis of these diseases involves the deposition of immune complexes around blood vessels, resulting in vascular damage. Collagen diseases are characterized clinically by overlap phenomena and immunologically by non-organ-specific autoantibodies, explaining why collagen diseases are classified among the systemic autoimmune disorders. Collagen diseases may be associated with inflammatory joint changes, bone necrosis, and soft-tissue calcifications (Thibièrge-Weissenbach syndrome) which, when accompanied by more or less specific skin changes, overlap the specialties of internal medicine (particularly rheumatology and immunology), clinical radiology, and dermatology and thus should be approached from a synoptic perspective.

At present the collagen diseases are considered to include the following:

- progressive systemic sclerosis (progressive scleroderma),
- systemic lupus erythematosus,
- polymyositis and dermatomyositis,
- Sjögren's syndrome,
- Jo-1 syndrome,
- Sharp's syndrome (mixed connective tissue disease),
- undifferentiated inflammatory systemic connective tissue disease,
- relapsing polychondritis? (see p. 85)

Collagen diseases can be extremely difficult to diagnose clinically, due in large part to the overlap phenomena mentioned above (e.g., coexisting rheumatoid arthritis or panarteritis nodosa). Thus, in a strict sense it is wrong to classify Sharp's syndrome as a separate entity, but this is justified on didactic grounds because the term "Sharp's syndrome" often denotes a highly characteristic and coherent set of clinical and radiologic features. Given the synoptic nature of this book, we can touch only briefly on special organic disease symptoms and the extremely complex laboratory evaluation of collagen diseases.

For the "outsider," it is interesting to note that new approaches are being taken to the classification of collagen diseases based on the identification of specific antibodies. A prime example of this is the Jo-1 syndrome. While the classic collagen diseases such as progressive scleroderma, systemic lupus erythematosus, and Sjögren's syndrome are defined mainly in terms of their clinical features, the characterization of the Jo-1 syndrome is based on the detection of the homonymous antibody (see p. 72)

References are listed at the end of Chap. 2, p. 75.

2.1 Progressive Systemic Sclerosis (PSS)

Synonym: progressive scleroderma

> Raynaud's phenomenon (initially); doughy edematous swelling of the fingers, hands, and forearms (edematous stage); indurated, tight, waxy, shiny skin (sclerotic stage); "claw hands"; "Madonna fingers"; "rat-bite necrosis"; fixed facial expression, microstomia, shortened frenulum of tongue; polyarthralgias.
>
> **Roentgen signs:** diffuse osteoporosis in the hands with resorption of distal phalanges and terminal tufts; osteolytic foci in other skeletal regions (ribs, spinous processes, etc.); fine osteolytic lesions ("cysts") in the wrists; interstitial calcinosis with ulceration of calcific masses through the skin.

Definition

Progressive systemic sclerosis (PSS) is a systemic, autoimmune connective tissue disease combined with an angiopathy that is marked by characteristic inflammatory, fibrotic, and degenerative changes in the skin, synovial membranes, and internal organs (gastrointestinal tract, heart, lungs, kidneys). The detection of anticentromeric antibodies and antibodies against the chromosomal antigen Scl-70 is a highly specific but not very sensitive test for PSS.

General Clinical Features

The diverse morphologic phenomena in scleroderma result from the excessive production of collagens and from obliterative changes in small blood vessels. Collagen overproduction is most likely triggered by activated T cells (mostly CD4 cells) and by activated monocytes and macrophages, whose production of various cytokines (interleukin-1 and -2) stimulates fibroblast proliferation leading to increased collagen synthesis. Apparently this is accompanied by damage to endothelial cells resulting in intimal proliferation ("onion-skin angiopathy"), which may culminate in an occlusive vasopathy. The vascular alterations that result from the occlusive angiopathy are responsible for the extensive infarcts and necrotic changes that occur in the kidneys, skin, bone (osteolytic lesions), and other organs.

The great majority of patients are women (20:1 ratio). The peak incidence is between 30 and 50 years of age, with an estimated prevalence of about 10 new cases per 1 million population per year.

The clinical symptoms involving the face include telangiectases and microstomia. Hand changes include Raynaud's phenomenon, sclerodactyly, and fingertip necrosis. Other key signs are sclerosis of the frenulum of the tongue and impaired esophageal motility, which can cause significant dysphagia. These changes, however, are actually late findings that would also include small-bowel hypomotility and paralytic ileus. Lung involvement may lead to pulmonary fibrosis (see Fig. 2.1 f), setting the stage for pulmonary arterial hypertension. Pleurisy may also develop. Occlusions of the small renal vessels induce hypertension and eventually lead to renal failure. In the heart, myocardial fibrosis and pericarditis may develop.

Several variants of scleroderma are listed below:

– *Localized scleroderma (morphea)*, characterized by circumscribed cutaneous sclerosis without involvement of the internal organs.
– *CRESTA syndrome*, an acronym for calcinosis, Raynaud's phenomenon, esophageal dysfunction, sclerodactyly, telangiectasis, and arthritis. This syndrome is believed to have a better prognosis than classic PSS.
– *Secondary PSS*, referring to scleroderma-like conditions that may be precipitated by exposure to certain chemicals (polyvinylchloride, solvents, etc.) or drugs (bleomycin, pentazocine, etc.).

Dermatology

One of the earliest dermatologic signs of PSS is Raynaud's phenomenon. The stages of painful ischemia, local cyanosis, and arterial hyperemia are seen most clearly in the upper extremity. Raynaud's phenomenon precedes or accompanies acral changes consisting of doughy – edematous, slightly erythematous swelling of the fingers, hands, and forearms (edematous stage). In-

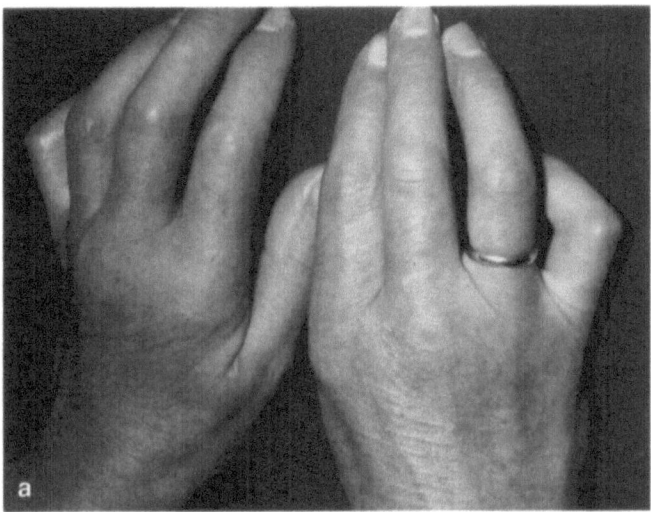

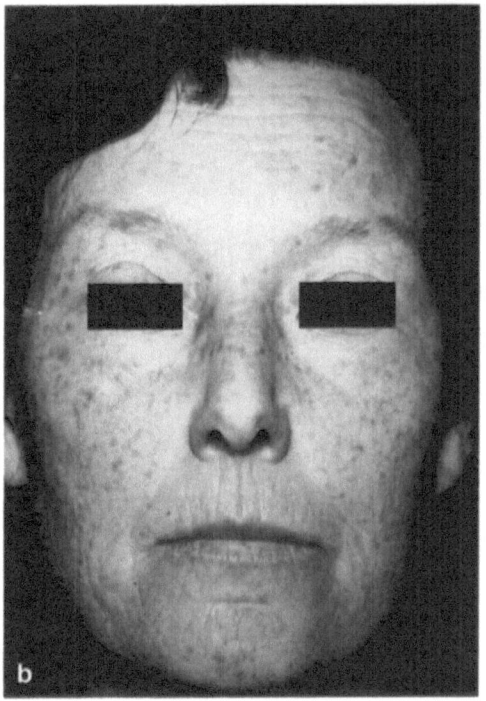

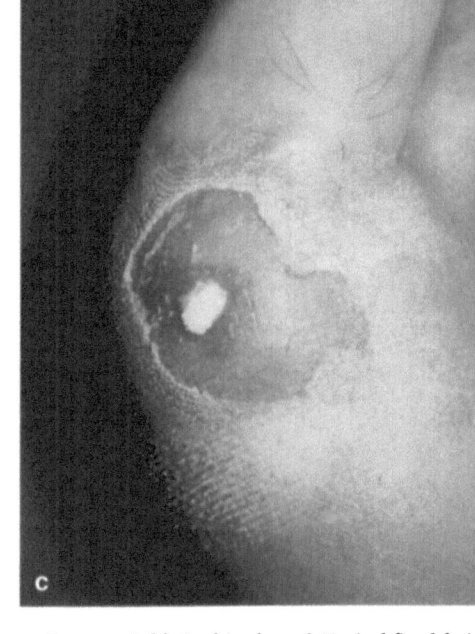

Fig. 2.1 a–j. Progressive systemic sclerosis (PSS). Typical examples of cutaneous and skeletal changes. **a** Sclerotic stage with wax-like skin that cannot be picked up in folds on the left side. Note the faint cyanotic discoloration of the fingertips. There is marked clawing of the third through fifth fingers of the left hand and the fourth and fifth fingers of the right hand. The patient also had small foci of necrosis on the fin-gertips, not visible in this photo. **b** Typical fixed facial expression (masklike face) and microstomia in scleroderma. This patient has CRESTA syndrome that includes conspicuous telangiectases. **c** A necrotic subcutaneous calcific mass has ulcerated through the skin, exposing a whitish, pasty material. There is secondary infection of surrounding tissues. **d–j** see pp. 64–66

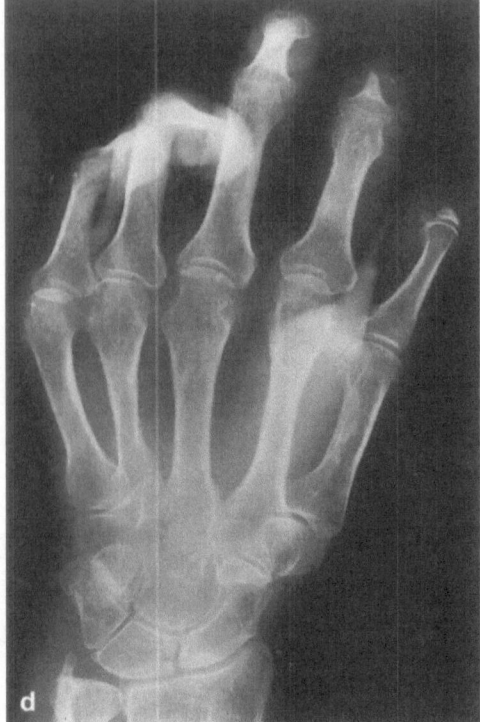
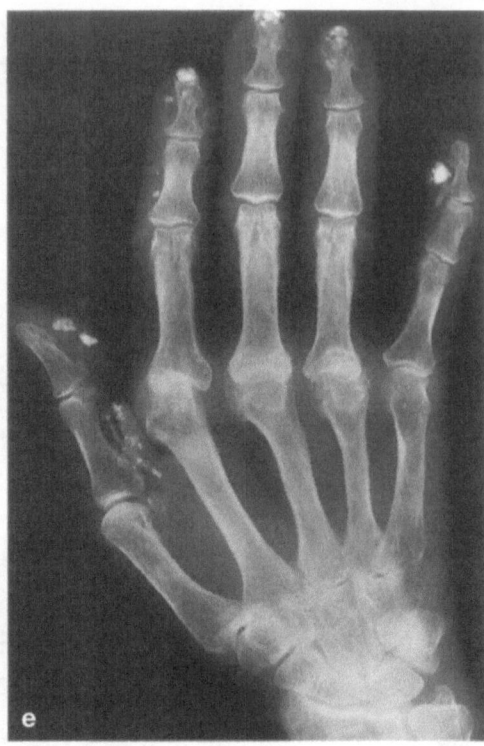

Fig. 2.1 (*continued*). **d** Typical clawhand deformity in scleroderma, with marked flexion deformity of the fourth and fifth proximal interphalangeal joints and extensive resorption (acro-osteolysis) involving the distal phalanx of the thumb, the distal and middle phalanges of the index finger, and the distal phalanges of the third through fifth fingers. Osteolytic changes are also visible on and around the ulnar styloid process. The heads of the second through fifth metacarpals show erosions suggestive of Sharp's syndrome, but the clinical, laboratory, and follow-up data refuted this diagnosis. Almost identical changes were seen in the op-posite hand. **e** In this true case of Sharp's syndrome, the sclerodermoid component is manifested by a diffuse osteoporosis and marked interstitial calcinosis (Thibièrge-Weissenbach syndrome). The conspicuous calcium deposits have already eroded the terminal tuft of the second digit and the medial side of the distal phalanx of the fifth digit. Clinically, pressure on the tip of the thumb extruded a pasty white material similar to that in **c**. This hand, unlike the one in **d**, shows no acro-osteolysis or clawing, making it less typical of pure scleroderma from a radiographic standpoint. **f–j** see pp. 65, 66

volvement of the feet is rare. Later the skin becomes tight, shiny, and wax-like and can no longer be picked up in folds (sclerotic stage, sclerodactyly, Fig. 2.1 a). The cutaneous sclerosis restricts the mobility of the joints, hands, and feet (dermatogenic contracture). The fingers develop a claw-like flexion deformity with severe limitation of movement (Fig. 2.1 a). Small "rat-bite" foci of necrosis develop in the fingertips and the skin around joints. In severe cases the distal phalanges are tapered ("Madonna fingers") or mutilated. The nails develop transverse striation and ridges. Punctate hemorrhages in the eponychium are an important diagnostic sign.

If the initial cutaneous manifestations are in the face, the facial expression becomes masked and fixed in a state of "sclerodermal amimia" (Fig. 2.1 b). The cutaneous sclerosis causes a diminished facial size with a pointed nose, tense cheeks, and small mouth (microstomia). The face exhibits a yellowish-white pallor. The sclerosis may spread to involve the neck, trunk, and proximal extremities, causing patients to appear "encased" within their board-hard sclerosed skin, as if in a suit of armur.

Other skin changes include telangiectases (Fig. 2.1 b) and spotty or linear areas of hypo- and hyperpigmentation resembling poikiloder-

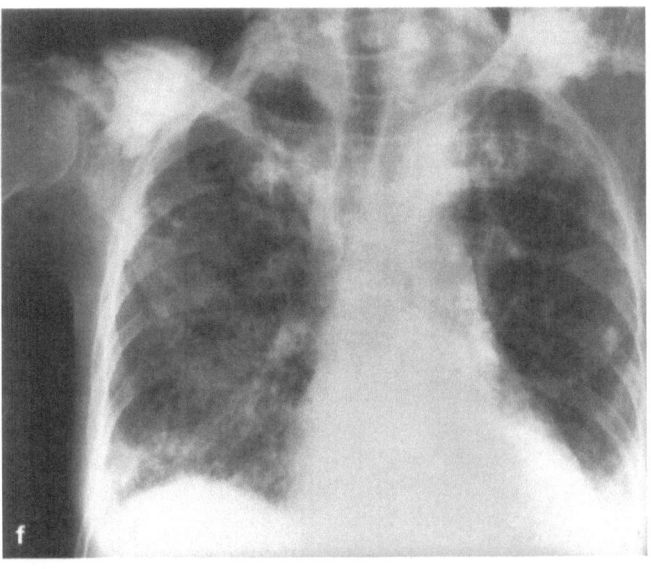

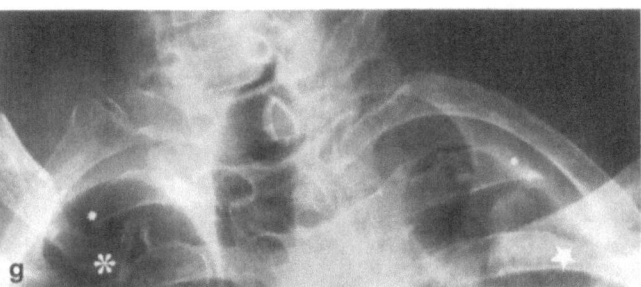

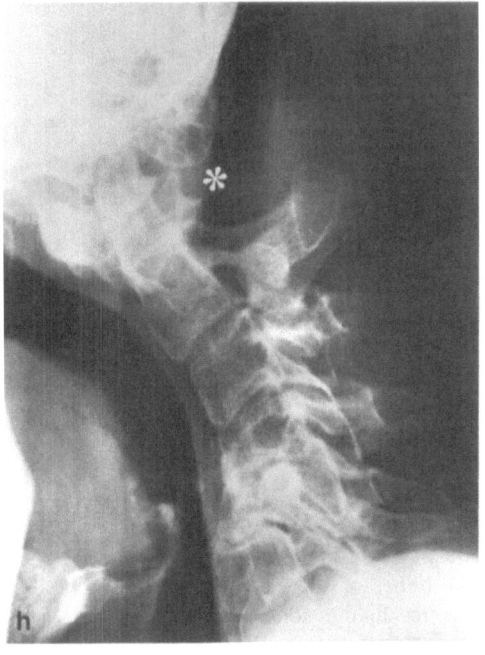

Fig. 2.1 (*continued*). **f** Extensive interstitial calcinosis involving the shoulder girdle and the soft tissues of the lower neck in a scleroderma patient. Note the advanced interstitial pulmonary fibrosis accompanied by pleural effusions. **g–j** Sharp's syndrome with a dominant sclerodermoid component. **g** Pure osteolysis has affected the posterior portions of the right second and third ribs, the posterior part of the left third rib, and the medial portions of both clavicles. The bone segments still intact proximal to the osteolytic areas show a typical tapered, conical shape. Early resorption of the posterior part of the left fourth rib appears as a scooped-out defect in the upper rib contour (*star*). **h** Acro-osteolysis in the spine involves the C1 lamina, the C2 lamina on one side, and the tips of the spinous processes of C3–C5. **i, j** see p. 66

ma. Atrophy of the cutaneous appendages leads to *sclerodermal alopecia*. Calcific deposits in the skin (Fig. 2.1 c) are described more fully under Radiology. The oral mucosa may show small foci of atrophy and sclerosis. The surface of the tongue is smooth and atrophic, and the *shortened frenulum* restricts tongue movements.

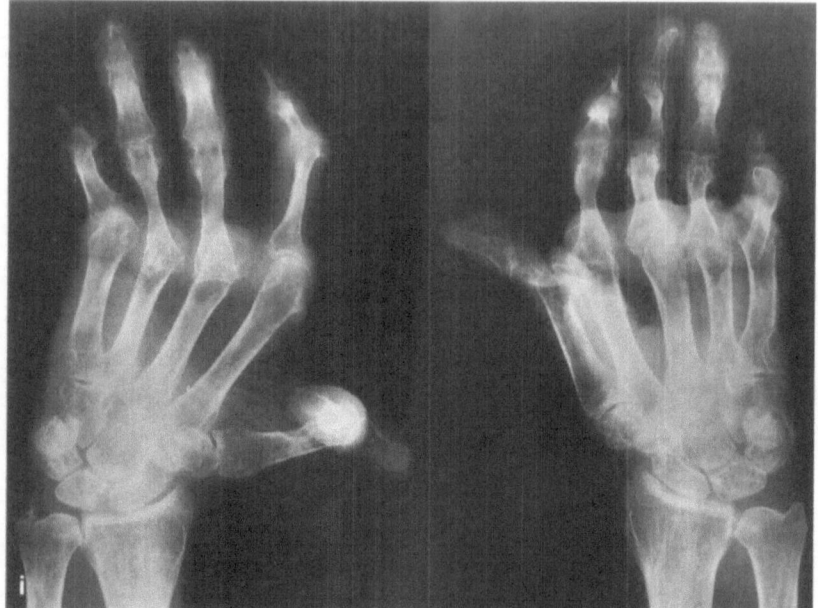

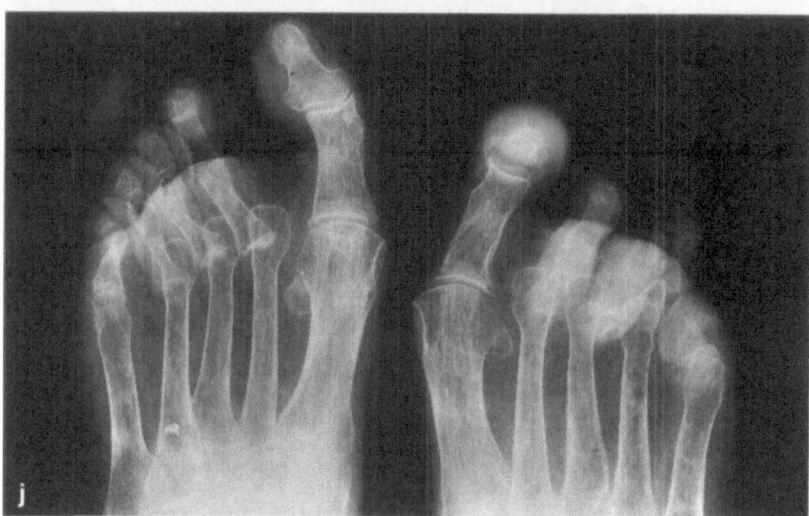

Fig. 2.1 (*continued*). **i, j** Radiographs of the hands and feet show extensive deformities due in part to dislocations of the metacarpophalangeal and metatarsophalangeal joints. Acro-osteolytic lesions are most pronounced in the second and fifth distal phalanges of both hands, the third middle phalanx of the right hand, and the second middle phalanx of the left hand. (Radiographs courtesy of Prof. H. Menninger, Bad Abbach)

Radiology

Patients often have concomitant polyarthralgia (due to synovitis) that rarely progresses to a florid or chronic inflammation, so usually there are no erosive changes or other radiographic signs of joint disease. Erosive arthritis is a very rare finding in PSS and should direct suspicion to Sharp's syndrome.

The bones of the hand display typical radiographic changes consisting of diffuse osteoporosis (Fig. 2.1 d) that is not predominantly articular and probably results from deficient blood flow to the bone due to surrounding soft-tissue changes. The soft-tissue shadow is initially thickened on radiographs and later appears thinned, particularly around the terminal tufts. The degree of soft-tissue thinning can be measured with the Yune index. The tapered configuration of the soft tissues at the fingertips is also referred to as the "candy-stick sign."

A rather characteristic sign seen in most patients is a *resorbing osteolysis of the terminal tufts* of the fingers that may also involve the distal phalanges and the distal parts of the middle phalanges (Fig. 2.1 d). Palmar or subungual foci of osteolysis are clearly visible only in lateral views. The acro-osteolytic lesions sometimes have a "nibbled" appearance. The pathogenesis of the lesions is probably based not just on vascular insufficiency due to occlusive angiopathy but also on strictural changes in the surrounding soft tissues. While the osteolytic lesions most commonly affect the bones of the hand, they may also involve the radius or ulna, clavicles, ribs, or mandible (Fig. 2.1 g–j). Pinstein et al. (1989) described osteolytic lesions of the cervical spine, mainly involving the facets and dorsal appendages (C4–C6 region), combined with more or less extensive paravertebral soft-tissue calcifications. The patients displayed clinical symptoms of cord and root compression.

Not infrequently, radiographs of the *wrist* show *very fine multiple osteolytic foci* surrounded by thin sclerotic margins and having a cyst-like appearance. These are circumscribed areas of necrosis like those seen in lupus erythematosus.

A typical feature of PSS is the presence of *interstitial soft-tissue calcifications* (localized interstitial calcinosis, Thibièrge-Weissenbach syndrome), which occur in at least 25% of all patients who have had the disease for 10–11 years and in patients with pronounced skin changes (Fig. 2.1 e, f). Scleroderma patients with significant internal organ involvement usually do not live long enough to develop soft-tissue calcinosis. The calcinosis results from a dystrophic process (subcutaneous necrosis) and appears as a disseminated pattern of thin plaques of variable size and thickness in the skin and subcutaneous tissues. Calcifications are particularly common in pressure areas such as the fingertips, the soles of the feet, the styloid process, and around joints.

Calcinosis between the deeper muscles can lead secondarily to muscular atrophy and contractures with corresponding limb deformities.

Calcifications in the fingers appear radiographically as stippled densities that often are arranged in clusters. Universal interstitial calcinosis is characterized by linear, band-like, or clumped calcifications located around large extremity joints (shoulders, hips) and in lateral portions of the chest and pelvis.

Occasionally the subcutaneous calcific masses erode through the overlying skin, either spontaneously or under compression, and discharge a grayish-white pasty material (Fig. 2.1 c). These sites are susceptible to secondary infection.

Radionuclide bone scans permit the very early and specific detection of interstitial calcinosis.

References are listed at the end of Chap. 2, p. 75.

2.2 Systemic Lupus Erythematosus (SLE)

Butterfly rash; diffuse erythema; discoid lupus with reddish, raised, scaly skin eruptions; Raynaud's phenomenon; alopecia areata; photosensitivity; oral and nasopharyngeal ulcerations; nonerosive polyarthritis.

Roentgen signs: osteoporosis in the hands and feet; small subarticular cysts in the bones of the hand.

Definition

Systemic lupus erythematosus (SLE) is an inflammatory rheumatic disease that involves the skin, joints, and internal organs. While SLE is known to show a genetic predisposition, its etiology is unclear. The pathogenesis involves inflammatory changes around small vessels with the deposition of autoimmune complexes in the vascular endothelium. Principally affected are the kidneys, heart, spleen, skin, muscles, mucous membranes, and central nervous system. The disease may be precipitated by various exogenous factors (e.g., hormonal changes, ultraviolet light). Patients are positive for numerous autoantibodies and antinuclear antibodies (ANA). The diagnosis is established by laboratory findings of anti-DNA, leukopenia, anemia, thrombocytopenia, ANA, and LE phenomenon.

Classic SLE requires differentiation from lupus-like syndromes that are associated with drug administration (e.g., sulfonamides, hydralazine).

General Clinical and Dermatologic Features

SLE has an estimated prevalence of about 50 cases per 100,000 population and is most common in young women. Its protean clinical features are based on the diverse reactions that are evoked by high titers of autoantibodies and antibodies directed against numerous ubiquitous antigens. The American Rheumatism Association (ARA) has established the following set of diagnostic criteria[1] for SLE:

---

[1] Slightly modified for nondermatologists.

- malar (butterfly) rash, diffuse erythema with telangiectases, keratoses, and atrophy (Fig. 2.2 a, b);
- discoid lesions with reddish, raised, scaly skin eruptions showing follicular keratosis and hyperesthesia; atrophic scarring;
- Raynaud's phenomenon;
- diffuse alopecia and scarring alopecia;
- photosensitivity;
- oral and nasopharyngeal ulceration;
- arthritis (nonerosive);
- antibodies against native DNA (ANA, LE cells);
- false-positive serologic test for syphilis;
- proteinuria (greater than 3.5 g/24 h);
- red cell hemoglobin, tubular, or mixed casts in the urine;
- serositis (pleuritis and/or pericarditis);
- hemolytic anemia (positive Coombs' test) or leukopenia or thrombocytopenia;
- psychosis or seizures.

This list covers the main clinical and dermatologic features of SLE. We shall dispense with a more detailed description, because radiologic studies of the musculoskeletal system are relatively unrewarding and the diagnosis of SLE does not fit within the framework of our radiologic-dermatologic synopsis.

It is worthwhile, however, to consider the articular manifestations of SLE. One of the first and most common symptoms is a polyarticular arthralgia that occurs in 80–90% of cases and involves both large and small joints, especially the metacarpophalangeal and proximal interphalangeal joints and the knee. In many cases polyarthralgia, myalgia *and* fever are the first and only symptoms, requiring differentiation from rheumatic fever and rheumatoid arthritis. This is particularly true when arthralgia progresses to a nonerosive arthritis causing local warmth and painful swelling.

Radiology

As mentioned earlier, the clinical articular manifestations of SLE are associated with few if any radiographic changes (e.g., poor delineation of the subchondral plate, erosions), and this may be considered a direct, typical sign of SLE. It is unusual for arthritic soft-tissue changes (thicken-

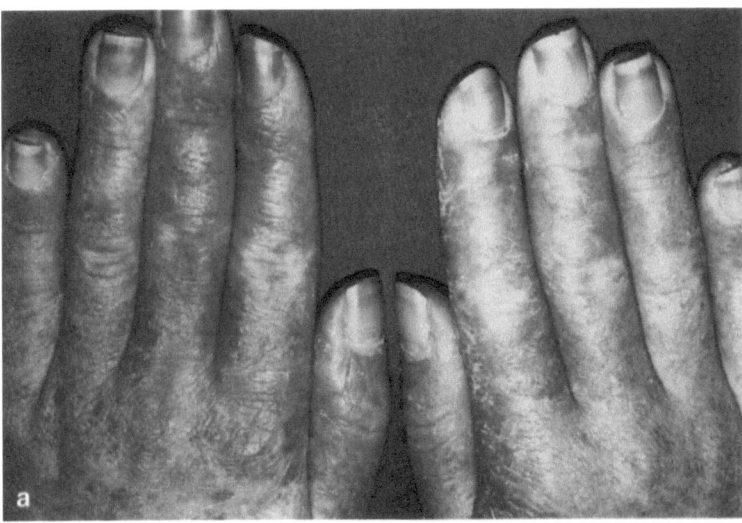

Fig.2.2a,b. Systemic lupus erythematosus (SLE). **a** Typical patchy areas of erythema with keratoses and telangiectases in the skin of the distal phalanges. **b** Diffuse erythematous eruption over the face and neck. The butterfly configuration of the rash was obvious when the patient was viewed from the front

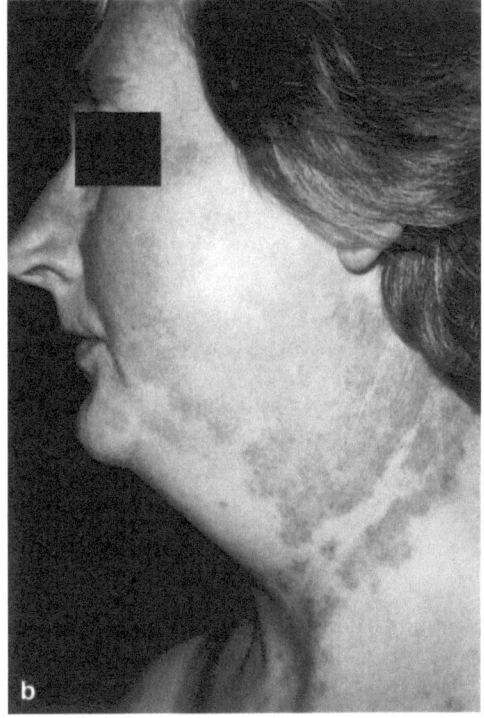

ing and increased density of periarticular soft tissues) to be accompanied by erosive changes. One-third to one-fourth of patients may exhibit *osteoporosis* in the bones of the hands and feet. Multiple, small subarticular cysts that tend to progress and mainly involve the hands have been reported (Leskinen et al. 1984). These cystic lesions are less common in the foot and almost never involve other joint regions. The cysts may be necrotic in nature.

Soft-tissue calcifications (as in Thibièrge-Weissenbach syndrome) and acro-osteolysis are very rarely seen in SLE.

References are listed at the end of Chap. 2, p. 75.

2.3 Polymyositis and Dermatomyositis

Depressive facial expression; patchy and diffuse areas of wine-red to lilac-colored erythema on the face (eyelids!) also involving the neck, upper chest, elbows, and knees; striate erythema on the dorsal surfaces of the hands and fingers; later, poikilodermal changes with telangiectases, porcelain-white atrophy, and pigmentary changes; pale pink or violet, lichenoid papules on the back of the neck; periungual erythematous edema with telangiectasis (Keining's sign).
Roentgen signs: osteoporosis near the joints of the hand, interstitial calcinosis.

Definition

Polymyositis (PM) is a progressive, inflammatory systemic disease of skeletal muscles characterized by symmetric muscle weakness involving the pelvis and/or shoulder girdle. Dermatomyositis (DM) refers to muscle weakness and soreness accompanied by typical skin changes. Bohen and Peter (1975) have distinguished five types of PM/DM:

Type 1: primary idiopathic PM
Type 2: primary idiopathic DM
Type 3: PM/DM associated with malignancy
Type 4: PM/DM in childhood
Type 5: PM/DM with an associated collagen disease (overlap syndrome).

General Clinical Features

Diseases of the PM/DM spectrum are rare, with an estimated incidence of 2 to 6 cases per year per 1 million population. Women over 50 years of age are most commonly affected. Following the above classification, PM alone accounts for about 34% of cases, DM alone for 29%, and overlap syndromes for about 21%.

PM and DM are classified as autoimmune diseases. The detection of an inclusion-body myositis may suggest a viral etiology with a pathologic immune response, probably based on a genetic predisposition (HLA-B8 and HLA-DR3). The cellular immune mechanisms presumed to be dominant in PM/DM have an electron-micro-

scopic correlate in the form of round cells (T cells) with spikes in their processes that penetrate deeply into the muscle fibers. The main clinical symptoms of PM and DM are muscle weakness and myalgia primarily involving the shoulder girdle, pelvic girdle, and proximal limb muscles. Later there is generalized muscular atrophy with all its clinical consequences. Involvement of the muscles of respiration leads to ventilatory impairment, while involvement of the esophageal, pharyngeal, and laryngeal muscles leads to dysphagia and dysphonia. About 30–50% of patients complain of arthralgia or transient arthritis. Less common is an acute joint inflammation with effusion, usually affecting the joints of the fingers. Thirty percent of patients develop interstitial myocarditis with corresponding symptoms. There may also be weight loss, lethargy, and fever as manifestations of the systemic illness. Typical cutaneous lesions are described below.

Laboratory tests show an elevated ESR, elevations of the CRP and γ-globulin fractions, high CK, LDH, GOT and aldolase levels, and increased urinary excretion of myoglobin and creatinine. From 30% to 50% of PM/DM patients have a positive rheumatoid factor, 40–80% have antinuclear antibodies, and 30–40% have anti-Jo-1 and anti-PM1 autoantibodies.

The diagnosis can be established by demonstrating specific EMG abnormalities or by muscle biopsy showing interstitial and perivascular round-cell infiltration along with degenerative muscle changes.

Dermatology

The skin changes occur in a symmetric pattern that mainly involves the face, periorbital area, eyelids, and cheeks as well as the elbows, knees, knuckles, nailfold, and nail bed. The face wears a typical downcast or sad expression and shows patchy and diffuse areas of wine-red to violaceous (lilac-colored) erythema (Fig. 2.3 a). The areas of erythema are always edematous. Affected areas show an adherent hyperkeratotic scale and telangiectases. An important diagnostic clue is periungual erythema with telangiectases, known as the Heuck-Gottron sign. As the disease progresses, areas of porcelain-white atrophy appear. These areas may have a parchment-like ap-

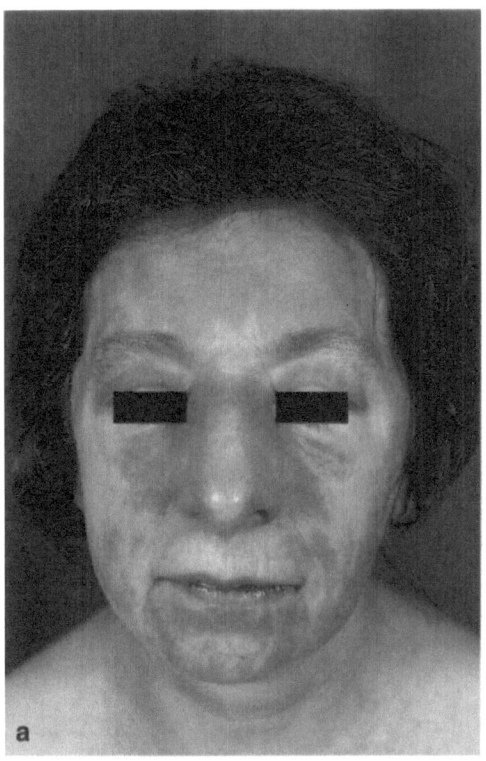

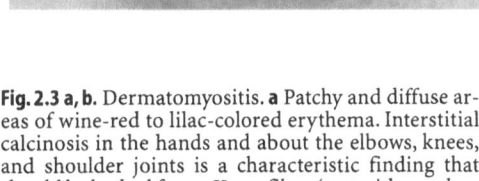

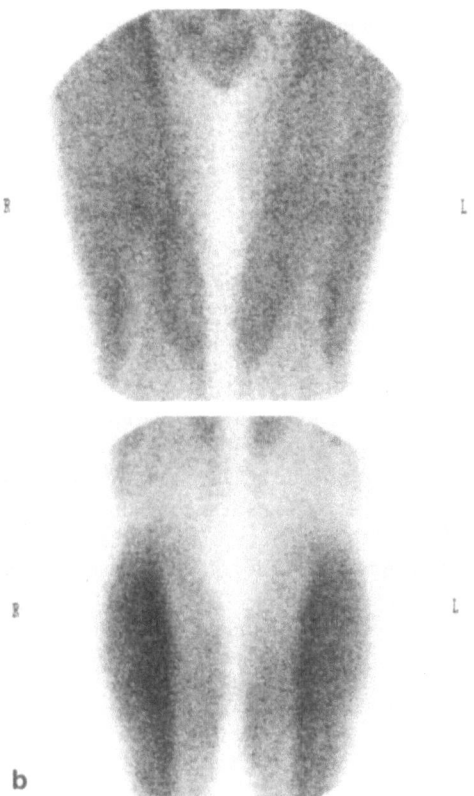

Fig. 2.3 a, b. Dermatomyositis. **a** Patchy and diffuse areas of wine-red to lilac-colored erythema. Interstitial calcinosis in the hands and about the elbows, knees, and shoulder joints is a characteristic finding that should be looked for on X-ray films (test with one dorsopalmar view of the hand). **b** Radionuclide images in dermatomyositis typically show massive radiotracer uptake in the soft tissues. This finding is highly specific for the disease. Note the minimal radiotracer uptake in the bones

pearance (colodion spots), particularly at the nailfold and over the knees and the interphalangeal joints of the hand. Diffuse cutaneous atrophy with telangiectases and areas of hyper- and hypopigmentation on the neck, shoulder, chest, and upper back create a motley picture (poikilodermatomyositis). Pale pink or violet lichenoid papules are particularly common on the back of the neck, and occasional hemorrhagic bullous or nodular eruptions with a tendency to necrosis may round out the clinical picture.

Intracutaneous calcifications may develop about the elbows, knees, and shoulder joints.

Diffuse alopecia can occur, but also hypertrichosis. The nails are corrugated and the groove of the nail bed becomes yellowish, hyperkeratotic, and painful if one tries to push it back (Keining's sign).

Radiology

Radiographs of the hand very often show a periarticular osteoporosis that later may become strand-like. A characteristic finding is interstitial calcinosis at subcutaneous or deeper sites (Thibièrge-Weissenbach syndrome). These calcifications may appear as flaky, granular, linear, or reticular deposits in the soft tissues. Their distribution pattern resembles that in scleroderma. Chronic arthritis is a somewhat rare finding whose radiographic manifestations consist of soft-tissue swelling, marked decalcification near joints, and erosions.

Besides showing interstitial calcinosis, *radionuclide scans* have a characteristic appearance in PM or DM. Areas involved by myositis absorb large amounts of radiotracer, producing areas of intense uptake in the soft tissues (Fig. 2.3 b).

References are listed at the end of Chap. 2, p. 75.

2.4 Sjögren's Syndrome

Sjögren's syndrome will not be discussed here in detail, as it lacks specific radiographic features, and radiographs are unnecessary in establishing the diagnosis. The occasional arthritis and arthralgia that accompany the cardinal symptoms of xerophthalmia and xerostomia are nonerosive and produce no radiographic changes. The sicca manifestations that occur in patients who develop *secondary Sjögren's syndrome* in a setting of rheumatoid arthritis or other collagen diseases are discussed under those headings.

2.5 Jo-1 (Antisynthetase) Syndrome

Onset with flulike symptoms, usually in the spring; fibrosing alveolitis; Raynaud's phenomenon plus signs of dermatomyositis and scleroderma.
Roentgen signs: periarticular osteoporosis in the hands; polyarthritis, usually nonerosive and producing no radiographic changes.

◼ Definition

Jo-1 syndrome is an overlap syndrome with myositis that is very often associated with a fibrosing pulmonary alveolitis and chronic polyarthritis and is sometimes associated with Raynaud's phenomenon, edema of the hands and lower legs, sicca syndrome, and dermatomyositic or scleroderma-like changes in the skin of the hands and face. Up to 70% of patients are found to have Jo-1 antibodies against the cytoplasmic enzyme histidyl-tRNA synthetase.

◼ General Clinical, Dermatologic, and Radiologic Features

In 1980, an antibody against a previously unknown antigen (histidyl-tRNA synthetase) was detected in a patient with polymyositis. Named for the first two letters in the patient's name, the Jo-1 antigen is found in approximately 30–40% of patients with polymyositis. According to Genth and Mierau (1993), the "Jo-1 (antisynthetase) syndrome" represents the first attempt to describe an inflammatory rheumatic condition based on the detection of autoantibodies (high titers of U1-nRNP antibodies) and distinguish it from established entities belonging to the spectrum of collagen diseases.

The disease may have a mono- or oligosymptomatic onset, usually with flulike symptoms (fever, cough, limb pains) that begin in the spring. This presentation suggests that the disease is incited by a previous infection – possibly a picornavirus infection involving the interaction of viral RNA with synthetases as in an autoimmune response. An association with HLA-DR3 and HLA-DRw52 suggests a possible genetic predisposition to this type of immune response. The fibrosing alveolitis and chronic polyarthritis serve to distinguish Jo-1 syndrome from other forms of myositis and dermatomyositis.

Women are affected almost three times as often as men. Following the mono- or oligosymptomatic onset mentioned above, the disease may take an episodic or chronic course, and years may pass before the overall symptoms suggest a diagnosis of Jo-1 syndrome. The presentation is relevant to the "interdisciplinary" theme of this book, as the main dermatologic features of the syndrome include Raynaud's phenomenon (see p. 62), dermatomyositic skin changes, and signs of scleroderma (see p. 62ff.) while its radiologic features are marked by polyarthritis. The latter is usually nonerosive, but periarticular osteoporosis is a common finding, and subluxations may be seen in the joints of the hand.

Löhr et al. (1993) described the case of a 67-year-old man whose disease began with the features of an exogenous allergic alveolitis. Initial treatment consisted of immunosuppressive therapy. Ten months later the symptoms recurred, followed 2 months later by facial erythema, sclerosis of the frenulum, sclerodactyly, and dorsal hand edema. These symptoms were accompanied by progressive weakness of the lower extremities and a markedly elevated CK. Several months later the patient presented again with progressive weight loss and weakness in all extremities. He also had dyspnea, fever, increasing pulmonary infiltration, an almost 30-fold elevation of C-reactive protein, and a continued rise in CK. Only at this stage were anti-Jo-1 antibodies detected in the patient's serum. A muscle biopsy showed the typical features of polymyositis. Another case published by Treher et al. (1993) illustrates the complexity of the Jo-1 syndrome. This case involved a 44-year-old woman who had a lengthy history of an indeterminate rheumatoid disease with pulmonary fibrosis. Because the patient also had psoriasis, previous doctors had attributed the patient's polyarticular symptoms to psoriatic arthritis, scleroderma, and an overlap syndrome. Examination by the authors revealed the classic signs of psoriasis, asymmetry of the mouth with a shortened and thickened frenulum, and sclerodactyly without skin thickening. There were contractures of all the proximal interphalangeal joints. Laboratory tests showed marked inflammatory signs, and the initial test for Jo-1 antibodies was positive. Radiographs showed subluxations at the metacarpophalangeal and interphalangeal joints of the left thumb, erosions of the metacarpophalangeal joint of the right thumb, and periarticular osteoporosis. Radionuclide scanning showed increased uptake (inflammatory) not only in the hands but also in the shoulders and knees. EMG showed definite signs of myositis.

Jo-1 syndrome mainly requires differentiation from other overlap syndromes. This syndrome, which apparently is not particularly rare, should be considered in patients with acute alveolitis and rheumatic complaints, and a search for Jo-1 antibodies (e.g., ELISA system) should be made.

References are listed at the end of Chap. 2, p. 75.

2.6 Sharp's Syndrome

Synonyms: mixed connective tissue disease (MCTD), mixed collagen disease

> Signs and symptoms depend on the nature of the overlapping collagen diseases.

Definition

Sharp's syndrome is a systemic disorder that combines features of other collagen diseases (progressive systemic sclerosis, systemic lupus erythematosus, dermatomyositis) with rheumatoid arthritis and is associated with high titers of an autoantibody against ribonucleoprotein (anti-RNP). Renal and CNS involvement are uncommon, so the disease usually has a favorable prognosis.

General Clinical and Dermatologic Features

As stated in the definition, Sharp's syndrome tends to take a benign course, and more than 90% of patients are alive 6 years after onset. Tests reveal circulating immune complexes as in systemic lupus erythematosus (SLE), but the complement serum concentrations are low. As a result, immune complex-induced tissue lesions very rarely occur. Some 50% of patients have positive rheumatoid factors as a result of polyclonal hyper-γ-globulinemia. Even very low doses of glucocorticoids are sufficient to ameliorate symptoms. The clinical presentation of Sharp's syndrome is relatively broad and depends on the influence of the individual overlapping collagen diseases. Overlaps with scleroderma are most common. The next most frequent combination consists of SLE, progressive scleroderma (PSS), and polymyositis. Overlap with rheumatoid arthritis is not uncommon, especially in patients with sicca manifestations. The clinical features of PSS (Raynaud's phenomenon, skin changes, dysphagia), SLE (erythema, serositis, fever, lymphadenopathy), polymyositis and dermatomyositis (muscle weakness, myalgia, muscular atrophy, violaceous erythema) are described fully under the corresponding headings.

Radiology

Radiographic findings reflect the diverse clinical symptoms of the overlapping collagen diseases and may include signs of scleroderma (see p. 66f.) with acral and periarticular osteolysis (see Fig. 2.1 g–j), particularly at the DIP joints, erosions and periarticular osteoporosis as in rheumatoid arthritis (see Fig. 2.1 e), and deformities, which may not be accompanied by significant erosion. Interstitial calcinosis is another typical finding (see p. 65). The radiographic manifestations are variable in their degree and can vary from region to region, at times making Sharp's syndrome extremely difficult to distinguish from rheumatoid arthritis and scleroderma (see Fig. 2.1 d, e).

References are listed at the end of Chap. 2, p. 75.

2.7 Undifferentiated Inflammatory Systemic Connective Tissue Disease

Many patients in the early stage of a collagen disease have isolated or nonspecific symptoms of an inflammatory connective tissue disease that may include malaise, fever, joint pain, Raynaud's phenomenon, hyper-γ-globulinemia, positive rheumatoid factors and antinuclear antibodies. If observation of these patients is continued, characteristic symptoms will appear that enable a particular collagen disease to be diagnosed. In cases where this is not possible, Le Roy et al. (1980) favor the term *"undifferentiated connective tissue disease."*

References

Bassett LW, Blocka KLN, Furst DE et al. (1981) Skeletal findings in progressive systemic sclerosis (scleroderma). Am J Roentgenol 136: 1121

Bleifeld CJ, Inglis AE (1974) The hand in systemic lupus erythematodes. J Bone Joint Surg Am 56: 1207

Bohan A, Peter JB (1975) Polymyositis and dermatomyositis. N Engl J Med 292: 344

Braun-Falco O, Plewig G, Wolff HH (1984) Dermatologie und Venerologie. Springer, Berlin Heidelberg New York

Freyschmidt J (1997) Skeletterkrankungen. Klinisch-radiologische Diagnose und Differentialdiagnose, 2. Aufl. Springer, Berlin Heidelberg New York

Genth E, Mierau R (1993) Jo-1-(Antisynthetase-)Syndrom – verbessern Autoantikörper die Klassifikation von Myositiden? Z Rheumatol 52: 259

Haverbush TJ, Wilde AH, Hawk WA (1974) Osteolysis of the ribs and cervical spine in progressive systemic sclerosis (scleroderma). J Bone Joint Surg Am 56: 637

Le Roy EC, Maricq HR, Kahalch MB (1980) Undifferentiated connective tissue syndroms. Arch Rheum 32: 341

Leskinen RH, Skrifvars BV, Laasonen LS et al. (1984) Bone lesions in systemic lupus erythematosus. Radiology 153: 349

Löhr HF, Böcher WO, Hermann E et al. (1993) Interstitial alveolitis as early manifestation of anti-Jo-1-positive polymyositis. Z Rheumatol 52: 307

Pinstein ML, Sebes JI, Leventhal M (1989) Progressive systemic sclerosis (PSS) with cervical cord compression syndrome, osteolysis and bilateral facet arthropathy. Case Report 579. Skeletal Radiol 18: 603

Treher E, Niederhoff A, Gellissen U et al. (1993) Polymyositis and Jo-1-Syndrom. Z Rheumatol 52: 301

Udhoff EJ, Genant HK, Kozin F, Ginsberg M (1977) Mixed connective tissue disease: The spectrum of radiographic manifestations. Radiology 124: 613

Weissmann BN, Rappoport AS, Sosman JL, Schur PH (1978) Radiographic findings in the hands in patients with systemic lupus erythematosus. Radiology 126: 313

3 Rheumatic Disorders

3.1 Rheumatoid Arthritis

Synonyms: chronic polyarthritis, primary chronic polyarthritis

Rheumatoid arthritis ranks with the seronegative spondyloarthropathies as one of the most common inflammatory joint diseases. Usually it is associated with highly characteristic radiographic features. Except for rheumatoid nodules, no specific skin changes are observed. Rheumatoid nodules, which occur subcutaneously or on periosteum, develop in approximately 20–30% of patients with advanced rheumatoid arthritis. They are firm, painless, and occur mainly over pressure areas such as the extensor surface of the elbow, the Achilles tendon, the extensor surface of the fingers, the ischial tuberosities, buttocks, knees, and head. Inflammation or mechanical trauma can lead to ulceration of the nodules.

Because rheumatoid arthritis is not a condition that appreciably overlaps the fields of dermatology and clinical radiology, it will not be discussed here in detail.

3.2 Fibroblastic Rheumatism

Reddish, papulonodular skin lesions occurring near joints.
Roentgen signs: symmetric erosive-destructive polyarthritis; rheumatoid factors always negative.

Fibroblastic rheumatism is a symmetric polyarticular arthritis (wrists, fingers, elbows, knees) that is associated with the formation of cutaneous nodules, especially on the hands, and with sclerodactyly and Raynaud's phenomenon.

Only a few cases of fibroblastic rheumatism have been described (e.g., Chaouat et al. 1980; Hernandez et al. 1989). The skin lesions are reddish and papulonodular, similar to the lesions of multicentric reticulohistiocytosis (see Sect. 5.5). Rheumatoid factors are invariably negative, providing a useful differentiating criterion from rheumatoid nodules.

The nodules of fibroblastic rheumatism and rheumatoid arthritis also show histologic differences. Fibroblastic rheumatism is characterized by a fibroblastic proliferation of the papillary layer resulting in fibrosis. Elastic fibers are absent, and there is no fibrinoid necrosis like that seen in rheumatoid arthritis.

Hernandez et al. (1989) described the case of an 8-year-old boy with a rapidly progressive, destructive polyarthritis involving the wrists, metacarpophalangeal joints, proximal and distal interphalangeal joints, elbows, and feet. Reddish papulonodular skin lesions were found over the right elbow, the knees, the dorsal aspects of the hands, and the fingertips. The main *differential diagnosis* to be considered in this case was juvenile rheumatoid arthritis, which the authors felt was excluded by the rapidly progressive course and the specific histologic features of the nodules. They noted that the nodules of juvenile rheumatoid arthritis are generally associated with positive rheumatoid factors. Differentiation from multicentric reticulohistiocytosis relied on histologic examination (see p. 153).

References

Chaouat Y, Aron-Brunetiere R, Faures B, Binet O, Ginet CI, Aubart D (1980) Une nouvelle entité: le rhumatisme fibroblastique. A propos d'une observation. Rev Rhum Mal Osteoartic 47: 345

Hernandez RJ, Headington JT, Kaufman RA (1989) Case report 511 (fibroblastic rheumatism). Skeletal Radiol 8: 43

3.3 Gouty Arthritis

Synonyms: uratic arthritis, gouty arthropathy

Acute gouty attack: gross swelling and redness about the affected joint.
Chronic gout: gouty tophi in the auricles and extremities in the form of yellowish-white nodules.
Roentgen signs (hands and feet): joint erosions, subchondral osteolytic areas (medullary tophi) that may extend far into the diaphysis; destruction of joint contours by erosive tophi; spiculated periosteal calcifications; osteoplastic reactions; calcified urate deposits in the soft tissues; long-standing cases show only features of degenerative arthritis in affected joints.

Definition

Gouty arthritis is based on a derangement of uric acid metabolism that is associated with hyperuricemia and acute attacks of arthritis subsequently progressing to chronic arthritis. Primary gout, which is congenital, is distinguished from secondary or symptomatic gout, which develops in diseases associated with a prolonged secondary elevation of uric acid levels in body fluids.

General Clinical and Dermatologic Features

A detailed discussion of the etiology and pathogenesis of gout is beyond our scope. Basically, when the solubility product of sodium urate is exceeded, urate crystals are deposited in the synovial fluid, tendon sheaths, bursae, subcutaneous tissues, and kidneys. The synovial membrane responds to the crystal deposition with a foreign-body reaction, inciting a synovitis. Additionally urate crystals apparently damage the articular cartilage directly. Thus, two components characterize the joint changes in gout: synovitis and cartilage damage.

The deposition of urate crystals in subchondral bone can cause focal bone destruction with osteolysis ("medullary tophus," see below) that may break into the joint or into paraosseous structures. *Tophus* refers to a heavy focal (bushy) deposition of sodium urate with the formation of a granulation tissue that contains foreign body giant cells. Tophi may form in auricular and other subcutaneous tissues, in bursae, and in tendon sheaths. The degree of pathoanatomic, clinical, and radiologic changes depends on the duration of the hyperuricemia and on its extent (i.e., the quantity of urate precipitation per unit time). Excessive urate deposition within a brief period incites a highly acute exudative gouty arthritis – as illustrated by the classic involvement of the metatarsophalangeal joint of the great toe ("podagra") – corresponding to a large quantity per time unit. Less intense urate precipitation that extends over a longer period will incite a primarily chronic proliferative arthritis or arthropathy. This milder process does not evoke an inflammatory response in the synovial membrane, but it does damage the articular cartilage, leading to degenerative arthritis. A uric acid level higher than 8 mg% will lead to gout in 36% of the individuals affected; a level higher than 9 mg% will almost invariably produce gout (Mertz 1983). Genetic predisposition, age, and physical constitution are all considered risk factors for gout.

Four clinical phases are recognized in the natural history of gout:

1. Asymptomatic familial (genetically determined) hyperuricemia.
2. Acute gouty arthritis.
3. Intercritical gout (symptom-free interval between attacks).
4. Chronic polyarticular gout.

If no treatment is given, the intercritical intervals become shorter, and gradually a chronic condition is established in which acute attacks become less severe while intervening complaints increase. But years or even decades may pass between the first and second attacks of gout, during which time the patient is free of complaints even without treatment. It is important to note that acute gout does not inevitably progress to chronic gout, particularly when adequate treatment is provided that decreases uric acid levels and creates a negative uric acid balance in the urine.

An *acute gouty attack* usually occurs abruptly while the patient is feeling well. It is marked by redness, swelling, heat, and exquisite tenderness of the affected joint to touch or vibration (Fig. 3.3 a). In about 75% of cases, the dominant site of clinical involvement is the metatarsophalangeal joint of the big toe ("podagra"). Primary manifestations in other joints are less common. Polyarticular manifestations (usually asymmetric) are also somewhat unusual initially but become common later in the course of the disease.

The dominant feature of *chronic gout* is a chronic destructive arthritis that often is accompanied by clinically palpable soft-tissue tophi at periarticular sites, in the auricular subcutaneous tissue, and in the extremities. *Auricular tophi* ("gouty pearls") appear as small, pale, pearl-like, mobile nodules usually located on the helical rim (Fig. 3.3 b). The dermatologic differential diagnosis of auricular tophi should include calcified nodules on the auricular border, granuloma annulare, basal cell carcinoma, and chondrodermatitis nodularis chronica helicis. Larger *acral tophi*, which appear as yellowish-white nodules on the fingers, heels, etc., may break through the overlying skin and discharge a white chalky or pasty material containing urate crystals. Interestingly, these gouty tophi are usually painless and are most commonly found after an acute attack. The dermatologic differential diagnosis of periarticular tophi should include rheumatoid nodules, nodules in multicentric reticulohistiocytosis, Heberden's nodes, and joint tumors.

We close this brief review of the clinical and dermatologic features of gout with a reference to the rare *Lesch-Nyhan syndrome*, an X-linked recessive disorder in which a deficiency of hypoxanthine-guanine phosphoribosyltransferase leads to excessive uric acid synthesis. Usually there is an initial asymptomatic phase in early childhood followed by nephrolithiasis and gout as well as characteristic neurologic signs, self-mutilation by biting, choreoathetosis, spasticity, and developmental disturbances.

Radiology

In brief, gout is characterized radiographically by a combination of marked soft-tissue swelling, with or without visible calcifications, erosions with subchondral osteolysis, and osteoplastic (osteosclerotic) changes without significant osteoporosis. Urate deposits in the periarticular

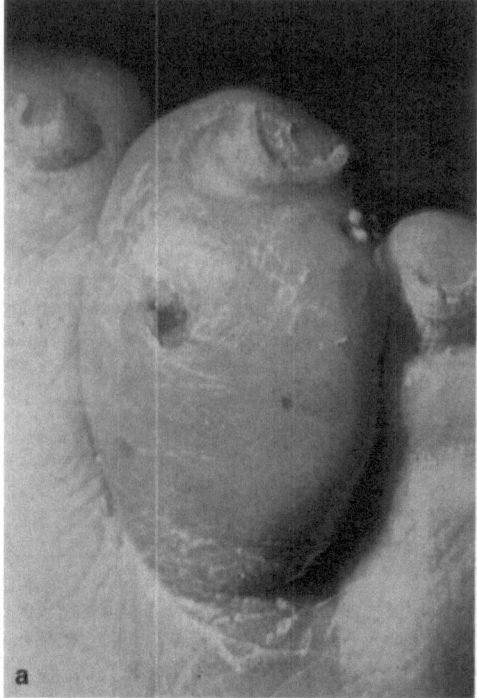

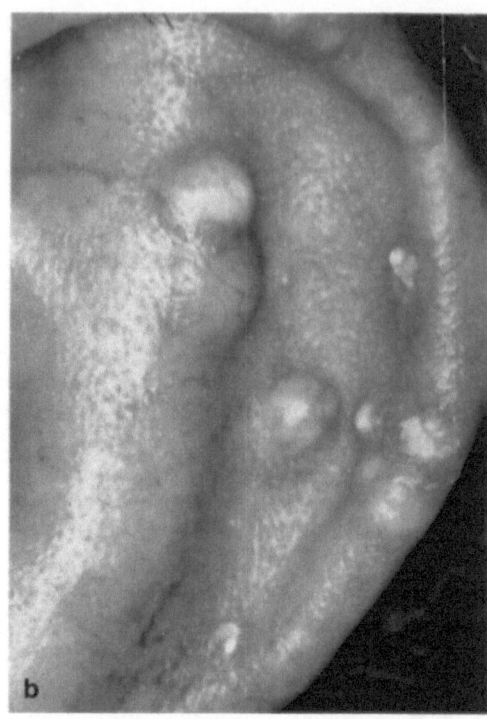

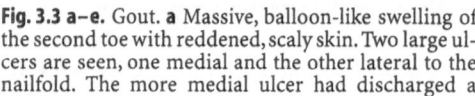

Fig. 3.3 a–e. Gout. **a** Massive, balloon-like swelling of the second toe with reddened, scaly skin. Two large ulcers are seen, one medial and the other lateral to the nailfold. The more medial ulcer had discharged a white, chalk-like material (sodium urate); similar material is still visible within the second lesion. **b** Gouty tophi on the auricle appear as small, pale, pearl-like nodules that are mobile on palpation. **c–e** see p. 81

soft tissues incite brush-like or spicule-like periosteal reactions known as *tophaceous spicules* (Fig. 3.3 c). This sign is most evident on the medial aspects of the first metatarsals and proximal phalanx. As the disease progresses, prominent calcifications may appear in the periarticular soft tissues, sometimes accompanied by intracortical erosions or faint irregularities. Radiographs typically show intraosseous *osteolytic lesions* (tophi) at the subchondral level that gradually spread to involve the shaft of the affected bone. These lesions can easily break into the adjacent joints and produce saucer-like defects in the small tubular bones (Fig. 3.3 d, e).

If the gout is untreated, the changes can progress to a late stage in which increasing destruction of the bones can produce mutilating defects, especially in the shafts of the tubular bones of the hands and feet, with pronounced tapering of the bone ends like that seen in rheumatoid arthritis (Fig. 3.3 d).

The radiologic features of gouty arthropathy also include progressive joint space narrowing due to cartilage destruction. This most commonly affects the bones of the foot, the carpal bones, and the joints of the hand and elbow. Generally it is not difficult to interpret the radiographic changes of gout if the disease takes an erosive, destructive course. Other destructive processes such as rheumatoid arthritis and psoriatic arthritis are usually distinguished by a different pattern of involvement. Advanced degenerative osteoarthritis that affects multiple joints can sometimes be difficult to distinguish from gouty arthritis. Foci of periarticular osteolysis that are difficult to classify should call to mind the adage, "If in doubt, think of gout."

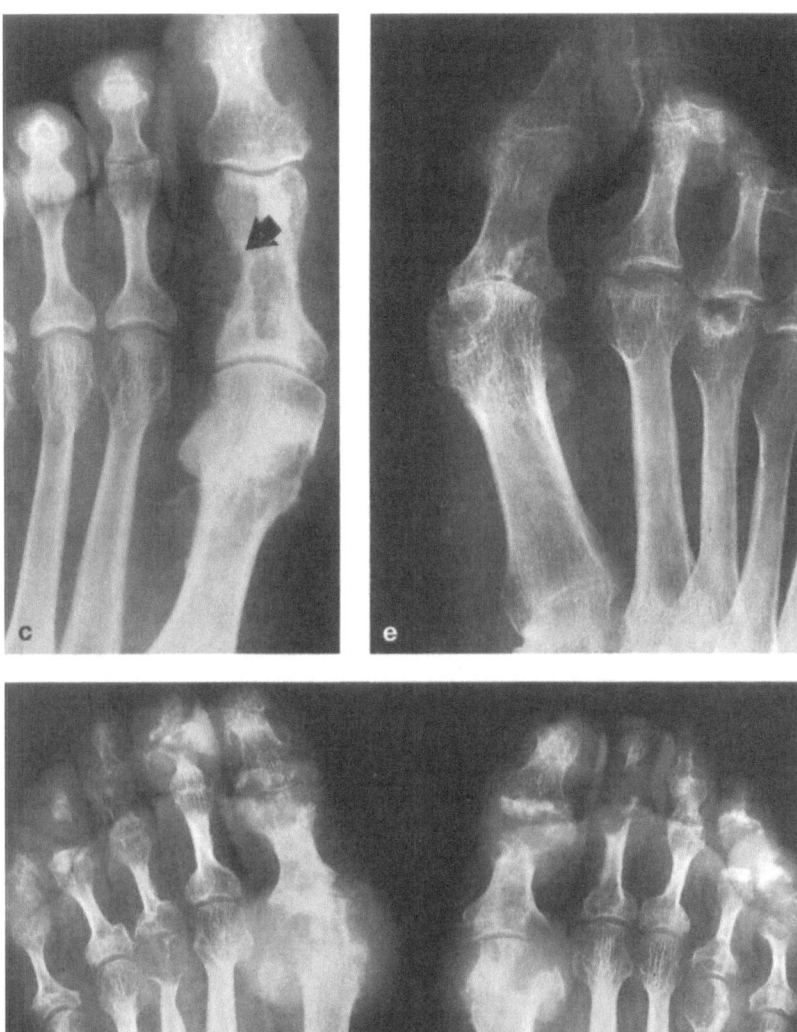

Fig. 3.3 (*continued*). **c** Severe radiographic changes of gout. The changes are particularly marked in the first ray of the left foot and were equivalent on both sides. Note the spiculated periosteal reactions, especially on the proximal phalanx ("tophaceous spicules"). Larger medullary tophi appear as osteolytic lesions in the proximal phalanx and in the distal shaft and metaphysis of the first metatarsal. **d** Grotesque destructive changes are visible about the metatarsophalangeal joints of the big toes. Medullary tophi have destroyed almost all of the head of the third metatarsal of the left foot and much of the head of the fourth metatarsal of the right foot. Severe destructive changes also appear in the second, fourth, and fifth middle and distal phalanges of the right foot and the second through fourth middle phalanges of the left foot. Note the calcifications in the soft tissues of the toes, especially the second toe of the left foot, corresponding to urate deposits in the soft tissues. **e** The metatarsophalangeal joint of the big toe shows severe gouty changes with extensive destruction of the articular cartilage and extreme joint space narrowing. Large medullary tophi are seen in the head of the first metatarsal and at the lateral base of the proximal phalanx of the big toe. Medullary tophi have also eroded the articular surfaces of the second and third metatarsals

References

Barthelemy CR, Nakayama DA, Carrera GF et al. (1984) Gouty arthritis: a prospective radiographic evaluation of sixty patients. Skeletal Radiol 11: 1

Bloch C, Hermann G, Ts'ai-Fan Y (1980) A radiological reevaluation of gout: a study of 2000 patients. Am J Roentgenol 134: 781

Dihlmann W, Fernholz HJ (1969) Gibt es charakteristische Röntgenbefunde bei der Gicht? Dtsch Med Wochenschr 94: 1909

Dihlmann W, Fernholz HJ (1974) Osteoplastische Reaktionen bei chronischer Gicht. Röfo 120: 216

Mertz DP (1983) Gicht. Grundlagen, Klinik und Therapie, 4. Aufl. Thieme, Stuttgart

Zöllner N (1982) Gicht. In: Gross R, Schölmerich P (Hrsg) Lehrbuch der Inneren Medizin, 6. Aufl. Schattauer, Stuttgart

3.4 Hemochromatosis

Increased skin pigmentation (bluish gray initially, later bronze), especially in exposed areas; testicular atrophy; hepatic cirrhosis, diabetes mellitus; loss of body hair; clinical polyarthralgia and swollen joints.

Roentgen signs (hands or other symptomatic regions): joint space narrowing, cartilage calcification, fine subchondral cysts, "dropping osteophytes" at the second and third metacarpophalangeal joints.

Definition

Primary hemochromatosis is an autosomal recessive disorder of iron metabolism characterized by an increasing accumulation of iron stores and the deposition of iron in the parenchymal cells of the liver, myocardium, pancreas, skin, synovial membranes, and other organs causing morphologic and functional damage to the parenchymal cells. In *secondary* hemochromatosis, the pathologic iron deposition is secondary to other diseases or an excessive iron uptake.

General Clinical and Dermatologic Features

The increased intestinal iron absorption in hemochromatosis is believed to result from the increased expression of a membrane-bound, iron-binding protein that acts as a transport carrier for iron in the mucosal cells of the proximal small bowel. The same protein is probably also responsible for the increased cellular absorption of non-transferrin-bound iron by hepatocytes and possibly by other organs. The iron overload in the hepatocytes leads to fibrosis and cirrhosis of the liver. Iron deposition in the pancreas, heart, and endocrine glands in the form of hemosiderin leads to functional insufficiency in these organs. Iron accelerates the enzymatic breakdown of vitamin C, resulting in a vitamin C deficiency that negatively affects collagen synthesis, particularly impairing the synthesis of cartilage and bone (see also p. 189).

The prevalence of hemochromatosis in the general population is approximately 1:4000 to 1:10.000, but it is estimated that about 1 person in 20 is a heterozygous carrier of the trait. The great majority of patients are males (about 80%), as females can compensate physiologically for the iron overload through menstrual bleeding. Secondary hemochromatosis may develop in patients with sideroblastic anemia or thalassemia, and it may occur rarely in *porphyria cutanea tarda*, late-stage alcohol abuse as well as by excessive iron uptake, i.e., by blood transfusion.

The *clinical presentation* is dominated by the features of hepatic cirrhosis, diabetes mellitus (bronze diabetes), and endocrine disorders due to *testicular atrophy*. The *increased skin pigmentation* in light-exposed areas is caused by increased amounts of melanin rather than iron deposition. In this respect, the above definition of hemochromatosis is not entirely correct. The hyperpigmented skin may appear bluish-gray, yellowish-brown, or bronze in more severe cases; the most commonly affected sites are the face (Fig. 3.4 a), hands, and flexural areas. The oral mucosa may develop a patchy hyperpigmentation similar to that in adrenal insufficiency. Braun-Falco et al. (1991) note that the skin appears sebostatic and sometimes slightly atrophic with a tendency to pityriasiform scaling. *Loss of body hair* in the axillary and pubic regions is a result of hepatotesticular insufficiency.

The joint changes of hemochromatosis are manifested by polyarthralgia and swelling with limitation of motion. The disease may be chronic from the onset, or it may take an intermittent, acute inflammatory course. Large joints are often clinically dominant.

The average age of patients with hemochromatosis-related arthropathy is about 56 years. Approximately 60% of patients develop hemosiderotic joint changes. The diagnosis of hemochromatosis is established histologically by liver biopsy and by finding an elevation of serum iron ferritin and increased transferrin saturation. If liver biopsy cannot be performed, CT scans may show increased attenuation values in the liver (> 72 HU).

Radiology

At least two components account for the radiologic changes of hemochromatosis: the synovial component resulting from iron deposition

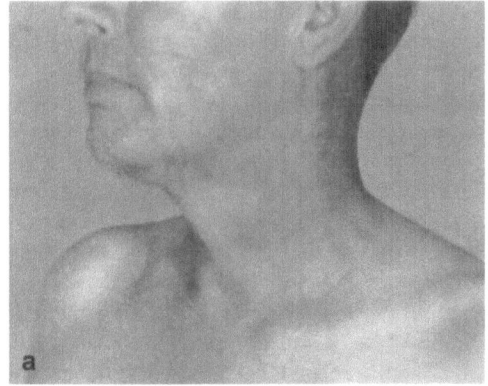

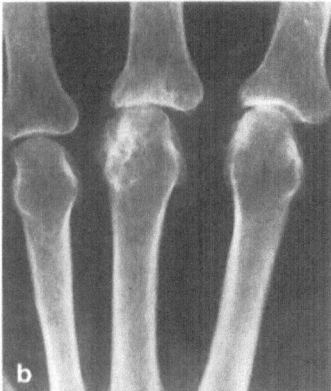

Fig. 3.4 a, b. Hemochromatosis. **a** Increased melanin deposition has produced bronze areas of hyperpigmentation that have a greenish- or bluish-gray tinge at the base of the neck. **b** Joint changes in hemochromatosis. An enlarged view of the second and third metacarpophalangeal joints of the left hand (same changes on the opposite side) shows marked joint space narrowing and small, subchondral, cyst-like rarefactions of the cancellous bone, especially at the third metacarpophalangeal joint. The structure of the subchondral cancellous bone has a generally nibbled appearance. Note the "dropping osteophyte" on the radial side of the head of the third metacarpal

(hemosiderotic synovitis) and a *secondary chondrocalcinosis* caused by a disturbance of ion equilibrium in the joint fluid due to the high local iron concentrations, leading to the deposition of calcium pyrophosphate dihydrate and other calcium compounds. It is very likely that the chondrocalcinosis that gradually destroys the cartilage is supported by the relative vitamin C deficiency (see above). The essential radiographic features of hemochromatosis closely resemble those of chondrocalcinosis with joint space narrowing and fine calcifications in the hyaline cartilage and fibrocartilage. Erosive and destructive changes are generally absent.

A distinctive and almost pathognomonic feature of hemochromatosis is the *involvement of the second and third metacarpophalangeal joints* (Fig. 3.4 b), where joint space narrowing, conspicuous subchondral cysts 1–6 mm in diameter, and marginal defects (due to breaks in marginal cyst walls) are observed. There may be disruption of the subchondral plate, and the subchondral cancellous bone may acquire a "nibbled" appearance as the disease progresses. The culmination of this process is a degenerative arthritis with sclerosis and osteophytosis ("dropping osteophytes"). Other sites of predilection for hemochromatotic arthropathy are the knees, wrists, hip joints, and the interphalangeal joints, which tend to show degenerative arthritis with chondrocalcinosis. Spinal changes may consist of intervertebral disk calcifications and longitudinal ligament ossification.

The differential diagnosis is straightforward in cases where the second and third metacarpophalangeal joints manifest the typical changes described above. Greater difficulties are encountered in cases that have an atypical primary site of involvement, e.g., an ankle joint with effusion and soft-tissue swelling, or in cases that show only features of degenerative arthritis, as there is little age difference between patients with secondary chondrocalcinosis and those with degenerative arthritis.

References

Braun-Falco O, Plewig G, Wolff HH, Winkelmann RK (1991) Dermatology, 3rd edn. Springer, Berlin Heidelberg New York

Bywaters EGL, Hamilton EBD, Williams R (1971) The spine in idiopathic haemochromatosis. Ann Rheum Dis 30: 453

Cartwright GE, Edwards CQ, Krawitz K et al. (1979) Hereditary haemochromatosis: Phenotypic expression of the disease. N Engl J Med 301: 175

Classen M, Diehl V, Kochsiek K (1993) Innere Medizin, 3. Aufl. Urban-Schwarzenberg, München, S 843 ff.

Dorfmann H, Solnica J, Mitrovic D, Dreyfuß P (1969) Veränderungen an Knochen und Gelenken bei der Hämochromatose. Münch Med Wochenschr 111: 1396

Dymock JW, Hamilton EB, Laws JW, Williams R (1970) Arthropathy of haemochromatosis. Clinical and radiological analysis of 63 patients with iron overload. Ann Rheum Dis 29: 469

Harrison TR (1977) Principles of internal medicine. McGraw-Hill, New York

Mall H, Zander W (1980) Arthropathie bei Hämochromatose. Röfo 132: 442

Strohmeyer G (1973) Hämochromatose. In: Hornbostel H, Kaufmann W, Siegenthaler W (Hrsg) Innere Medizin in Klinik und Praxis, Bd. 4. Thieme, Stuttgart

Walker RJ, Dymock JW, Ansell JP et al. (1972) Synovial biopsy in haemochromatosis. Ann Rheum Dis 31: 98

3.5 Relapsing Polychondritis (RP)

Synonym: chronic atrophic polychondritis

> Bilateral pain, swelling, redness, tension involving the helix, antehelix, and tragus with subsequent floppy- or cauliflower-ear deformity; nasal swelling and discharges, later saddle nose; tracheitis, bronchitis, hoarseness, and aphonia with eventual inspiratory and expiratory stridor; scleritis, episcleritis, iritis, keratitis; psoriasis; vasculitis.
>
> **Clinical and radiologic signs:** oligo- or polyarticular arthralgia and seronegative arthritis, rarely erosive; calcifications in necrotic areas; association with rheumatoid arthritis, autoimmune diseases, etc.

collagen fragments that finally precipitate an autoimmune disease.

Polychondritis is characterized histologically by regressive cartilage changes with asbestos-like degeneration, swelling, hyalinization, and cartilage necrosis. The destroyed cartilage may be replaced by a fibroblastic granulation tissue.

The dominant clinical feature of this still very rare disease is *bilateral auricular inflammation* (Fig. 3.5). Auricular chondritis is the initial manifestation in about one-third of cases, but about 85% of patients develop this condition later in the course of the disease. They complain of sudden pain, swelling or tension in the helix, antehelix, tragus, and occasionally the external auditory canal (bilateral in more than 90% of cases). Local redness may also be observed. Progression of cartilage destruction leads to "floppy ear" or "cauliflower ear" deformity.

Definition

Relapsing polychondritis (RP) is a generalized, recurring inflammatory disease of cartilaginous structures (ears, nose, tracheobronchial tree, joints) that may involve cartilage as well as biochemically related structures (in the eyes, inner ear, etc). There may be involvement of the skin, kidneys, cardiovascular system, and central nervous system, especially in patients with associated systemic diseases such as rheumatoid arthritis, collagen diseases, and vasculitides.

General Clinical and Dermatologic Features

RP is probably an immunopathologic disorder belonging to the class of collagen diseases and vasculitides. This relationship is suggested by the extracartilaginous organ manifestations noted in the definition and by the association with HLA-DR4, the presence of type II collagen antibodies, other autoantibodies, and the occasional presence of other autoimmune disorders (Benning et al. 1993). It has been postulated that a previously unknown exogenous or endogenous agent or trigger acts through humoral factors to incite the inflammation of cartilaginous structures. The proteinases and oxygen-derived radicals released by this process destroy proteoglycan-rich tissues and type II collagen, in turn leading to the release of biochemically altered

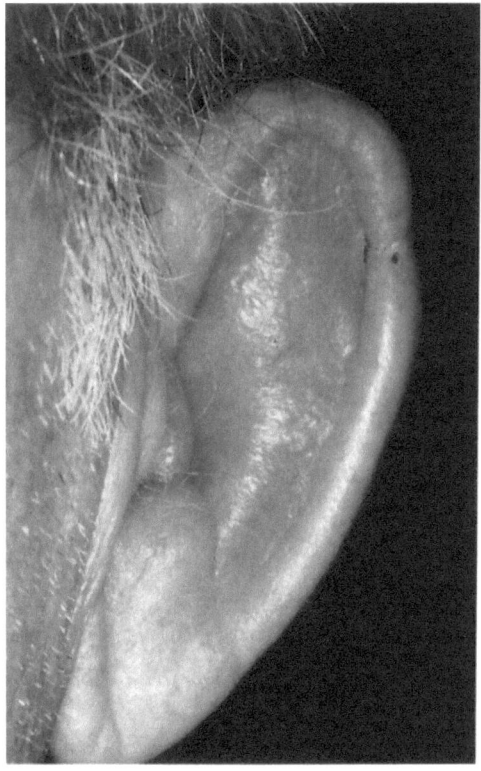

Fig. 3.5. Auricular redness and swelling in polychondritis. The earlobe is typically spared. (Photo courtesy of Prof. Dr. H. H. Wolff, Department of Dermatology and Venerology, Lübeck Medical University)

The second most common symptom of the disease is *arthralgia* and seronegative arthritis, which are the initial symptoms in 23–35% of cases. The fine survey work by Benning et al. (1993) states that 70–80% of patients experience joint symptoms during the course of the disease. This involvement is oligo- or polyarticular with a predilection for small and medium-size joints. About 50% of cases show concomitant involvement of the costochondral, sternoclavicular, and manubriosternal joints. The arthropathy is usually nonerosive and is often spontaneously remitting, but destructive or mutilating changes are occasionally observed.

Nasal chondritis is present in about 15% of cases at diagnosis and eventually develops in about 75%. The chondritis, marked by mucosal swelling, nasal discharge, and epistaxis in rare cases, leads to saddle nose deformity in one-third of patients. This differs from syphilitic saddle nose in that it destroys only the anterior, cartilaginous part of the septum.

The *cartilaginous structures of the respiratory tract* are involved initially in 14% of cases and show subsequent involvement in 55–70%. The dominant clinical features are tracheitis and bronchitis with inflammatory edema. Laryngitis causes hoarseness, aphonia, dry cough, and dyspnea. Eventually the process weakens the walls of the affected structures, leading to collapse, obstruction, and inspiratory-expiratory stridor. One-third of these patients will require tracheostomy.

Potential involvement of the *cardiovascular system* (valvular dysfunction due to dilatation of the valve ring, aortitis with aneurysms, etc.), the kidneys (microhematuria, proteinuria), the inner ear (cochleovestibular dysfunction), and the central and peripheral nervous systems (due to vasculitis) cannot be discussed here in any detail. It should be noted, however, that *ocular inflammation* is present initially in up to 19% of cases and supervenes in 50–65%. The most common ocular manifestations are scleritis and episcleritis, iritis, keratitis, and keratoconjunctivitis sicca.

Cutaneous manifestations reportedly occur in up to 40% of patients with RP. Benning et al. (1993) mention psoriasis vulgaris, pustular psoriasis, psoriatic arthropathy, occasional leukocytoclastic vasculitis and, in rare cases, erythema nodo-sum, thrombophlebitis, urticaria, livedo reticularis, panniculitis, and erythema multiforme.

As mentioned, one-third of cases are associated with rheumatic polychondritis, autoimmune diseases, or vasculitis ("secondary polychondritis"). Vasculitis is the most common of these, occurring in 10% of cases. Rarely, Churg-Strauss syndrome or Wegener's disease may precede clinically apparent RP. About 5–8% of patients have concomitant rheumatoid arthritis or juvenile arthritis, and 3–6% have an associated Sjögren's syndrome. Rare associations exist with lupus erythematosus, Hashimoto's thyroiditis, progressive scleroderma, and overlap syndrome. A rare association with seronegative spondyloarthropathies has also been described. The *prognosis* of the disease is uncertain. The average length of survival after diagnosis is 7 to 11 years, averaging 9 years for males and 16 years for females. The 5-year survival rate is 74%, the 10-year survival rate 55%. The disease usually takes an episodic course. The prognosis may worsen considerably as a result of associated diseases or the involvement of vital structures.

McAdam et al. (1976) state that three or more of the following criteria must be met to support a clinical diagnosis of RP:

– recurrent bilateral auricular chondritis,
– nonerosive polyarthritis,
– nasal chondritis,
– ocular involvement,
– respiratory tract chondritis involving laryngeal and tracheal cartilaginous structures,
– cochlear or vestibular damage.

The *differential diagnosis* of RP can be extremely difficult in cases that do not present initially with auricular and nasal chondritis. Wegener's disease or a necrotizing vasculitis would have to be considered in cases of this kind. The differential diagnosis would also include the rare *Cogan's syndrome* (keratitis, deafness, vertigo, mild polyarthritis, and possible systemic vasculitis), but cartilaginous structures are not destroyed in this disease. An *hereditary degenerative chondropathy* (autosomal dominant with congenital saddle nose, myxoid degeneration of thyroid and cricoid cartilage with laryngeal stenosis and stridor) should also be considered in patients 9 to 12 years of age. Other differential diagnostic possibilities would depend on the relative prominence of the various clinical symptoms.

Radiology

Irregular regressive calcifications are seen in areas of cartilage necrosis, raising the possibility of sequelae to frostbite, repetitive trauma (e.g., boxing), gout, chondrocalcinosis, ochronosis, or acromegaly. Reference was made earlier to rare erosive arthritis with destructive and mutilative changes. Cartilage destruction tends to incite an irritative synovitis that is manifested radiographically by soft-tissue swelling, periarticular osteoporosis, and gradual joint space narrowing.

References

Bachman F, Foroutan R, Hartl PW (1976) Der informative Fall: Rezidivierende Polychondritis. Therapiewoche 26: 6306

Benning K, Müller-Ladner U, Rauh G, Lang B (1993) Die chronisch rezidivierende Polychondritis. Z Rheumatol 52: 142

Brinkmann J, Yang C, Müller PK, Wolff HH (1993) Rezidivierende Polychondritis. Nachweis von Antikörpern gegen Kollagen IX. Aktuelle Dermatol 19: 154

Johnson TN, Mital N, Rodnan GP, Wilson RJ (1973) Relapsing polychondritis. Radiology 106: 313

McAdam LP, O'Hanlan MA, Bluestone R, Pearson CM (1976) Relapsing polychondritis: prospective study of 23 patients and a review of the literature. Medicine 55: 193

Spritzer HW, Weaver AL, Diamond HS, Overholt EL (1969) Relapsing polychondritis. Report of a case with vertebral column involvement. JAMA 208: 355

3.6 Seronegative Spondyloarthropathies

Synonym: seronegative spondylarthritides

The seronegative spondyloarthropathies are a group of joint disorders that have certain characteristics in common: negative rheumatoid factors, a "variegated" type of sacroiliitis, and a variable but definite association with HLA-B27. The original classification of Wright and Moll (1976) has undergone modifications during the past decade, and today the seronegative spondyloarthropathies are considered to include the following diseases (according to Calin 1981)[1]:

- ankylosing spondylitis;
- psoriatic spondylarthritis;
- pustulotic arthro-osteitis;
- Reiter's syndrome;
- reactive arthritis other than Reiter's syndrome;
- oligoarticular juvenile rheumatoid arthritis (type II);
- enterospondylarthritis (Crohn's disease, ulcerative colitis, etc.);
- undifferentiated spondyloarthropathy.

The essential features of the seronegative spondyloarthropathies are as follows:

- oligo- or polyarthritis;
- involvement of the axial skeleton with sacroiliitis and/or spondylitis;
- absence of rheumatoid nodules *and* rheumatoid factors;
- inflammatory changes at the insertions of ligaments or tendons (enthesopathy);
- tendency for extra-articular manifestations such as anterior uveitis, aortitis, and cutaneous lesions;
- onset usually in young adults; less common in children and older adults;
- definite familial occurrence and a strong association with the genetically determined histocompatibility antigen HLA-B27 (Table 3.6.1).

---

[1] Some authors classify inflammatory enthesopathy as a separate spondylarthritis, but we feel that this is illogical since enthesopathy is an integral component of most seronegative spondyloarthropathies.

Table 3.6.1. HLA-B27 in rheumatic diseases. (Modified from Calin 1981)

Disease	HLA-B27 positive (%)
Ankylosing spondylitis	90–100
Reiter's disease	70–90
Reactive arthritis	
Post-*Yersinia*	80
Post-*Salmonella*	80–90
Post-*Shigella*	80
Intestinal arthropathies	
With sacroiliitis	50–70
Without sacroiliitis	6
Psoriatic arthropathy	
With sacroiliitis	35–100[a]
Without sacroiliitis	14–24[a]
Juvenile rheumatoid arthritis	
With sacroiliitis	40–60
Iritis	40–50
Rheumatoid arthritis	6–10
Healthy controls	6–8

[a] Data from Wright 1985.

The criteria used by European authors for the classification of seronegative spondyloarthropathies are listed in Table 3.6.2.

Table 3.6.2. Criteria for spondyloarthropathies (European Spondyloarthropathy Study Group 1991)[a]

Inflammatory spinal pain

  or

Synovitis (asymmetric or predominantly in the lower limbs)

together with at least one of the following criteria:

- positive family history
- psoriasis
- inflammatory bowel disease
- urethritis, cervicitis, or acute diarrhea within 1 month prior to arthritis
- alternating buttock pain
- enthesopathy
- sacroiliitis

[a] The criteria are based on a study of 403 patients with all forms of spondyloarthropathy and 674 controls with other rheumatic diseases. The criteria resulted in a specificity of 88.7% and a sensitivity of 87%. The inclusion of HLA-B27 did not significantly improve the accuracy of the criteria (specificity 89.2%, sensitivity 82.6%). This supports the recommendation to avoid diagnosing a seronegative spondyloarthropathy in a patient with, say, unexplained oligoarthritis accompanied by lumbar pain (perhaps due to degenerative disease) simply because the patient is positive for HLA-B27. Conversely, the absence of HLA-B27 by no means excludes the presence of a seronegative spondyloarthropathy.

Almost all of these diseases may progress to ankylosing spondylitis, or one may give way to another (e.g., Reiter's dermatosis to a psoriasiform skin condition). The common genetic basis (HLA-B27 association) is expressed by a familial aggregation in which, for example, some family members may develop ankylosing spondylitis while others develop Reiter's syndrome, psoriatic arthritis, or ankylosing spondylarthritis. The common pathogenic principle probably lies in a genetic (B-locus-associated) defect in the immune response to urogenital and enteral infections. It is common to elicit a prior history of urogenital infection in patients with ankylosing spondylitis. Discoveries from clinical and epidemiologic studies on the etiology and pathogenesis of seronegative spondyloarthropathies were recently confirmed by experiments in transgenic HLA-B27 rats (Märker-Hermann et al., 1996): seronegative spondyloarthropathies did not occur in animals that were kept under more or less sterile conditions but did develop in animals that had normal infectious contacts. It is unclear why most seronegative spondyloarthropathies are associated with a mixture of destruction and bony proliferation primarily affecting the axial skeleton, and why the sacroiliac joints are so frequently involved. Many diseases in this group are prime examples of entities that can be correctly diagnosed only when viewed from a synoptic perspective that takes into account clinical, dermatologic, and radiologic findings. The importance of a correct diagnostic classification becomes clear when we consider *that approximately 2–3% of the population have some type of seronegative spondyloarthropathy.*

Seronegative HLA-B27-associated rheumatic disorders show a high prevalence in *HIV-infected and AIDS patients* (psoriatic arthropathy is 10 to 40 times more prevalent than in the normal population, and Reiter's syndrome is 144 times more prevalent). The reason for this is obscure, but the known genetic predisposition (HLA-B27 locus!) combined with a pathologic immune response (in connection with seronegative spondyloarthropathies) is perhaps significant in that the HIV-related immune deficiency may "trigger" the development of Reiter syndrome or psoriasis in genetically predisposed individuals. It is also conceivable that the weakened host defenses in HIV-infected patients may heighten their susceptibility to bacterial, parasitic, and viral infections of the urogenital and gastrointestinal tract, which in turn catalyzes arthritic processes in genetically predisposed patients.

References

Calin A (1981) Ankylosing spondylitis. In: Kelly W, Harris E, Ruddy L, Sledge C (eds) Textbook of rheumatology. Saunders, Philadelphia, p 691

Dougados M, van der Linden S, Juhlin R (1991) The European spondylarthropathy study group preliminary criteria for the classification of spondylarthropathy. Arthritis Rheum 34: 1218–1227

Freyschmidt J (1985) Gelenkerkrankungen. Röntgenologische Diagnose und Differentialdiagnose. Springer, Berlin Heidelberg New York

Freyschmidt J (1997) Skeletterkrankungen. Klinisch-radiologische Diagnose und Differentialdiagnose, 2. Aufl. Springer, Berlin Heidelberg New York

Märker-Herrmann E, Sucké B, Meyer zum Büschenfelde KH (1996) Neue Aspekte zur Pathogenese des Morbus Bechterew. Z Rheumatol 55: 4

Salomon G, Brancato LJ, Itescu S et al. (1988) Arthritis, psoriasis and related syndromes associated with HIV infection (abstr). Arthritis Rheum 31 [Suppl 4]: 12

Wright V (1985) Psoriatic arthritis. In: Kelley W, Harris E, Ruddy S, Sledge C (eds) Textbook of rheumatology. Saunders, Philadelphia, pp 1021–1031

Wright V, Moll JMH (1976) Seronegative polyarthritis. North-Holland, Amsterdam

3.6.1 Ankylosing Spondylitis (AS)

Synonyms: rheumatoid spondylitis, Bechterew's disease, spondylitis ankylopoetica, Marie-Strumpell arthritis

Iritis, iridocyclitis, conjunctivitis, nonspecific urethritis; low back pain, oligoarthritis, enthesopathy.

Roentgen signs: "variegated" type of sacroiliitis, syndesmophytes bridging between vertebral bodies; destructive and proliferative changes involving the anterior spine; eventual ossification of paraspinal ligaments and apophyseal joints; fibro-osteitis with "spiculation" at ligament and tendon attachments.

Radiographic test view: AP projection of the lumbar spine in the lithotomy position including the sacroiliac joints and both lower thoracic vertebrae.

Definition

Ankylosing spondylitis (AS) is a destructive and proliferative systemic disease of the spine and its joints, including the pelvic and thoracic articulations, that may involve ligament and tendon insertions, bursae, synchondroses, extremity joints, and may have extra-articular manifestations involving the eyes, heart, aorta, and lungs.

General Clinical Features

Previous reference was made to the genetically determined defect in the immune response to urogenital and enteric infections as the critical etiologic factor leading to destructive and proliferative changes in the spine and synovial joints.

Ankylosing spondylitis has an estimated prevalence of up to 1.8% in the general population. Studies in HLA-B27-positive blood donors have shown that the disease takes a subthreshold clinical course in up to 30–40% of patients. Only about one-third of cases develop fully established AS from a preceding sacroiliitis. Some 80% of patients remain able to work even after a protracted course; only about 5% develop a rapidly progressive, debilitating illness. The disease may become arrested at any stage. At least the clinical presentation of AS is predominantly a disease of males, occurring about four times as often as in females. In more than 80% of cases the onset of AS symptoms occurs between 16 and 40 years of age. Only 10% of patients are over age 40 at onset, and 7% of all cases start as a juvenile form between age 8 and 16 years.

The earliest clinical symptoms usually consist of nocturnal or early-morning low back pain, causing the patient to stand up and pace the floor until the pain subsides. Some patients, however, may initially experience a nonspecific lumbago and pseudoradicular symptoms. In almost 50% of cases the sacroiliitic symptoms are accompanied by a mono- or oligoarticular arthritis primarily involving the large joints of the lower extremity (hip, knee, and ankle). These arthritides tend to be fleeting and rarely progress to a chronic destructive or ankylosing process. There may be a very early inflammatory enthesopathy with pain and swelling chiefly involving the calcaneus (Achilles bursitis) as well as the greater and lesser trochanters, iliac spines, etc. These may be the predominant symptoms in some cases.

If the disease spreads from the sacroiliac joints to the spine, it will cause a painful limitation of motion with associated objective changes (positive Schober and Ott test, decreased finger-to-floor distance, increased occiput-wall distance and chin-manubrium distance). Finally the spine may become painful even at rest. Involvement of the costotransverse, costovertebral, sternoclavicular, and intersternal joints and enthesopathy at the junctions of the sternum and rib cartilages lead to a girdling chest pain that is felt on deep inspiration or vibration. If ossifications limit chest expansion, breathing becomes increasingly diaphragmatic and progressive abdominal protrusion may occur. In some cases the limited chest expansion may adversely affect respiratory mechanics, causing progressive impairment of ventilatory function with cor pulmonale.

In the *eye*, there may be an unilateral or alternating inflammation of the anterior uvea (iritis, iridocyclitis) with pain, photophobia, and accompanying conjunctivitis. Only a small percentage of cases manifest aortic insufficiency, cardiac conduction disturbances (first or second degree AV block), pericarditis, or upper lobe fibrosis in the lung.

Laboratory tests show that 90–100% of patients are positive for HLA-B27. The ESR is elevated in about two-thirds of patients, C-reactive protein is increased, and rheumatoid factor tests are negative. Joint effusions are bacteriologically sterile.

Dermatology

No cutaneous manifestations are pathognomonic for AS. Not infrequently, however, iritis and iridocyclitis with symptomatic conjunctival injection or a nonspecific urethritis will lead the patient to consult a dermatologist. In rare cases these symptoms may predominate. But if they occur in conjunction with low back pain and perhaps with mono- or oligoarticular arthritis in the lower extremities, the dermatologist should consider the possibility of AS or at least some form of spondyloarthropathy. *It is important for the dermatologist to know that AS may represent an end stage of other seronegative spondyloarthropathies*, inasmuch as Reiter syndrome, psoriatic arthritis, undifferentiated spondyloarthropathy, and enteropathic spondylarthritis may progress to fully established AS.

Radiology

The radiologic features of AS cannot be described fully in this interdisciplinary monograph. The radiologic diagnosis of AS is extremely difficult in its early stages and requires a great deal of experience.

In almost 99% of all cases, radiologic changes appear first in the sacroiliac joints. Less than 1% of cases show initial, disease-specific radiologic changes in the spine *before* sacroiliac manifestations appear.

The simultaneous radiologic occurrence of joint destruction, subchondral sclerosis, and bony ankylosis is pathognomonic for sacroiliitis in AS (Fig. 3.6.1 a). This bilateral triad occurs in at least 90% of all cases. Dihlmann (1976) described this as the "variegated (in German: multicolored)" type of sacroiliitis. In contrast to bacterial sacroiliitis, which usually is unilateral and is marked by *consecutive* destruction, sclerosis, and ankylosis, the three cardinal features of AS-related sacroiliitis always occur *simultaneously*. Typical cases show multiple lacunar defects in the radio-

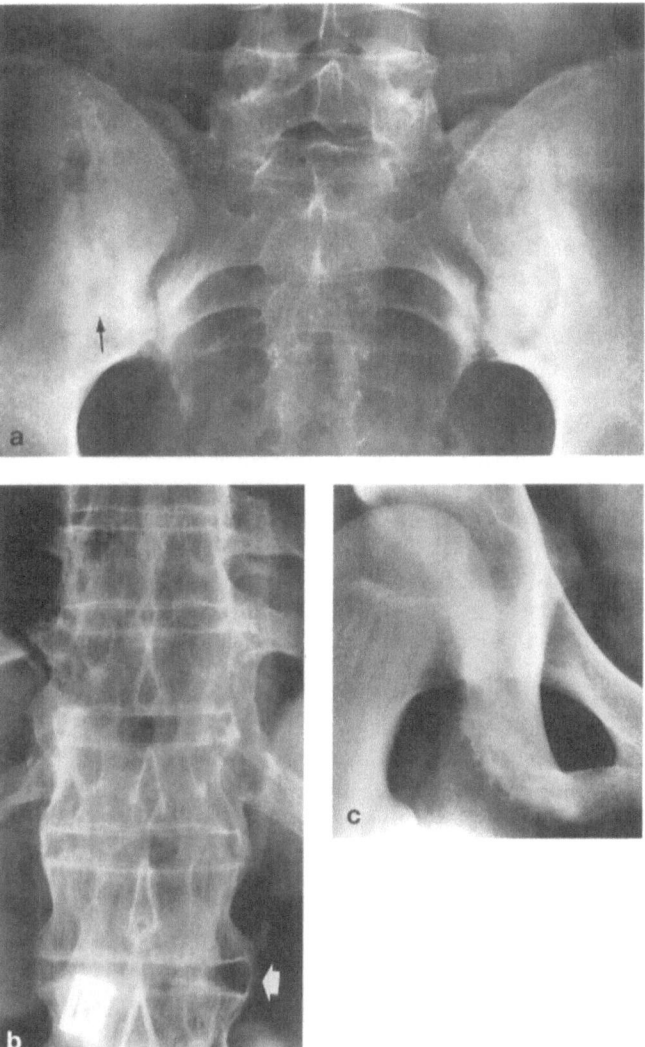

Fig. 3.6.1 a – c. Typical radiographic features of ankylosing spondylitis. **a** Bilateral sacroiliitis shows the concomitant triad of joint destruction (serrated and blurred contour of left posterior sacroiliac joint margin), dense marginal sclerosis, and ankylosing processes (*arrow*). The clinical picture included low back pain, alternating buttock pain, and severe aching pain in the right heel. The patient presented initially with iritis and conjunctivitis. **b** Advanced stage of ankylosing syndesmophyte formation. The *arrow* indicates a syndesmophyte that has formed a lateral bony bridge between the corners of adjacent vertebrae. Note also the complete destruction and obliteration of the costotransverse joints. **c** Typical appearance of ischial fibro-osteitis in a young man with ankylosing spondylitis. Concomitant destructive changes and proliferative new bone formation have caused "whiskering" or "serration" of the ischial contour, combined clinically with marked local tenderness. Other fibro-osteitic changes were found on the calcaneus, with clinical manifestations of achilles bursitis (see also Fig. 3.6.4 i)

graphic contours of the sacroiliac joints combined with marginal sclerosis and a variable amount of ossification in the joint space later leading to ankylosis. In the great majority of cases, these changes are clearly appreciated on standard X-ray films. But if there is strong clinical suspicion of AS and X-ray findings are equivocal, CT should be performed as it will provide a non-superimposed, high-definition view of all the changes. MRI is reserved for special indications. These changes may be accompanied or followed by the formation of *syndesmophytes* (Fig. 3.6.1 b), spur-like bony proliferations at the corners of the vertebral bodies. Unlike spondylophytes, these outgrowths develop from the outer layers of the anulus fibrosus or intervertebral disk and "grow" longitudinally toward the adjacent vertebral body. Ankylosis ensues as extensive lateral bony bridges are formed between the vertebral bodies. In almost two-thirds of cases, the syndesmophytes first appear in the area of the thoracolumbar junction, usually involving segments T11 – L2. This is useful for the primary radiologic diagnosis of AS, as a *single* sagittal projection of the lumbar spine including the sacroiliac joints and thoracolumbar junction will demonstrate these changes. Syndesmophytes are rarely a primary finding in patients under 20 years of age, while syndesmophytes in patients over 45 often have an atypical appearance because they coexist with degenerative marginal spondylophytes ("mixed osteophyte" pattern). The costotransverse joints of the lower thoracic spine are a very early site of destructive and proliferative changes that are sometimes difficult to distinguish from degenerative processes that are associated with subchondral sclerosis and the ossification of capsules and ligaments.

The anterior borders of the vertebral bodies may be affected by destructive and proliferative changes, called "anterior or marginal spondylitis" or Romanus lesions. Radiologically they correspond to defects in the anterior marginal and subdiscal portions of the vertebral bodies especially at the L3 – L5 level. These defects may be preceded by a circumscribed increase in cancellous bone density – the "shiny corner" sign. The anterior spondylitis may cause a loss of normal anterior concavity with *vertebral body squaring*. Further progression of the destructive inflammatory changes may round off the edges of the vertebral bodies, producing *barrel-shaped vertebrae*.

A potential complication of the ankylosing spinal changes is the "Andersson lesion," which usually is a fatigue fracture but sometimes may represent inflammatory destruction due to spondylodiscitis.

In adolescent patients with AS, the restriction of spinal mobility is due less to the formation of syndesmophytes than to ankylosis of the apophyseal joints and ossification of the ligamenta flava, sometimes producing a "tramline" pattern as a very early radiographic sign.

Ossification of the anterior and posterior longitudinal ligaments occurs relatively late in the course of the disease. The "bamboo spine" once considered so typical of AS has become an infrequent finding.

Rarefying or productive fibro-osteitis (see Figs. 3.6.1 c, 3.6.4 i), usually with bilateral ischial and calcanean involvement, may present radiographically as small lacunar defects in the bony contours of the affected regions or as ill-defined pencil-, flame- or vesicle-shaped ossifications. Other sites of predilection for fibro-osteitis besides the trochanters are the insertions of the abductor hallucis, abductor digiti minimi, flexor digitorum brevis muscles, the long plantar ligament, and the calcaneocuboid ligament.

Differential Diagnosis

The differential diagnosis of AS is based on the nosologic criteria presented above (see p. 87f.). Criteria for the early diagnosis of AS are reviewed in Table 3.6.3. The well-known New York criteria are used in the assessment of later changes. Essential differential diagnostic criteria are summarized in Table 3.6.4.

Radiographically conspicuous hyperostotic changes suggestive of *hyperostotic spondylosis deformans* (DISH syndrome) with pronounced ankylosing spondylophytosis and no disk space narrowing require strict differentiation from the metaplastic-ossifying changes in AS. Patients with the former condition generally do not have low back pain or any other signs of an inflammatory rheumatic process. The hyperostotic changes are often associated with a latent or overt diabetes mellitus or with gout.

Table 3.6.3. Early diagnosis of ankylosing spondylitis. (According to Mau and Zeidler 1990)

Criteria	Points
Genetic	
HLA-B27-positive	1.5
Clinical	
Spinal pain (inflammatory type)	1
Ischialgiform spontaneous pain and/or positive Mennell sign	1
Spontaneous or compression pain in the bony thorax and/or limited respiratory excursions (≤2.5 cm)	1
Peripheral arthritis and/or heel pain	1
Iritis or iridocyclitis	1
Restricted mobility of the cervical and/or lumbar spine at all levels	1
Laboratory	
Elevated ESR	
• age <50: male >15 mm/h, female >20 mm/h	1
• age ≥50: male >20 mm/h, female >30 mm/h	
Radiographic	
Spinal signs: syndesmophytes, squared or barrel-shaped vertebrae, Romanus-Andersson lesion, arthritis of costo-vertebral and/or intervertebral joints	1

A score of 3.5 or more warrants an early diagnosis of ankylosing spondylitis.

Criteria excluding a diagnosis of AS
• traumatic, degenerative, or other noninflammatory spinal disorders;
• psoriatic arthritis or reactive arthritis;
• malignant, infectious, metabolic, or endocrine disorders;
• other reasons for an elevated ESR or positive rheumatoid factor.

Sternocostoclavicular hyperostosis with *destructive and proliferative changes in the sternocostoclavicular region* does occur in AS but usually coexists with other typical manifestations described above. If two or three vertebral segments also display inflammatory changes with dense reactive sclerosis accompanied by predominantly proliferative changes in other skeletal regions and there is a prior history or visual evidence of palmoplantar pustulosis, then pustulotic arthro-osteitis should be considered in the differential diagnosis (see p. 101).

References

Bollow M, Braun I, Kannenberg J et al. (1997) Normal morphology of sacroiliac joints in children: magnetic resonance studies related to age und sex. Skeletal Radiol 26: 697

Dihlmann W (1976) Röntgendiagnostische Basisinformation: Das „bunte" Sakroiliakalbild. Aktuelle Rheumatol 1: 17

Mau W, Zeidler H (1990) Spondylitis ankylosans. In: Gerok W et al. (Hrsg) Innere Medizin der Gegenwart, Bd. 7 Rheumatologie, Teil C. Urban & Schwarzenberg, S 404

Table 3.6.4. Differential diagnosis of spondyloarthropathies (extravertebral and extra-articular manifestations). (According to Mau and Zeidler 1990)

	Idiopathic ankylosing spondylitis	Spondylitis in reactive arthritis	Psoriatic spondylarthritis	Spondylitis in enteropathic arthritis
Age at onset	16–40	variable	variable	variable
Male:female ratio	3–1:1	9–1:1	2:1	1:1
HLA-B27	~90%	~80%	~50%	50–80%
Diarrhea	–	++ OR	–	++
Urethritis	–	++	–	–
Prostatitis	+	++	–	–
Conjunctivitis	+/–	++	+	+/–
Acute iritis	+	+	+	+
Aortic insufficiency	+	–	–	–
Mucocutaneous lesions	–	+	++	+
Enthesopathy	++	++	++	+

3.6.2 Psoriatic Spondylarthritis and Psoriatic Arthritis

Synonyms: psoriatic spondyloarthropathy/psoriatic arthritis, psoriatic osteoarthropathy

> Erythematous macules with a silvery-white scale; nail changes (oil spots, pitting, crumbling); sterile pustules.
> **Roentgen signs:** erosive, mutilating, and ankylosing joint changes, mainly involving the hands and feet, with a typical axial, transverse, or mixed pattern of involvement; proliferative changes (periosteal ossification, protuberances); spondylarthritis with sacroiliitis, pasasyndesmophytes, etc; enthesopathy.

Definition

Psoriatic spondylarthritis and psoriatic arthritis are seronegative erosive-destructive joint disorders, prone to osteoproliferation, that are causally related to psoriasis. The bone and joint changes have an oligo- or polyarticular distribution and principally involve the hands and feet, the sacroiliac joints, and the spine.

General Clinical Features

The etiology of psoriatic spondylarthritis and psoriatic arthritis is as poorly understood as that of psoriasis itself. It is reasonable to speculate that the proteoglycan loss found in association with the keratinization and proliferation disorders in the skin *and* bone (see below) is a shared etiopathologic factor. Today psoriasis is widely regarded as a polygenic, multifactorial disease with a definite familial occurrence. The psoriatic arthropathies in particular are known to have a genetic association via the HLA-B27 antigen. It has been estimated that up to 6% of the Western European population have some clinical degree of psoriasis vulgaris, and that up to 7% of these patients develop a clinically and radiographically variable degree of psoriatic arthritis. Psoriatic spondylarthritis accounts for almost 20% of the seronegative spondyloarthropathies. Psoriasis has no known sex predilection, and its peak incidence is between 30 and 50 years of age.

Skin disease antedates joint changes in the great majority of cases, but 15–30% of patients develop joint changes *before* skin lesions are observed (Fig. 3.6.2 k, l). This is probably due to different methods of skin examination. It is not unusual for examiners to miss a subtle psoriatic eruption in an inconspicuous location such as the perineal or umbilical area (Fig. 3.6.2 c). Because psoriatic skin lesions are variable in their expression, a careful history should be taken if there is clinical or radiologic suspicion of psoriasis. The family history is also important, as the presence of overt psoriasis in blood relatives is considered a highly significant diagnostic factor (see p. 87 and Table 3.6.2).

Initial joint complaints are usually mono- or oligoarticular. Rare cases are primarily chronic with an insidious onset, but typically the onset is acute or subacute. The monarthritic form generally has an acute onset, producing symptoms that mimic gout (pseudogouty arthritis). Psoriatic arthritis takes a more eventful course than rheumatoid arthritis, and the individual episodes are more severe. The prognosis is relatively good, however, with 80% of patients experiencing a mild form of the disease (versus only about 20% in rheumatoid arthritis). In 50–70% of cases the arthritis is confined to a few joints. Interestingly, involvement of the axial skeleton in psoriatic arthritis often causes minimal complaints, although spinal involvement may ultimately progress to the full presentation of ankylosing spondylitis (see p. 88 and Fig. 3.6.2 k, l). The severity of the psoriasis and the acuteness of the skin changes very often correlate with the

Fig. 3.6.2 a–l. Psoriasis. The dermatologic photos illustrate "minimal lesions" rather than the well-known features of psoriasis in its fully developed presentation. The examiner should look for these lesions in cases where skeletal changes raise suspicion of psoriatic arthritis-spondylarthritis. **a** Relatively subtle psoriatic eruption behind the ear, unaccompanied by other changes. **b** Typical nail changes in psoriasis: pitting (*small arrow*) and oil spots (*asterisk*). **c** Subtle psoriatic eruptions around the umbilicus are the only cutaneous manifestation in this patient. This type of lesions should be sought in etiologically unclear cases of arthritis and spondylarthritis with negative rheumatoid factor. **d** Psoriatic eruption on the glans penis. **e** Erythemosquamous and pustular lesions on the soles of the feet. **f–l** see pp. 96, 98, 99

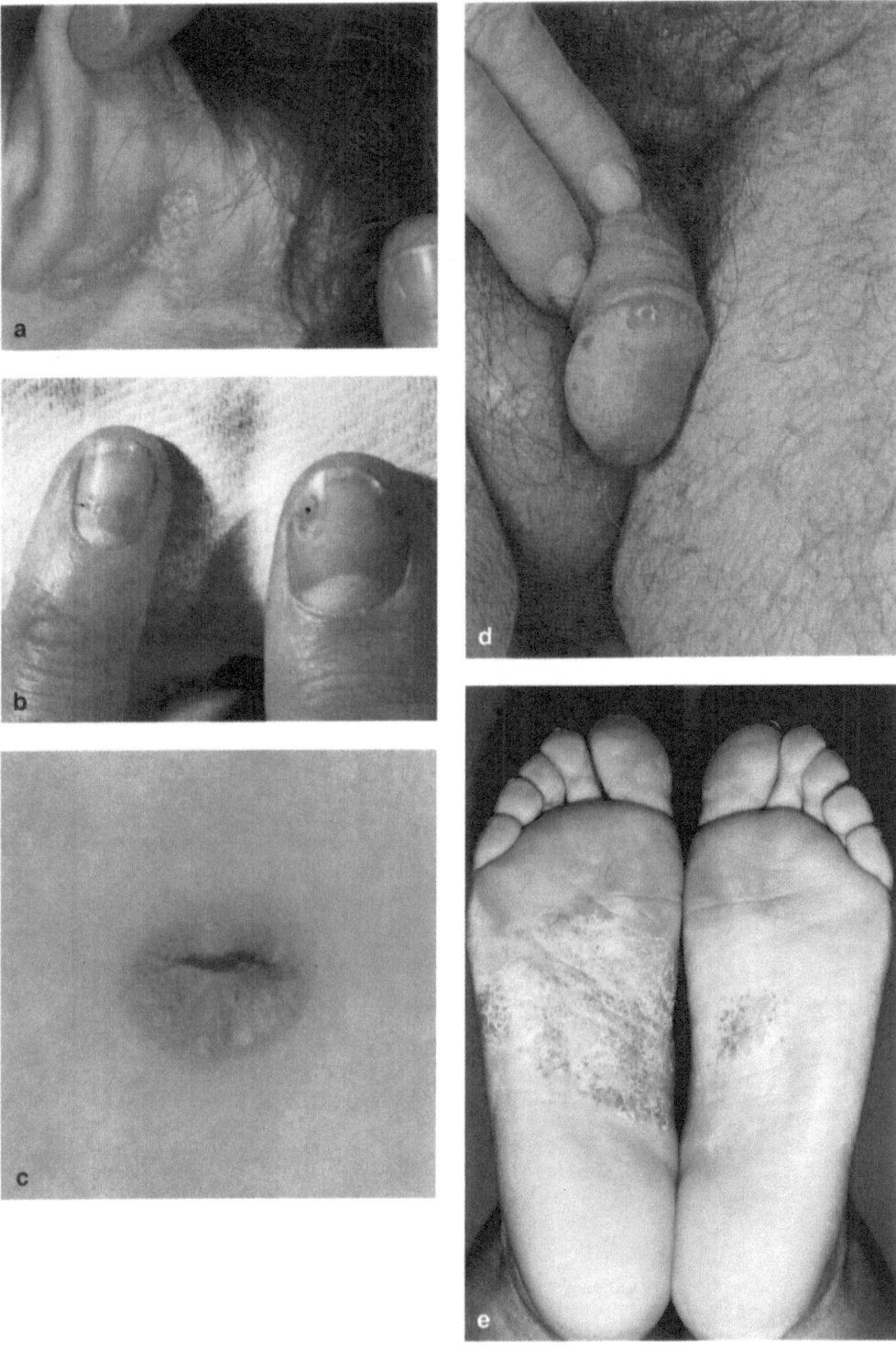

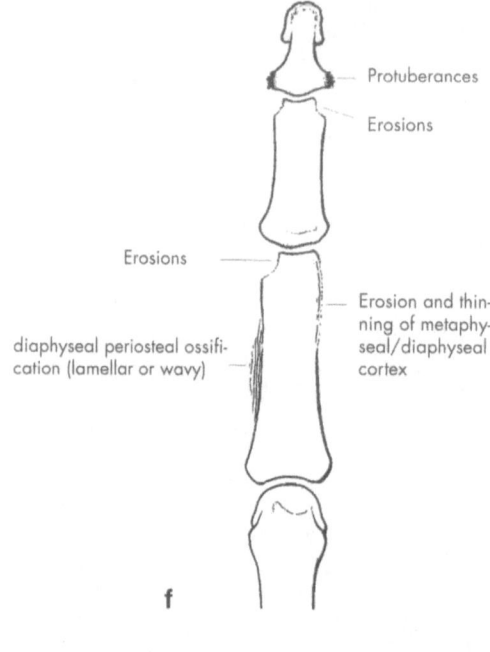

Protuberances

Erosions

Erosions

diaphyseal periosteal ossification (lamellar or wavy)

Erosion and thinning of metaphyseal/diaphyseal cortex

f

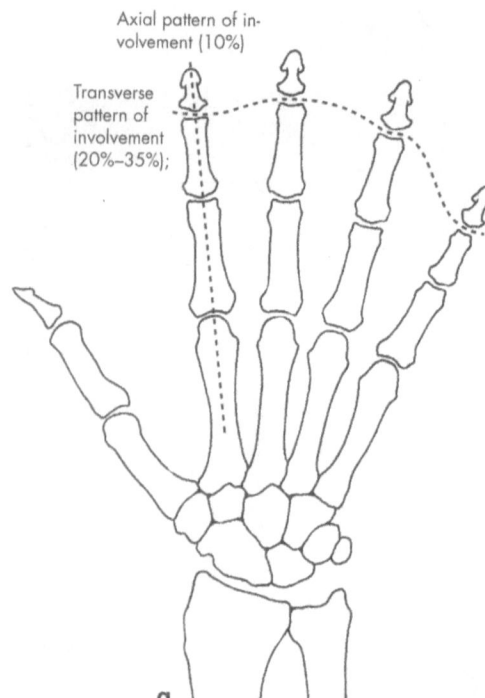

Axial pattern of involvement (10%)

Transverse pattern of involvement (20%–35%);

g

Fig. 3.6.2 (*continued*). **f** Primary radiologic findings in psoriatic arthritis. **g** Characteristic pattern of involvement in psoriatic arthritis. Joint involvement is asymmetric in more than 50% of cases, with oligo- or polyarticular involvement of the DIP, PIP and MCP joints. **h–l** see pp. 98, 99

severity of the arthritic episodes. Psoriatic arthritis shows a predilection for the distal interphalangeal joints of the fingers and the interphalangeal joints of the toes. Involvement of the joints along one ray is known as *axial* or *ray involvement*. Significant associated involvement of the extra-articular soft tissues is termed *psoriatic dactylitis*. The affected fingers or toes have a sausage-shaped appearance (sausage digits). These changes suggest a high likelihood of eventual diaphyseal-metaphyseal periosteal new bone formation and of osteolytic lesions developing in the diaphyseal or metaphyseal segments of one or more small tubular bones.

Laboratory tests show a slight elevation of the ESR. Rheumatoid factor tests are usually negative, with positive tests signifying a concomitant rheumatoid arthritis. This is most commonly seen in cases of long-standing psoriasis.

According to Mathies (1974), psoriatic arthritis should be diagnosed if three or more of the following criteria are met, including at least one of criteria 5, 6, or 8. If rheumatoid factors are positive, two additional criteria must be fulfilled. Criteria for the exclusion of psoriatic arthritis are evidence of Reiter's disease, Bechterew's disease, or polyarthritis of the fingers with Heberden's nodes.

1. Involvement of the distal interphalangeal joints.
2. Involvement of the metacarpophalangeal and interphalangeal joints of the same finger.
3. Early involvement of the joints of the toes.
4. Heel pain.
5. Dermatologically confirmed psoriatic lesions of the skin or nails.
6. Close relative with confirmed psoriasis.
7. Negative rheumatoid factor.
8. Radiographs of the hands and/or feet showing typical osteolytic changes along with bony proliferation and no periarticular osteoporosis.
9. Clinical and/or radiographic involvement of the sacroiliac joints.
10. Typical paravertebral ossifications on spinal radiographs.

The incidence of psoriatic arthropathy is 10 to 40 times higher in HIV-infected and AIDS patients than in the normal population (see p. 88).

Dermatology

Three dermatologic signs of psoriasis are helpful in making a diagnosis:

1. The candle sign.
2. The last skin layer sign (last cuticle phenomenon).
3. The pinpoint bleeding sign (focal bleeding phenomenon).

The basic skin eruption of psoriasis vulgaris is erythemosquamous, i.e., an erythematous patch or macule covered by a silvery-white scale that can be scraped off in layers (like the wax shavings from a stearin candle: the "candle sign"). When all of the scale is removed, further scraping exposes a coherent moist tissue comprising the lowest layers of the epidermis above the dermal papillae. This "last epidermal layer" is regarded as the most telling sign of psoriasis. Removing that layer finally exposes capillaries, and spotty bleeding appears (the "pinpoint bleeding sign" or Auspitz sign).

The morphology of psoriatic lesions is highly variable (punctate, nummular, patchy, circinate, gyrate) and need not be discussed here in detail. It is more important to consider the *sites of involvement:*

The chronic, stationary form of psoriasis chiefly involves the sacral region, elbows, and knees. Another common site is the hair-bearing scalp, where heavily scaled erythematous lesions often develop and spread 1–2 cm past the frontotemporal hairline onto bare skin. Inconspicuous psoriatic eruptions should be looked for in intertriginous areas such as the axillary, inframammary, umbilical (Fig. 3.6.2 c), inguinal, and perianal regions. The differential diagnosis of lesions at these sites should include eczema and tinea, although the sharply defined borders of psoriatic lesions are an important differentiating feature. The palms and soles of the hands and feet are an extremely important site of occurrence (Fig. 3.6.2 e). Areas affected by palmoplantar psoriasis show a yellowish, firmly adherent scale, often with fissuring, that is difficult to distinguish from hyperkeratotic rhagadiform eczema and tinea. Not infrequently, a sharply marginated, reddened, slightly infiltrated lesion on the glans penis may be the only cutaneous manifestation of psoriasis vulgaris (Fig. 3.6.2 d).

Nail changes are present in 30–50% of patients with psoriasis and in up to 70% of patients with psoriatic arthritis. The most common nail change is pitting (dimple-like indentations in the nail plate, pinhead-size or smaller, caused by punctate foci of psoriasis in the nail matrix, Fig. 3.6.2 b). More severe matrix involvement leads to rounded or linear depressions and undulations (psoriatic onychodystrophy). With *nail bed psoriasis*, punctate or lentiform foci of subungual psoriasis cause a yellowish discoloration of the nail plate called a *psoriatic oil spot* (Fig. 3.6.2 b). This parakeratotic scale lifts the nail plate from its bed, discharging a crumbly material that, when removed, leaves an air space beneath the nail. The elevated part of the nail appears white, creating a condition of *partial onycholysis*. With concomitant involvement of the nail matrix and nail bed, only a crumbly parakeratotic material is produced, and the picture of *crumbling nails* emerges. Psoriatic arthritis is commonly associated with paronychial psoriasis and nailfold psoriasis leading to secondary onychodystrophy and longitudinal and transverse ridging of the nails.

Pale, arcuate lesions of the oral mucosa are seen only in pustular psoriasis, but involvement of the vermilion of the lips is known to occur in psoriasis vulgaris. A particularly severe form of psoriasis is psoriatic erythroderma, characterized by widespread inflammatory skin reddening with psoriasiform and pityriasiform scales. Intense pruritus is present, and the lymph nodes may be slightly enlarged.

Another special form is *pustular psoriasis*, in which increased exudative changes cause pustules to erupt on the erythematous plaques. These pustules are *always sterile*. Here we shall mention only two forms of pustular psoriasis: generalized and palmoplantar.

1. *Generalized pustular psoriasis* (Zumbusch type) is marked by disseminated inflammatory erythema with innumerable pustules involving all of the cutaneous organ including the palms of the hands, soles of the feet, oral cavity, and genital mucosae. It is associated with fever and malaise.
2. *Palmoplantar pustular psoriasis* (Barber-Königsbeck type) is marked by erythematous plaques on the palms and soles of the hands

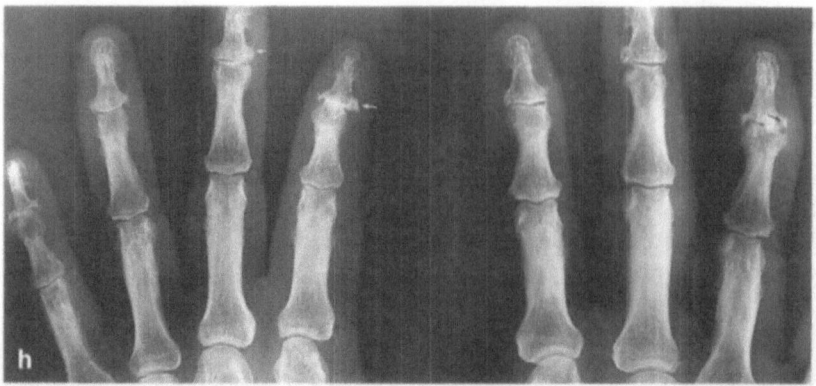

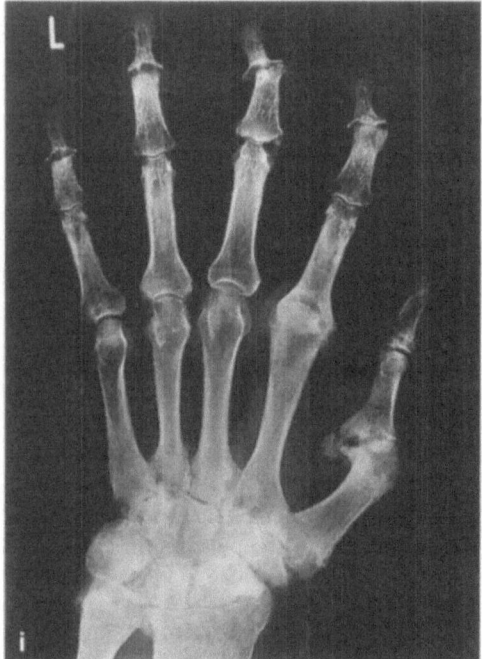

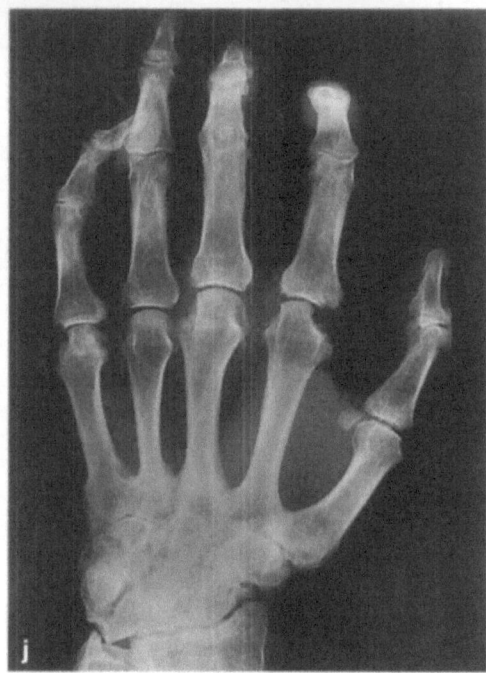

Fig. 3.6.2 (*continued*). **h** Transverse pattern of psoriatic arthritis involving the distal interphalangeal joints. Note the sites of bony proliferation ("protuberances," *arrows*) at the bases of the distal phalanges on each side and the fine erosions on the articular side of the proliferations. The erosions reflect the activity of the disease process, and protuberances are most conspicuous at eroded sites. **i** Very advanced destructive, mutilating form of psoriatic arthritis with complete destruction of the distal interphalangeal joints and coarse erosions about the proximal interphalangeal joints. Erosions are also seen at the first, second, and fourth metacarpophalangeal joints. Note the incipient ankylosis of the second metacarpophalangeal joint. Coarse erosive-destructive changes are also seen in the carpus. **j** Advanced erosive-destructive psoriatic arthritis of the hand, already with some ankylosis, accompanied by extensive spondylarthritic changes (not shown here). The second, third, and fifth metacarpophalangeal joints show coarse destructive changes, while the carpal joints show erosive-destructive changes and sites of ankylosis. The proximal interphalangeal joint of the third digit is completely ankylosed. Even greater deformity was present in the opposite hand. **k,l** see p. 99

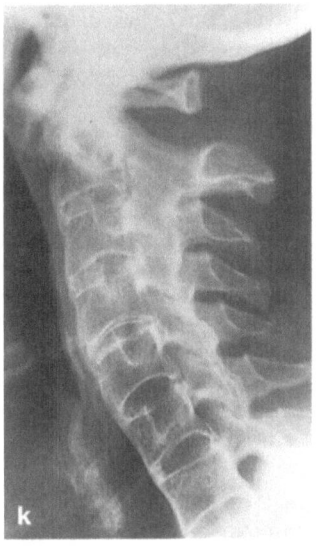
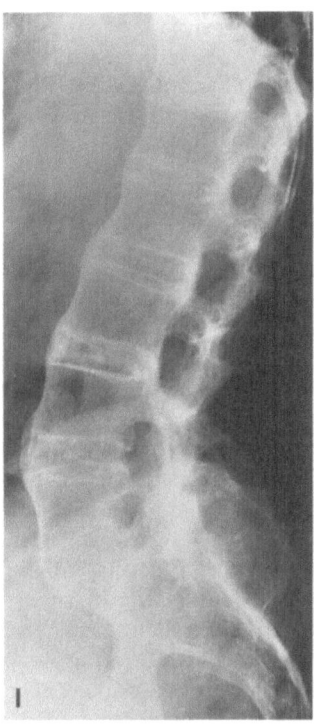

Fig. 3.6.2 (*continued*). **k, l** Full presentation of Bechterew's disease in a 58-year-old man. The patient was known to have psoriasis for only a few years, and definite changes of psoriatic arthritis were noted in the bones of the hand. Ankylosing spinal changes had been present for about 30 years. It is clear that, from the outset, this patient had a psoriatic spondylarthritis that progressed to fully established Bechterew's disease; it took several decades, meanwhile, for the dermatologic and manual arthritic changes to appear. This type of course is unusual but not unknown. Note the complete fusion of the apophyseal joints and the ossification of the anterior and posterior longitudinal ligaments, especially at the lumbar level. The sacroiliac joints (not shown here) also were completely ankylosed

and feet with shallow, sterile pustules forming "lakes of pus." There is an alternation of fresh and drying pustules. Occasionally pustules develop on normal-appearing skin.

When looking for psoriatic lesions, we should always assume that we are dealing with a *minimal form* of psoriasis that will require close inspection of the scalp, auricle, ear canal, retroauricular area (Fig. 3.6.2 a), nuchal area, eyelids, lips, umbilicus (Fig. 3.6.2 c), genital region (Fig. 3.6.2 d), perianal region, hands, feet, nails, elbows, and knees.

Radiology

Psoriatic arthritis is characterized radiographically by a *combination of destruction and bony proliferation*. Studies by Fassbender (1994) show that the course of pathoanatomic changes in psoriatic arthritis is quite different from that in rheumatoid arthritis. Whereas the destructive changes in rheumatoid arthritis result from a "tumorlike proliferation" (TLP) of the diseased synovial membrane, the changes in psoriatic arthritis appear to start in the bone. Fassbender (1994) noted a breakdown of proteoglycan in the subchondral cancellous and cortical bone, causing the collagen fibers to assume a ragged, herringbone appearance. This evokes a process of osteoblastic osteoid formation in which osteoid is laid down over the exposed collagen fibers, producing a "caricature" of the original bone. Because the process of proteoglycan breakdown and reactive-reparative new bone formation occurs in phases while mechanical loading of the structures continues, more heavily stressed sites apparently undergo bony surface fractures that contribute to the destructive process while other sites show bony proliferation, especially at joint margins ("protuberances"). The process of proteoglycan breakdown and reactive new bone formation may spread to the articular cartilage and then to the opposing bone, causing ankylosis of the joint. This mechanism may well account for the *ankylosing component* that is so typical of psoriatic arthritis. The clinically apparent synovitis is interpreted as a reaction to the destructive and remodeling processes in the bone and apparently does not initiate the process, as was once believed.

The typical radiographic features of psoriatic arthritis (Fig. 3.6.2 f) consist of partial or complete nondelineation of the *subchondral plate*, a combination of erosive and destructive changes, and eventual *joint space narrowing* that may progress to *ankylosis* (Fig. 3.6.2 h–j). *Mutilative changes* are a pronounced feature in many cases. Bony proliferative processes appear as irregular or spiculated ossification sites at capsuloligamentous insertions on the metaphyses and diaphyses, especially on small tubular bones. Spicular ossifications at joint margins, occurring mainly at the bases of the distal phalanges, are also known as *protuberances* (Fig. 3.6.2 h). Periostitic ossifications on the shafts of tubular bones usually have a layered or wavy appearance. With passage of time, these sites may become integrated into the cortical bone. Very early changes often consist only of fine whiskery or woolly sites of epiphyseal ossification that are visible only with a magnifying lens. These changes most commonly occur on the distal phalanges, and the radiologist should look for them in patients who have clinical arthritic symptoms. Acral osteolysis may also be observed.

The *pattern of involvement* is of key importance in the radiographic assessment and classification of visible changes (Fig. 3.6.2 g). The lesions tend to be asymmetric with an oligo- or polyarticular distribution. The pattern of involvement may be classified as *axial*, affecting all the joints of one finger or toe, or as *transverse*, affecting all the DIP joints of a hand or foot. There are also *mixed patterns*, which tend to be asymmetric. Involvement of the DIP and PIP joints is generally a more common pattern than combined involvement of the DIP, PIP, and MCP or MTP joints.

There seems to be a definite predilection for the great toe. Large joints are involved in fewer than 10% of cases, suggesting that the most efficient screening strategy would be to obtain *dorsopalmar and dorsoplantar radiographic views of the hands and feet whenever there is clinical suspicion of psoriatic arthritis.*

Approximately 50% of cases show sacroiliac joint involvement consisting of a *"variegated" sacroiliitis* (see p. 90). This involvement tends to be asymmetric and unilateral. It may be accompanied by *spinal changes* (psoriatic spondylitis) in the form of marginal erosions and paravertebral ossification. The latter may consist of an isolated lesion next to the disk space or adjacent vertebral body, or there may be an initial outgrowth that extends several millimeters horizontally from the vertebral end plate and then turns upward and projects past the adjacent vertebral body or establishes partial contact with it, forming a "parasyndesmophyte" (see Fig. 3.6.4 e). True syndesmophytes also may occur as in ankylosing spondylitis (see p. 92) and may coexist with degenerative spondylophytes to form a "mixed osteophyte" pattern (see p. 92). L1 to L3 is an area of predilection for parasyndesmophyte and syndesmophyte formation. Involvement of the cervical spine can lead to atlantoaxial subluxation.

A very important extra-articular feature of psoriatic arthritis and spondylarthritis is an *enthesopathy* consisting of ossification at the insertions of tendons, ligaments, and articular capsules (see Fig. 3.6.1 c). These sites appear radiographically as flame-shaped, fluffy, or spiculated ossifications on the ischium or other pelvic bones, the greater and lesser trochanters, the calcaneus, etc.

The radiologic features of pustular palmoplantar psoriasis are described on p. 101.

▪ Differential Diagnosis

The diagnostic criteria for psoriatic arthritis and psoriatic spondylarthritis are listed on p. 96. Despite these criteria, problems of differentiation continue to arise in diagnostic practice, especially if the history and clinical findings are equivocal. Cases with involvement of the sacroiliac joints and spine can be extremely difficult to distinguish from Reiter's syndrome (see p. 110), and either disease may progress to a classic ankylosing spondylitis (Fig. 3.6.2 k, l). Another very important differential diagnosis is rheumatoid arthritis. Whereas psoriatic arthritis usually has an acute or subacute onset, rheumatoid arthritis tends to have a more insidious onset. And while psoriatic arthritis tends to pursue a mild, irregular course, rheumatoid arthritis is progressive and episodic. Temperature elevation is a common feature of rheumatoid arthritis. Unlike rheumatoid arthritis, which is usually symmetric and polyarticular and mainly involves the proximal interphalangeal joints, psoriatic arthritis is usually mono- or oligoarticular and predominantly involves the distal interphalangeal joints or one ray, causing asymmetric rather than symmetric changes. Sacroiliitis, spondylitis, and enthesopathy are extremely rare in rheumatoid arthritis.

References

Fassbender HG (1994) Inflammatory reactions in arthritis. In: Davies ME, Dingle JT (eds) Immunopharmacology of joints and connective tissue. Academic Press, London, pp 165–198
Mathies H (1974) Arthritis psoriatica. Acta Med Austriaca 1: 3

3.6.3 Pustulotic Arthro-osteitis (PAO)

Synonyms: SAPHO syndrome (synovitis, acne, pustulosis, hyperostosis, osteitis); acquired hyperostosis syndrome; pustulopsoriatic hyperostotic spondylarthritis

> Predominantly productive sclerotic changes involving the vertebral bodies and long tubular bones, with or without sternocostoclavicular hyperostosis. Palmoplantar pustulosis or pustular psoriasis.
> **Basic imaging study:** radionuclide bone scans. Bullhead sign in the sternocostoclavicular region, often associated with hot spots in other locations.

Definition

Pustulotic arthro-osteitis (PAO) is an etiologically obscure disease that is associated with palmoplantar pustulosis (PPP) and with destructive and proliferative skeletal changes, especially in the sternocostoclavicular region. The letter "A" in the SAPHO acronym stands for "acne." We agree with Ellis et al. (1987), however, that the pattern of bone and joint involvement in acne-associated cases is different than in PPP, which is why we devote a separate section to acne-associated skeletal changes (see p. 127). In any event, PPP is a completely different dermatologic entity from acne fulminans or acne conglobata. The term "acquired hyperostosis syndrome," coined by Dihlmann (1993), refers to inflammatory, mostly hyperostotic changes in the supportive and gliding tissues of the axial and appendicular skeleton and joints characterized by sternocostoclavicular hyperostosis. Two-thirds of cases are associated with psoriasiform or acneiform skin lesions or show overlap with ankylosing spondylitis. We feel that Dihlmann's term is somewhat too general and imprecise, inasmuch as "acquired hyperostosis" is only *one* feature of other clinically and radiologically well-defined entities such as ankylosing spondylitis or psoriatic arthritis. We prefer the term "pustulotic arthro-osteitis" (PAO), now widely used in the international literature, to denote an etiologically related combination of PPP with inflammatory destructive *and* proliferative changes in the bones and joints, with or without sternocosto-clavicular hyperostosis. Disease entities are always best described by a name that reflects their cardinal features.

General Clinical Features

The etiology and pathogenesis of PAO are unclear. It has been well established that the pustular lesions on the palms and soles, like the destructive and proliferative skeletal lesions, are sterile in conventional microbiologic analysis. As in the classic seronegative spondyloarthropathies, however, the pathogenesis may involve a faulty or atypical immune response to viral or bacterial antigens. An HLA-B27 association has been found in several cases of PAO, but more precise data are not yet available.

PPP probably represents a special presentation or variant of psoriasis vulgaris. This manifestation may be at the extreme end of a spectrum that includes classic psoriasis and pustular psoriasis. In our own series of almost 60 cases, we have found a definite association between "pure" PPP and a positive family history of classic psoriasis. As stated in Sect. 3.6.2, classic psoriasis is known to be associated with characteristic destructive and proliferative changes in the appendicular joints and spine, and it is reasonable to assume that PPP, as a special clinical presentation of psoriasis, would also have special bone and joint manifestations like those seen in PAO. It is interesting to note that while the axial skeletal changes in classic psoriasis mainly involve the sacroiliac joints, those in PAO involve their anatomic counterpart, the sternocostoclavicular joints. Also, the prevalence of skeletal involvement is approximately 10% in both classic psoriasis and PPP, supporting the assumption that PPP is a variant of psoriasis.

Most patients with PAO have a very long history of illness, suffering, and medical confusion and uncertainty.

An essential feature of PAO is *sternocostoclavicular hyperostosis*. About two-thirds of our patients with sternocostoclavicular hyperostosis were found to have either PPP (about 50%) *or* classic psoriasis, often with a pustular component. Since we must assume that, as in classic psoriasis, the initial skeletal changes may antedate palmoplantar lesions, it is likely that the true prevalence of PPP in patients with sternocostoclavicular hyperostosis is significantly higher. The earliest clinical signs of sternocostoclavicular hyperostosis are swelling and redness mainly localized to the manubrial region. This may gradually increase and spread to involve the clavicles and anterior rib segments (see Fig. 3.6.3 e). These changes are extremely painful and restrict movements about the shoulder girdle, especially arm raising. In many patients we found that the severity of the pustular lesions of the hands and feet increased with the acuteness of the inflammatory changes in the sternocostoclavicular region.

Underlying the swelling and redness is a destructive inflammatory process involving the sternum, the medial ends of the clavicles, and ligament and tendon insertions, especially between the ribs and clavicles (see Fig. 3.6.3 f–i). Spread of this inflammatory process to the retrosternal region can exert pressure and cause impaired venous return with secondary venous thrombosis (thoracic inlet syndrome). Meanwhile, progressive reactive-reparative and ankylosing ossification can increasingly restrict the mobility of the joints between the manubrium and clavicles, and nonspecific spondylitic processes in one or more vertebral bodies can lead to back pain. Localized pain can also occur over large tubular bones as well as flat bones (e.g., scapula, pelvis) as a result of destructive and proliferative bone changes (see Fig. 3.6.3 n–r). Patients generally experience a moderate degree of malaise, and the ESR may be elevated.

The association of skeletal changes with HLA-B27 is difficult to evaluate at present but may be a factor in up to 50–60% of cases.

The therapeutic options in PAO have not been clearly defined. Nonsteroidal anti-inflammatory drugs are of limited benefit. The authors have achieved significant clinical and radiographic improvement in 12 patients treated with cyclosporine, but we do not yet have any long-term results to report.

Dermatology

Palmoplantar pustulosis (PPP) is a chronic disease of the palms of the hands and soles of the feet characterized by recurring eruptions of sterile pustules on initially normal skin. It predom-

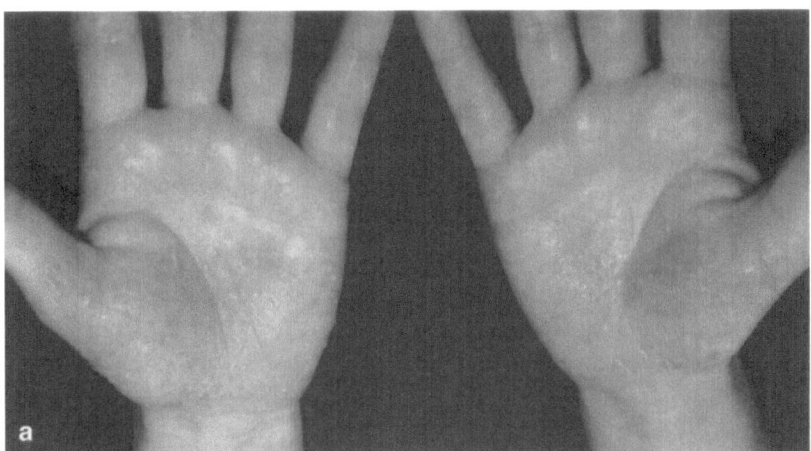

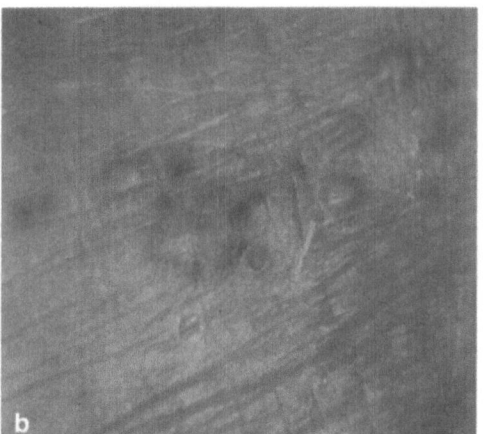

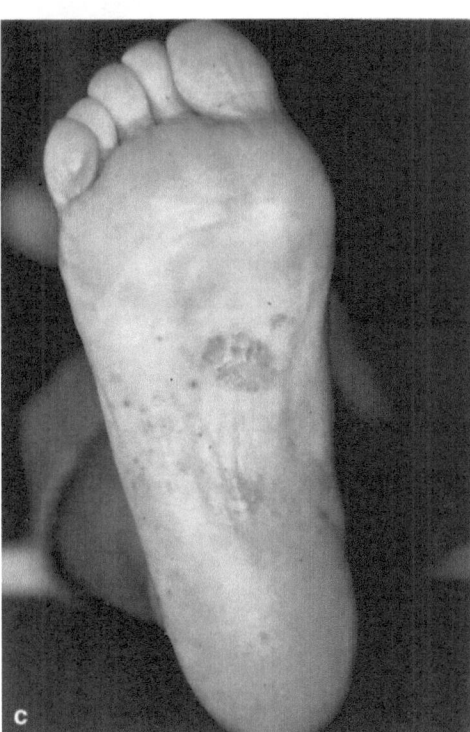

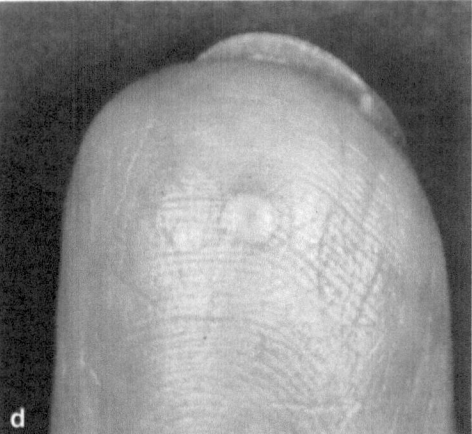

Fig. 3.6.3 a–u. Spectrum of dermatologic and radiologic findings in PAO. **a–d** Typical manifestations of PPP. The small pustules on the hands (**a**) are clustered mainly around the thenar and hypothenar eminences. The close-up in **b** illustrates the polymorphism of PPP, with florid pustules occurring next to dried, hemorrhagic lesions encrusted with a brown scale. Note the mild inflammatory erythema of the surrounding skin. **e–u** see pp. 104, 106–109

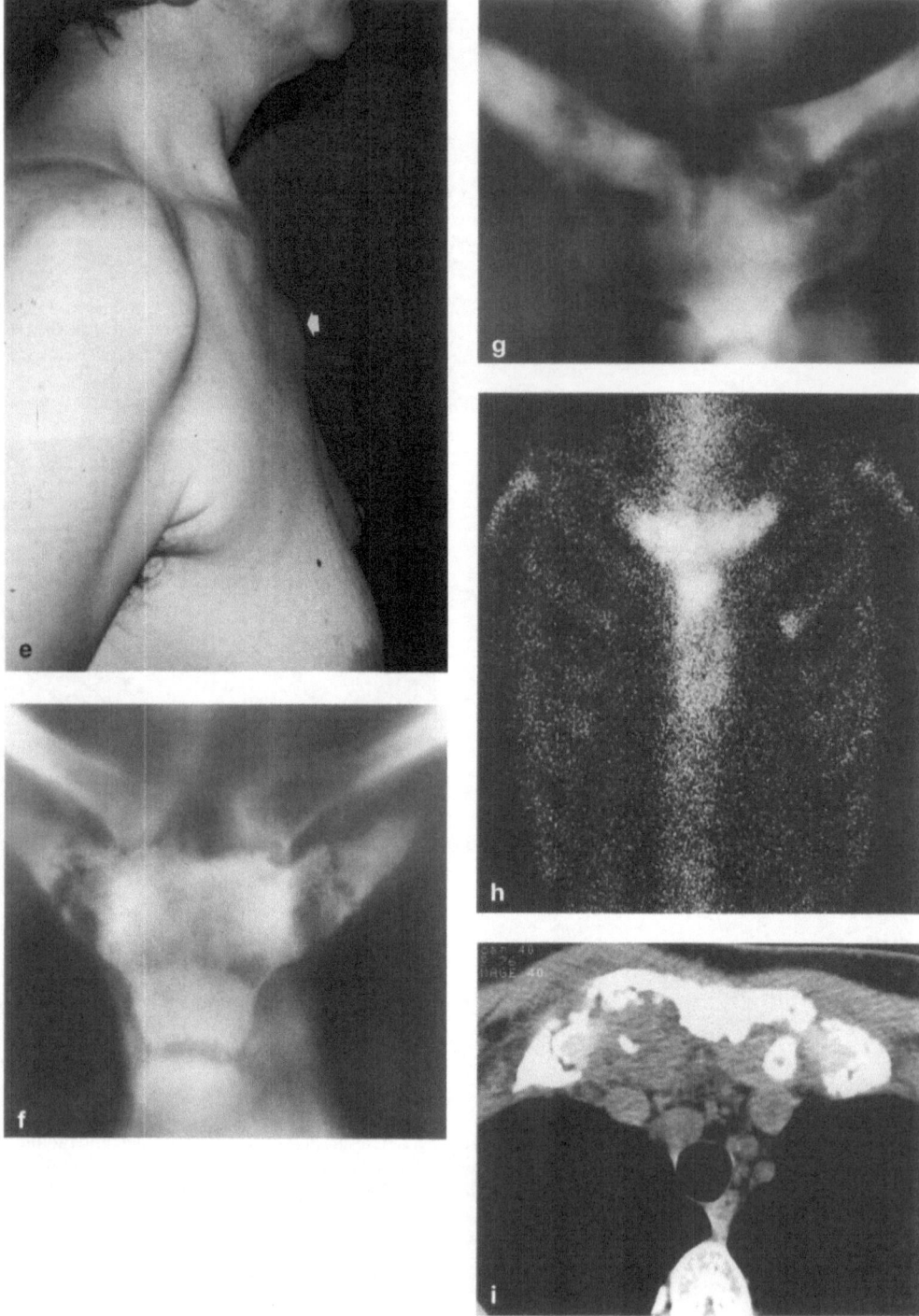

inantly affects the central areas of the palms and soles (Fig. 3.6.3 a, c). The lesions consist of pin-head- to rice-grain-size pustules (Fig. 3.6.3 b, d) that dry up and desquamate, leaving a heterogeneous pattern of dried yellowish pustules and small, brown, scaly crusts (Fig. 3.6.3 c). Only a mild inflammatory reaction is seen around fresh pustules, and later the skin shows only *slight* erythematous inflammatory change. Moderate pruritus occurs. As noted earlier, the correct diagnostic classification of PPP is the key to recognizing PAO, so it is essential to differentiate the pustular lesions from *dyshidrosis, dyshidrotic eczema*, and *dyshidrotic tinea*.

Radiology

The spectrum of radiologic changes in PAO is extremely broad and often misleading. As a result, many patients go through a long odyssey before a correct diagnosis is made. Almost every case that we discovered had involved years of evaluation by various specialties (dermatology, radiology, orthopedics, rheumatology, general medicine, etc.) and costly diagnostic procedures (CT, MRI, incisional biopsies, etc.) that did not advance the diagnosis as long as the case was not approached from a synoptic, interdisciplinary perspective. Initially we, too, had serious diagnostic difficulties, even in differentiating PAO from malignant tumors, until we learned to con-

sider that entity in the face of certain radiographic and scintigraphic changes and began conducting a thorough search for cutaneous lesions, especially on the hands and feet. Conversely, we learned to inquire about "rheumatic" complaints in patients who were seeking medical attention for PPP.

We believe that the *radionuclide bone scan* is a highly specific study in the diagnosis of PAO. If there is involvement of the sternocostoclavicular joints, as there is in most of our patients, the bone scan will show a characteristic *bullhead pattern* of intense radionuclide uptake in that region (Fig. 3.6.3 h, k, p, s). If additional areas of intense uptake are seen in a thoracic or lumbar vertebral body or in multiple segments (Fig. 3.6.3 k) and the cutaneous findings are confirmed, the diagnosis of PAO may be considered established and there is no need for further studies other than simple X-ray views. In patients who present initially with paraosseous new bone formation on the femur (Fig. 3.6.3 q) or tibia, for example, or with mixed destructive and sclerotic changes in the scapula or other bones (Fig. 3.6.3 r), PAO should be diagnosed if the bone scan shows increased uptake at those sites along with a bullhead pattern of sternocostoclavicular uptake, and the patient has coexisting cutaneous lesions or a positive family history. Above all, there is no need for "bloody" diagnostic procedures in cases of this kind (Dihlmann 1993).

The radiographic features of *sternocostoclavicular hyperostosis* consist of destructive changes in the manubrium and medial clavicular segments combined with reactive-reparative zones of sclerosis (Fig. 3.6.3 f, g, i). These sclerotic zones spread to involve the clavicles and upper anterior rib segments. Meanwhile, ossification of the interosseous ligaments (e.g., the costoclavicular ligaments) creates a platelike effect over those areas (Fig. 3.6.3 f). Periosteal new bone formation may lead to a marked enlargement of the medial ends of the clavicles. It is also common to find inflammatory destruction of the synchondrosis between the manubrium and body of the sternum, with joint space widening (Fig. 3.6.3 f, g). CT scans in acute stages generally show a soft-tissue mass developing behind the manubrium (Fig. 3.6.3 i).

If the disease involves a *vertebral body* or two or more vertebral segments including the disk

◁ **Fig.3.6.3** (*continued*). **e** Lateral view of sternocostoclavicular hyperostosis with marked swelling and redness (and local warmth) over the manubrium sterni. **f–i** Examples of sternocostoclavicular hyperostosis. In **f** note the pronounced sclerotic areas in the manubrium and manubriocostal synchondrosis. Note also the destructive changes with incipient sclerosis about the synchondrosis between the manubrium and body of the sternum. The radiograph in **g** shows coarse destructive changes in the manubrioclavicular joints with dislocation and marked clavicular sclerosis. Later the clavicles may undergo a clublike expansion. Bony ankylosis has commenced between the eroded ends of the manubrium and clavicles. Platelike areas of sclerosis have formed between the manubrium and the first ribs, and again there is destruction of the synchondrosis between the sternal body and manubrium. The bone scan in **h** shows the typical bullhead pattern of radiotracer uptake in the sternocostoclavicular region. Increased uptake is also seen in the anterior part of the third left rib. **i** CT scan through the sternocostoclavicular region defines the soft-tissue structures anterior and posterior to the manubrium and manubrioclavicular joints. **j–u** see pp. 106–109

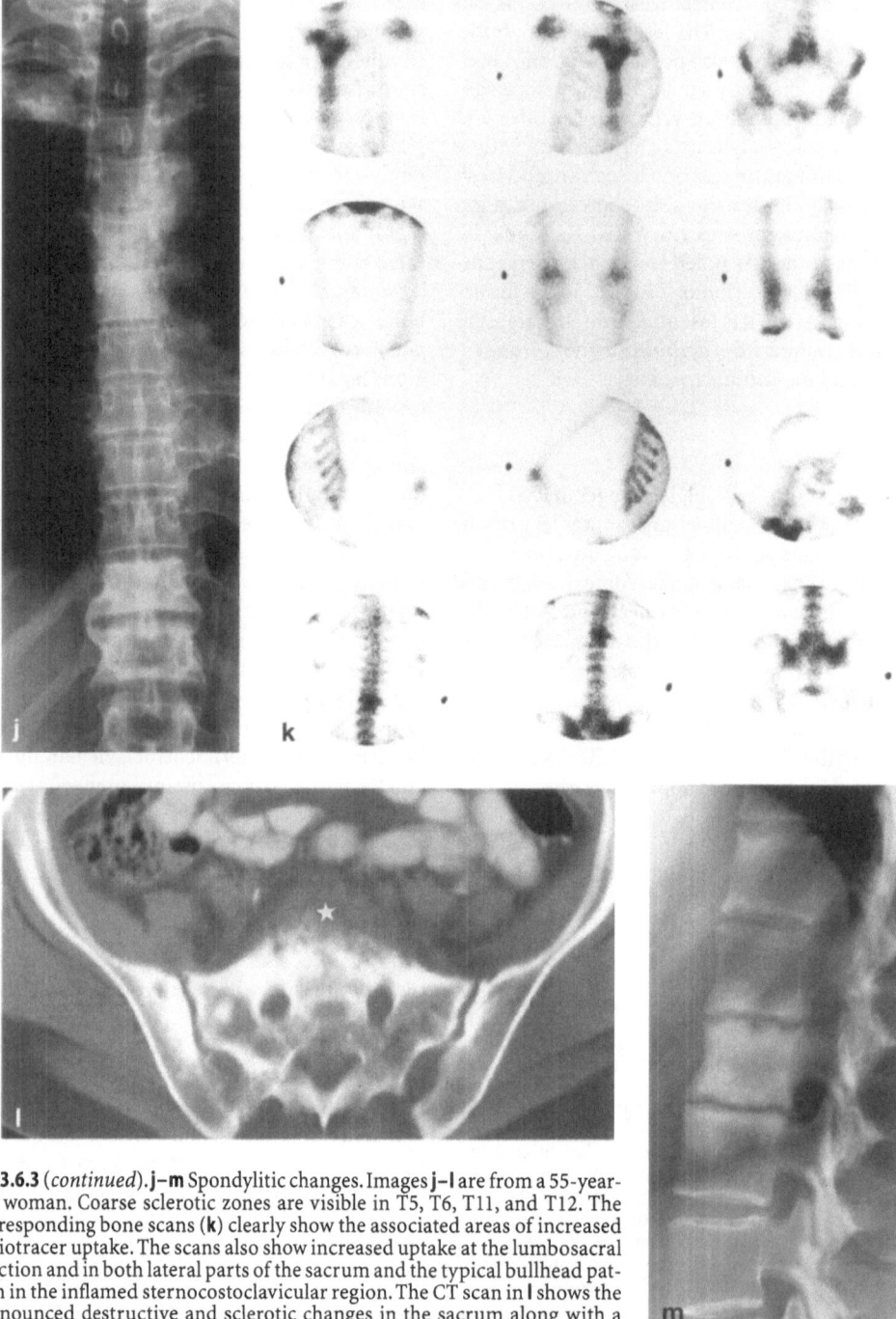

Fig.3.6.3 (*continued*). **j–m** Spondylitic changes. Images **j–l** are from a 55-year-old woman. Coarse sclerotic zones are visible in T5, T6, T11, and T12. The corresponding bone scans (**k**) clearly show the associated areas of increased radiotracer uptake. The scans also show increased uptake at the lumbosacral junction and in both lateral parts of the sacrum and the typical bullhead pattern in the inflamed sternocostoclavicular region. The CT scan in **l** shows the pronounced destructive and sclerotic changes in the sacrum along with a prominent anterior, tumor-simulating soft-tissue mass (*star*) as in retroperitoneal fibrosis (Pseudo-Ormond's disease). It is common to find syndesmophytes bridging between the sclerosed vertebral bodies (in **j**, between T11 and T12 and at the inferior margins of T12). In **m** note the destruction of the end plate of the vertebral body showing the most severe sclerotic changes. Incipient sclerosis is also visible in the second vertebral body from the top. **n–u** see pp. 107–109

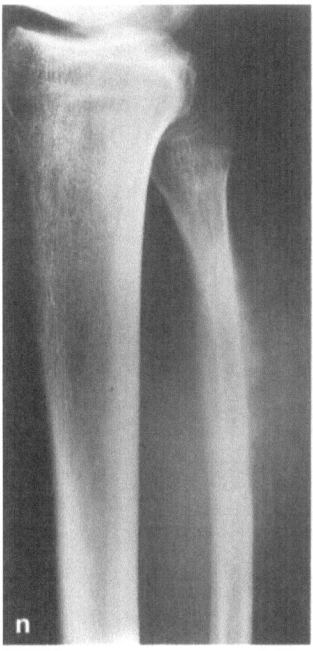
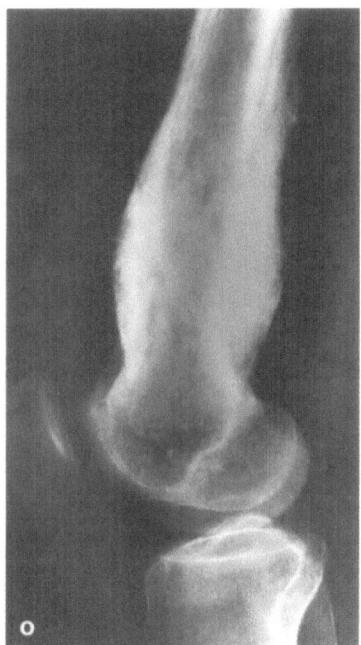

Fig. 3.6.3 (*continued*). **n, o** Examples of destructive and proliferative changes in the tubular bones. The young man in **n** presented initially with a coarse, spiculated area of periosteal ossification on the distal contralateral fibula that was interpreted as a periosteal osteosarcoma. Biopsy showed only a nonspecific inflammation. The lower third of the contralateral fibula was later resected because of severe pain, but new periosteal reactions soon appeared on the ipsilateral tibia and contralateral fibula (**n**), also associated with severe pain. Radionuclide imaging showed marked abnormal tracer concentration in the sternocostoclavicular region. The young woman in **o** presented with coarse proliferative changes on the distal femur, mimicking an osteosarcoma but accompanied by symmetric changes on the opposite side. There were severe concomitant sclerotic changes in several vertebral bodies (not shown). The patient had a long history of hospitalizations and outpatient visits, and previous physicians had suggested various possibilities including multicentric osteosarcoma. The affected areas were quite painful, and the patient had recurring outbreaks of palmoplantar pustulosis that seemed to coincide with the more severe episodes of skeletal pain. Some time passed before the patient developed sternocostoclavicular hyperostosis, leading us first to consider an association between the PPP and chronic recurring multifocal osteomyelitis. **p–u** see pp. 108, 109

space, radiographs will usually show *sclerotic changes* that may be accompanied by syndesmophyte- or mixed-osteophyte-type outgrowths (Fig. 3.6.3 j, m, t, u). These bony outgrowths prove the relationship of PAO to ankylosing spondylitis and justify its inclusion in the group of seronegative spondyloarthropathies (Fig. 3.6.3 t). Viewed in isolation, the sclerotic changes in the vertebral bodies and the destructive changes in the intervertebral disk space are indistinguishable from a primary subacute to chronic bacterial spondylitis or spondylodiscitis. This accounts for the many unnecessary biopsies and other "bloody" procedures that are performed when physicians fail to recognize the systemic nature of the changes prior to surgery.

Some patients additionally show the classic signs of a "variegated" sacroiliitis, which may be asymmetric.

Involvement of the extra-axial skeleton is manifested chiefly by *periosteal proliferative changes* (Fig. 3.6.3 n–q), usually accompanied by slight atrophy of the underlying cortex. In one patient we observed extensive sclerotic changes and circumscribed areas of destruction involving the scapula (Fig. 3.6.3 r, s). The proliferative processes on the outer surface of the bone are sometimes indistinguishable from juxtacortical osteosarcoma, especially if other features of the disease are ignored or if the patient presents only with that manifestation. In the latter case, there is no alternative to incisional biopsy. It is not unusual in

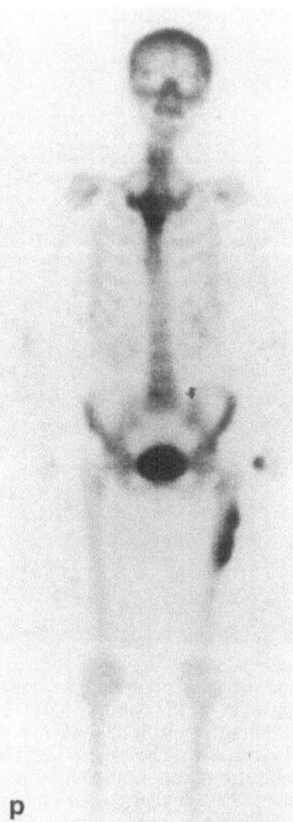

p

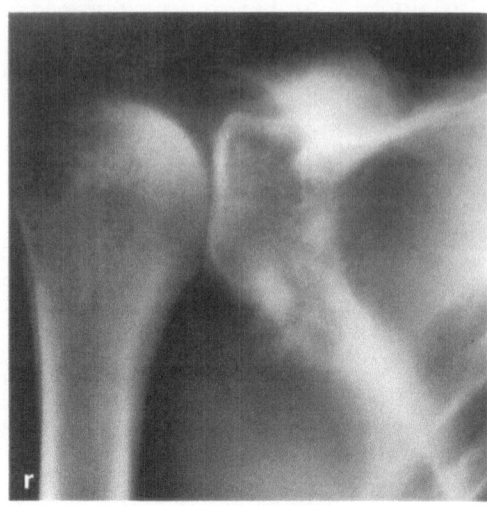

r

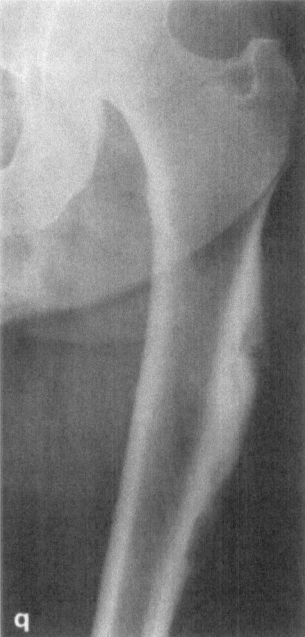

q

Fig. 3.6.3 (*continued*). The images in **p** and **q** show a solid hyperostotic lesion on the lateral aspect of the proximal femur in a 70-year-old woman, simulating a juxtacortical osteosarcoma. The patient also had pronounced sternocostoclavicular hyperostosis with a bullhead pattern of radionuclide uptake and incipient spondylitis in the first sacral segment. **r, s** Man 40 years of age with severe pain in the right scapula. The destructive changes in the lower scapula shown in the tomogram (**r**), combined with sites of bony proliferation (spiculations), first led us to suspect an osteosarcoma at an atypical site, but biopsy revealed a nonspecific osteitis. Subsequent bone scans (**s**) plus visual inspection of the hands and feet yielded the correct diagnosis of PAO. Note the typical bullhead pattern of intense radiotracer uptake in the sternocostoclavicular region, correlating with clinical and radiographic changes. Increased uptake is also seen in L5 and S1 and in both lateral parts of the sacrum, where radiographs showed marked sclerotic changes. **t, u** This 45-year-old man presented with destruction and paraosseous new bone involving the left femur and resembling a juxtacortical osteosarcoma or a sclerosing metastasis from bronchogenic carcinoma. A pathologist inexperienced in osteology interpreted the first biopsy as juxtacortical osteosarcoma, but a second, more extensive biopsy indicated a nonspecific inflammation consistent with calcifying tendinitis. Only then were bone scans ordered, demonstrating the classic features of sternocostoclavicular hyperostosis with sites of intense tracer uptake at the C4–C6 level. The radiograph at that level (**t**, *left side*) shows extensive sclerosis and a syndesmophyte on the anterosuperior corner of C6. CT scan (**u**) shows a conspicuous prevertebral soft-tissue mass (*asterisks*) consistent with a nonspecific tissue inflammation. Compare this soft-tissue mass with that in Fig. 3.6.3 l. Thirteen years later (**t**, *right side*) there is complete ossification of the anterior longitudinal ligament and ankylosis of intervertebral joints between C2–C4; a complete picture of Bechterew's disease!

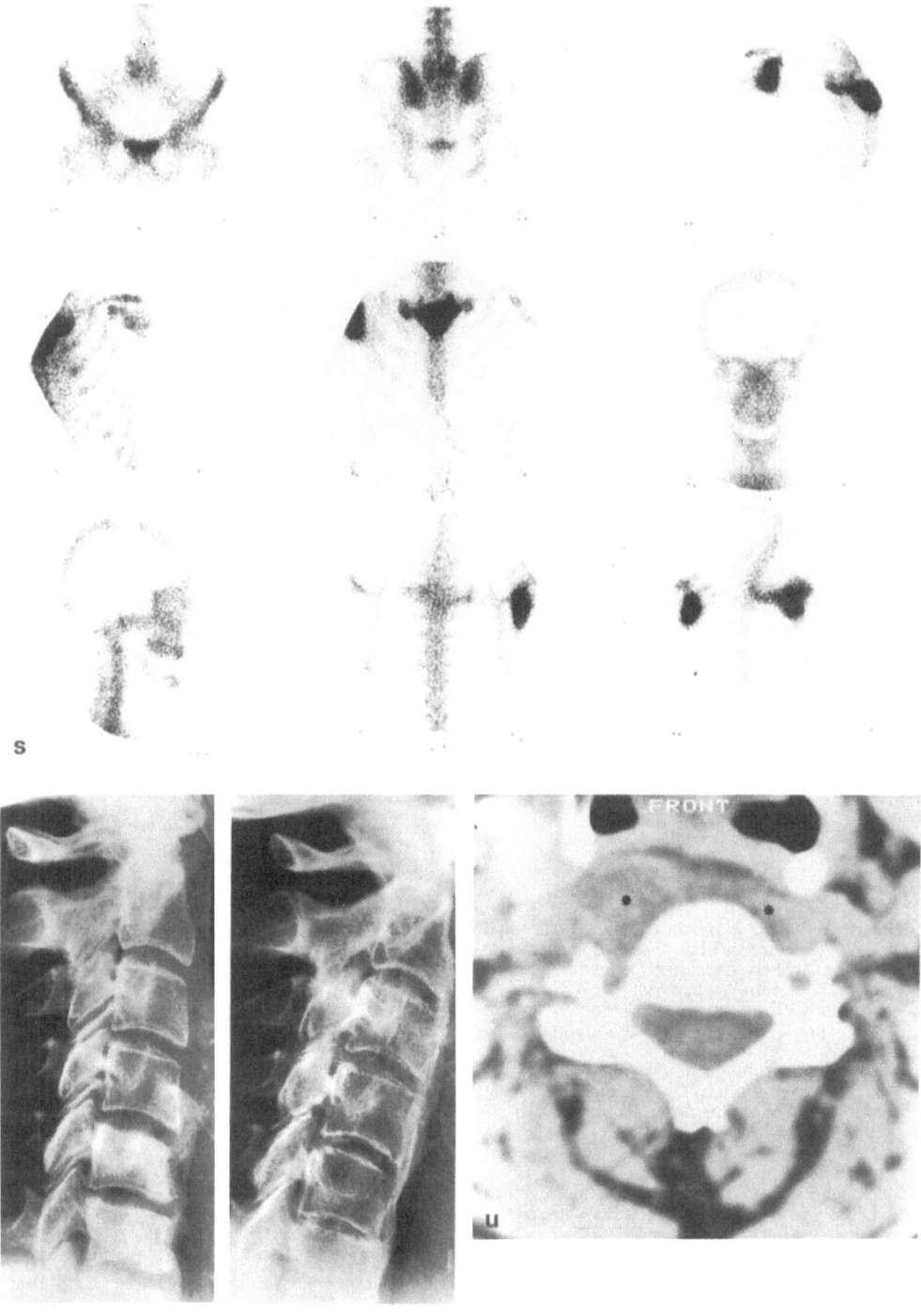

PAO to find sites of inflammatory destruction at the bony insertions of ligaments or tendons (e.g., gluteus maximus, adductor insertions on the femoral linea aspera), and subsequent ossification at these sites may prompt a diagnosis of *calcifying tendinitis*. This process is correctly classified as an enthesopathy, i.e., one feature (and occasionally the only feature) of a seronegative spondyloarthropathy.

Reports published to date indicate that the *skeletal changes in chronic acne* are similar to those in PAO. These changes should be distinguished, however, from the skeletal changes that tend to occur in patients with acne fulminans or acne conglobata (see p. 127).

In our own case material, we have been unable to find arthritic involvement of the upper and lower extremities in patients with chronic acne, although this has definitely been described in cases of acne fulminans.

In adolescents with palmoplantar pustulosis, we have observed three cases of *chronic recurring multifocal osteomyelitis*. The association between chronic recurring multifocal osteomyelitis and palmoplantar pustulosis is well known. Radiographs show destructive and proliferative changes predominantly involving the metaphyses and diaphyses of the large tubular bones. These lesions may appear and recur concomitantly or sequentially.

References

Dihlmann W (1993) Akquiriertes Hyperostose-Syndrom (sogenannte pustulöse Arthroosteitis). Literaturübersicht einschließlich 73 eigener Beobachtungen. Wien Klin Wochenschr 105: 127

Ellis BJ, Shier CRK, Leisen JJC et al. (1987) Acne-associated spondyloarthropathy: Radiographic features. Radiology 167: 541

Freyschmidt J, Sternberg A (1998) The bullhead sign – scintigraphic pattern of sternocostoclavicular hyperostosis and pustulotic arthro-osteitis. Eur Radiol 8: 807

Kahn MF, Chamot AM (1992) SAPHO syndrome. Rheum Dis Clin North Am 18: 225

Kasperczyk A, Freyschmidt J (1993) Pustulotic arthro-osteitis: Spectrum of bone lesions with palmoplantar pustulosis. Radiology 191: 207

Kasperczyk A, Freyschmidt J, Ostertag H (1990) Tumorsimulierende Knochenläsionen bei sternokostoklavikulärer Hyperostose und Pustulosis palmoplantaris. Röfo 152: 10

Schilling F (1986) Spondarthritis hyperostotica pustulo-psoriatica. In: Schilling F (Hrsg) Arthritis und Spondylitis psoriatica. Steinkopff, Darmstadt, S 289–296

Sonozaki H, Mitsui H, Miyanaga Y et al. (1981) Clinical features of 53 cases with pustulotic arthroosteitis. Ann Rheum Dis 40: 547

3.6.4 Reiter's Syndrome and Other Forms of Reactive Arthritis

Erythema nodosum; conjunctivitis, iridocyclitis; psoriasiform rash (scalp, umbilicus); lesions of oropharyngeal mucosa; nonspecific urethritis, erosive circinate balanitis.

Clinical features: mono- or oligoarticular arthritis of the lower extremity, Achilles bursitis.

Roentgen signs: mixed proliferative and destructive fibro-osteitis; erosive and nonerosive arthritis with asymmetric involvement of the lower extremity; "variegated" sacroiliitis, parasyndesmophytes.

Radiologic workup: symptomatic joints, sacroiliac joints and lumbar spine (same as in ankylosing spondylitis). If necessary, radionuclide bone scans may be added to the basic workup.

Definition

Reactive arthritis (ReA) is a postinfectious disease that follows within about 1–2 months of a bacterially induced urogenital or gastrointestinal infection. It occurs distant to the primary focus of infection and is associated with an acute or subacute, often self-limiting mono- or oligoarticular arthritis (asymmetric, most commonly affecting the lower extremity) and an often transient sacroiliitis. Reiter's syndrome is defined as a combination of more severe sacroiliitis with additional changes in the axial skeleton, inflammatory mucocutaneous lesions, and conjunctivitis.

General Clinical Features

While it was once believed that an infectious agent could not be isolated from affected joints and that this was characteristic of reactive arthritis in general, today the use of more sophisticated methods (e.g., polymerase chain reaction, PCR) can detect minute surface structures from bacteria such as *Campylobacter, Salmonella, Shigella,* and *Yersinia* (in post-enteritis cases) as well as *Chlamydia, Gonococci,* and *Ureaplasma* (in post-urethritis cases). It is assumed that the bacterial fragments enter the synovium by way of circulating immune complexes (e.g., *Yersinia* cell fragments as an antigen).

"Many organisms can trigger one syndrome, and *one organism can trigger many syndromes"* is a rule that applies to the various forms of reactive arthritis.

It is known that chlamydia can trigger reactive arthritis including classic Reiter's syndrome, enteropathic spondylarthritis, and uveitis. The genetic susceptibility to reactive arthritis linked to the presence of HLA-B27 was mentioned in the introductory chapter.

Reactive arthritis develops in an estimated 3% of patients with the urogenital and enteric bacterial infections noted above. An incidence of 30% has been estimated in patients with *Yersinia* enterocolitis.

Several important forms of reactive arthritis are discussed below in greater detail.

Posturethritic Reactive Arthritis and *Chlamydia*-Induced Arthritis

Arthritis develops in 1–4% of all patients with nongonorrheal urethritis, and 50% of these cases are triggered by *Chlamydia trachomatis.* A full one-third of patients may develop the full presentation of Reiter's syndrome (see below), which predominantly affects young men. The arthritis begins 2–4 weeks after the urogenital infection and lasts about 4 months. In about two-thirds of patients the arthritis recurs, but long-standing cases are uncommon. Hence it is very rare to find radiographic evidence of erosive inflammatory joint changes.

Yersinia-Induced Arthritis

The causative organism of this most common postenteritic arthritis is *Yersinia enterocolitica*. As mentioned, reactive arthritis is estimated to occur in up to 30% of patients with *Yersinia* enterocolitis. The arthritis takes an acute or subacute course, may be oligo- or polyarticular, most commonly involves the knees and ankles, and tends to resolve spontaneously without residual damage. Patients may develop *erythema nodosum*. Sacroiliitis is not uncommon in patients with HLA-B27 and may progress to Reiter's syndrome or eventual ankylosing spondylitis.

Salmonella-Induced Arthritis

Reactive arthritis develops in approximately 1–2% of patients with *Salmonella* enteritis. This arthritis occurs 2–4 weeks after the infectious episode (nonspecific gastroenteritis, enterocolitis, or even typhus), shows an oligoarticular distribution, and most commonly affects the lower extremity. Patients positive for HLA-B27 may develop Reiter's syndrome or ankylosing spondylitis.

Shigella-Induced Arthritis

An oligoarthritis, usually of the lower extremity, may occur 1–4 weeks after a *Shigella* infection, especially with *Shigella dysenteriae*. The incidence of this reactive arthritis is approximately 1.5%. Usually the joint changes resolve completely. *Shigella* enteritis is believed to be a relatively common trigger of Reiter's syndrome.

Campylobacter-Induced Arthritis

Campylobacter has increasingly been implicated as a causative organism of human gastrointestinal infections in recent years. Reactive arthritis develops in approximately 1–10% of patients with *Campylobacter* enteritis and may progress to a complete Reiter's syndrome.

Reiter's Syndrome

Reiter's syndrome affects men nine times more often than women. The peak age of onset is between 20 and 30 years. About 1.5% of postvenereal and postenteritic infections lead to Reiter's syndrome.

HLA-B27 is positive in 90–100% of cases. Patients give a history of gonorrheal or nongonorrheal urethritis or a gastrointestinal infection (e.g., *Shigella dysenteria, Salmonellae, Yersinia* infections, etc.). The disease usually begins acutely with arthralgia, joint swelling, and effusion. Usually there is asymmetric involvement of the knees and ankles, but various patterns of involvement may occur.

Heel pain and swelling due to fibro-osteitis, periostitis, or Achilles bursitis may be present as an early manifestation. The acute phase, which may be febrile, is commonly associated with marked conjunctivitis and/or iridocyclitis and nonspecific urethritis. In some cases this classic *Reiter triad* of arthritis, urethritis, and conjunctivitis may extend over a prolonged period in a dissipated form.

Sometimes urethritis and conjunctivitis are so mild that they are unnoticed by the patient and physician. The mucocutaneous lesions (see below) may consist of erythema nodosum, a psoriasiform rash, aphthous mouth ulcers, or circinate balanitis. The coexistence of cutaneous lesions with the classic triad is known as *Reiter's tetrad*.

In about 50% of cases, the foregoing symptoms last a minimum of 3–6 weeks and no more than 6 months. In other cases the disease enters a chronic stage whose dominant feature are joint symptoms with increasing polyarticular involvement of the feet, chronic sacroiliitis and spondylitis.

The prevalence of Reiter's syndrome is increased by a factor of 144 in the HIV-infected and AIDS population (Salomon et al. 1988).

Dermatology

All forms of reactive arthritis mentioned so far may be associated with erythema nodosum.

Erythema nodosum is a morphologic term denoting an acute, symmetric, nodular, erythematous (polychological) hypersensitivity reaction of the skin. Accompanied by general malaise and fever, it is marked by the bilateral appearance of firm, exquisitely tender, livid red cutaneous or subcutaneous nodules primarily on the anterior aspect of the lower legs including the knees, ankles, and shins (Fig. 3.6.4 a); involvement of the forearms and buttocks can also occur. As the lesions age, they progress – by hemoglobin destruction – from a livid red to greenish-yellow color, finally fading to a postinflammatory hyperpigmentation. Liquefaction or ulceration does *not* occur. The lesions require differentiation from erythema induratum (Bazin's disease), which involves the calves and is prone to liquefaction. Differentiation is also required from panniculitis, nodular vasculitis, and cutaneous periarteritis nodosa, all of which take a chronic course.

The specific dermatologic manifestations of Reiter's syndrome are as follows:

Ocular involvement may consist of an iridocyclitis and/or conjunctivitis (see Fig. 3.6.4 b).

Psoriasiform eruptions primarily involve the palms and soles of the hands and feet, the scalp, and the umbilical region (Fig. 3.6.4 c), but erythemosquamous skin changes ranging from coin-sized lesions to extensive areas of involvement may occur anywhere on the body. The callus-like lesions of keratoderma blennorrhagicum appear in about 10% of patients. The distal phalanges of the fingers and toes are commonly involved, and the region around the nails (paronychium) often shows dystrophic changes or complete nail loss. These dermatologic findings have the same clinical and histologic features as exudative psoriasis vulgaris or pustular psoriasis.

Lesions of the *oral and pharyngeal mucosae* consist of diffuse redness, erythematous macules, papules, erosions, and hemorrhages.

Erosive circinate balanitis is manifested initially by grayish-white macules on the glans penis that later progress to rounded, red, weeping lesions. These lesions enlarge and form maplike areas of bizarre shapes on the glans and the inner layer of the prepuce (Fig. 3.6.4 d).

Radiology

Reactive arthritis usually has an asymmetric distribution involving large and small joints of the lower extremity. Because the arthritis resolves in a matter of weeks, it generally does not produce characteristic radiographic changes. But Reiter's syndrome is different, with 50% of cases entering a chronic stage that displays characteristic radiographic features. These include a "variegated" sacroiliitis (see p. 88) and the coexistence of destructive and proliferative bone changes in the affected joints, usually involving the lower extremity. The joint changes may be mono- or oligoarticular, less commonly polyarticular, and often are associated with a very marked periarticular osteoporosis with erosive and occasional destructive changes and with periosteal ossification on the meta- and diaphyseal portions of

Fig. 3.6.4 a–j. Reiter's syndrome. **a–d** Dermatologic manifestations: **a** typical lesions of erythema nodosum; **b** conjunctivitis in the right eye; **c** typical psoriasiform eruptions; **d** circinate balanitis. **e–j** see p. 114

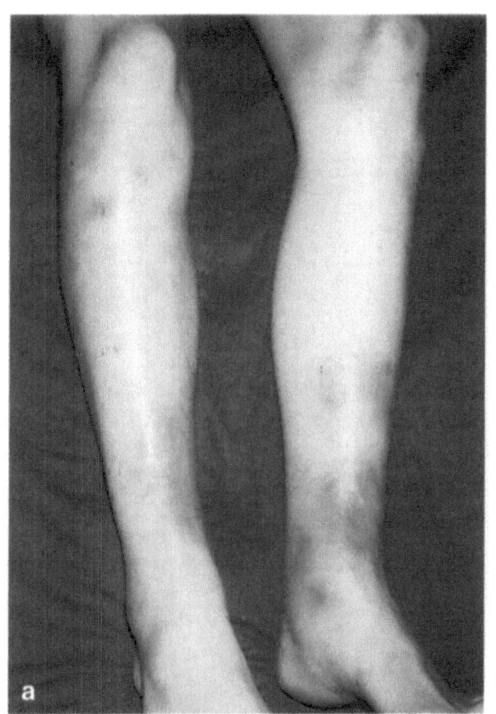

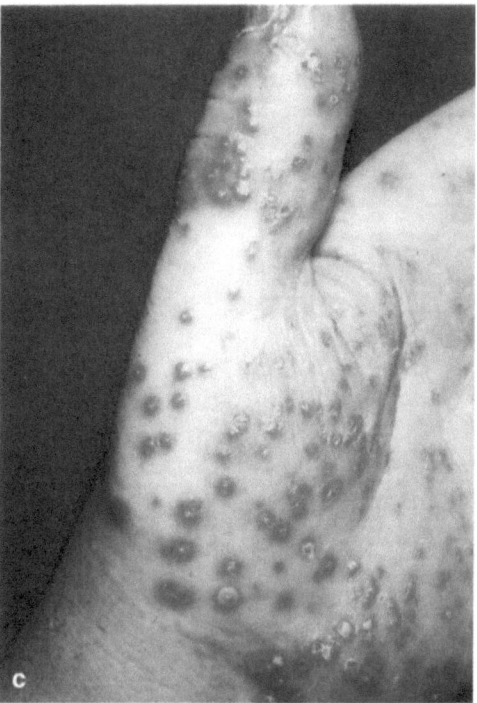

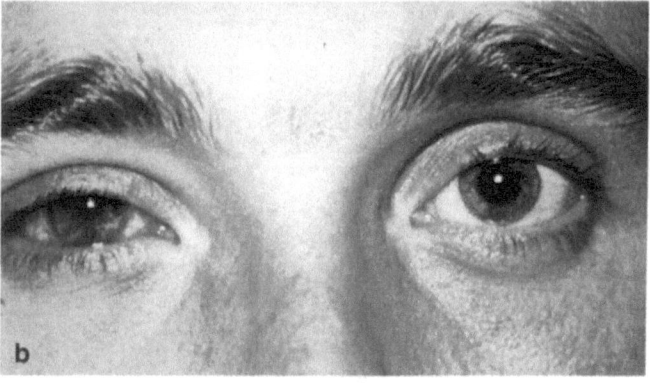

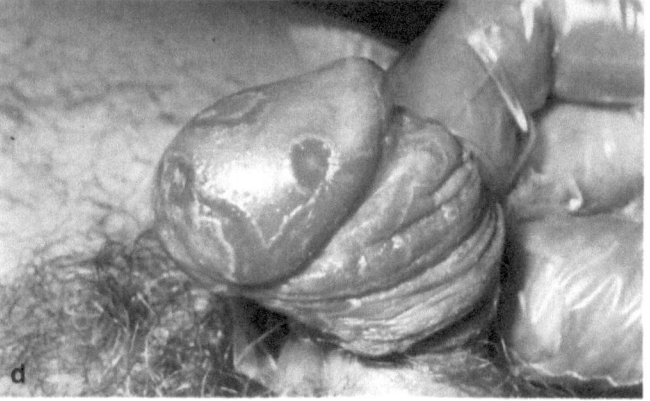

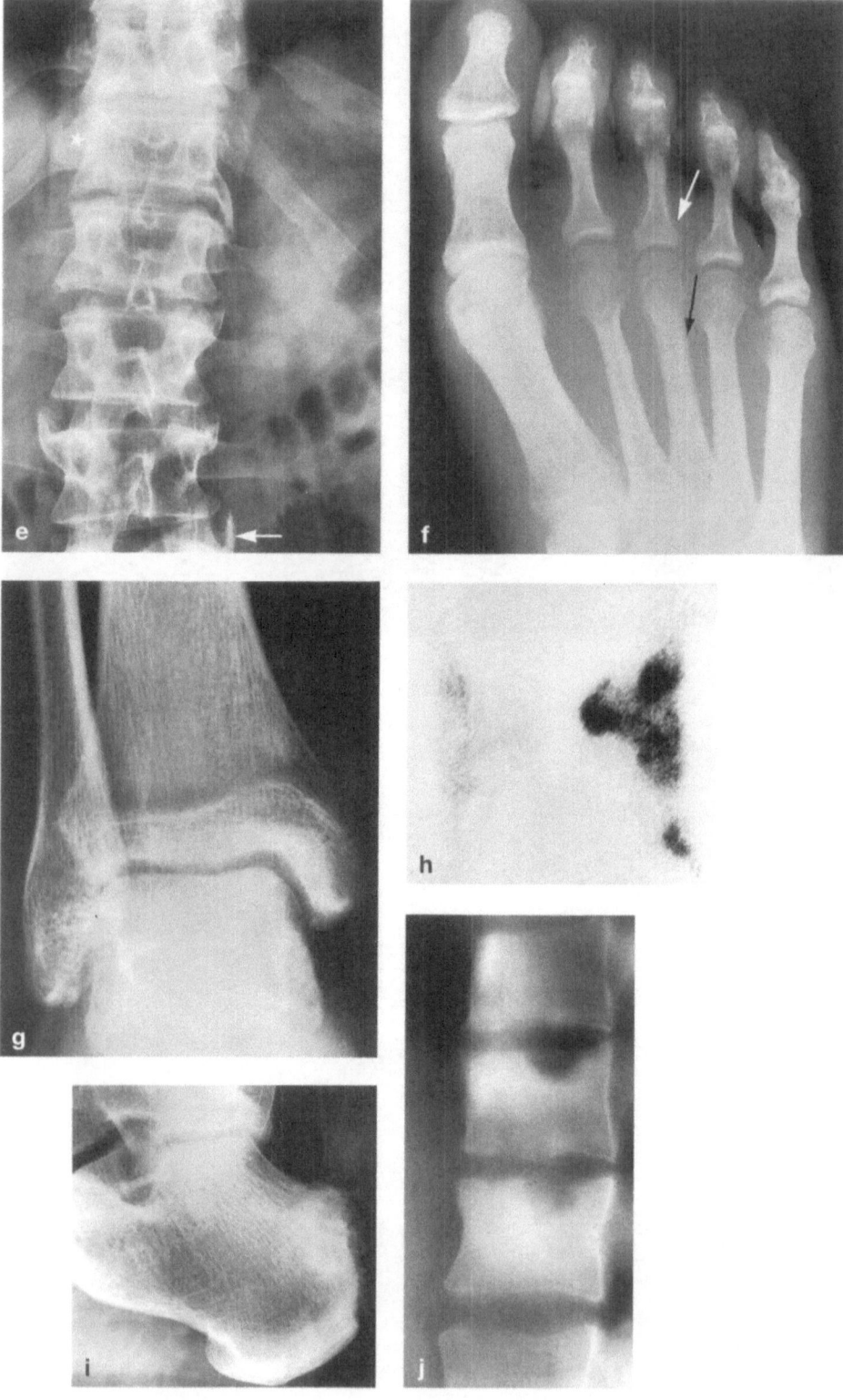

articulating tubular bones (Fig. 3.6.4 f, g). The latter changes tend to involve the feet rather than the hands, appear after the clinical onset of acute or subacute arthritis, and antedate periarticular decalcification. Chronic cases of Reiter's syndrome that progress for years or decades show increasing destruction, mutilation, and deformity similar to that seen in rheumatoid arthritis, except that Reiter's arthritis is also accompanied by sites of periosteal ossification. The rare *spinal involvement* is usually confined to the lower thoracic and upper lumbar region and consists of parasyndesmophyte formation as in psoriatic spondylarthritis (Fig. 3.6.4 e) and, less commonly, syndesmophyte formation as in ankylosing spondylitis. Rare cases may develop true ankylosis resembling Bechterew's disease. Involvement of the cervical spine (spondylarthritis with apophyseal joint ankylosis, anterior ossification near the disk spaces, anterior atlantoaxial subluxation) is seen in only about 3–4% of cases. *Spondylodiscitis* is also observed and may lead to relatively coarse destructive changes in the adjacent vertebral end plates with narrowing of the intervertebral spaces (Fig. 3.6.4 j).

Consistent with the clinical symptoms, radiographs show signs of *fibro-osteitis* principally involving the ischia, the greater and lesser trochanters, and the calcaneus. The latter shows typical erosive changes resulting from Achilles bursitis and/or periostitis (Fig. 3.6.4 i).

The main diseases to be considered in the *radiologic differential diagnosis* are psoriatic arthritis and psoriatic spondylarthritis. The primary differentiating criterion is the *distribution pattern*: while Reiter's arthritis mainly affects the joints of the lower extremity, psoriatic arthritis tends to involve the upper *and* lower extremities. Also, Reiter's syndrome has a special predilection for the interphalangeal joint of the big toe, whereas psoriatic arthritis involves other interphalangeal joints of the hands and feet with equal frequency and severity. Differentiation is also required from rheumatoid arthritis, especially seronegative cases. Reiter's syndrome is distinguished from rheumatoid arthritis by the sites of periosteal new bone formation that occur in Reiter's syndrome and by the typical bilateral symmetry of the joint changes, with involvement of the hands, that occurs in rheumatoid arthritis.

◁ **Fig. 3.6.4** (*continued*). **e–j** Examples of skeletal changes in Reiter's syndrome. **e** Typical parasyndesmophyte formation. Parasyndesmophytes are visible at lower left (*arrow*) and on the left side of T12, appearing as hornlike projections that arise from the vertebral body and extend up past the next higher vertebral body. The patient, a 38-year-old man, had about a 15-year history of Reiter's syndrome. The apophyseal joints of the cervical spine were completely ankylosed as a result of previous erosive-destructive inflammatory processes. Note the destructive changes in the right 12th costotransverse joint (*asterisk*). Images **f–h** are from a 22-year-old man who presented clinically with a recent history of urethritis and conjunctivitis and with gross swelling of the right foot and ankle. He also had low back pain referable to a "variegated" type of sacroiliitis. The swelling of the right foot correlated with a very severe erosive arthritis involving the ankle joint and all the metatarsophalangeal and interphalangeal joints. Note the pronounced demineralization about the ankle joint with subtle erosion of the medial malleolus and the extreme demineralization at the metatarsophalangeal joints. Layered periosteal reactions are clearly visible along the shafts of the third metatarsal and corresponding proximal phalanx (**f**, *arrows*). Massive radiotracer uptake in the foot and ankle region (**h**). The radiograph in **i** shows relatively coarse destructive changes with erosions of the posterior calcanean border and spicules of new bone formation. Note also the structural heterogeneity of the adjacent upper and central cancellous bone with areas of lucency and sclerosis. **j** Typical spondylodiscitis with coarse erosions of the vertebral end plates and very dense sclerosis of the cancellous bone, similar to the findings in PAO (see p. 106, Fig. 3.6.3 j, m)

References

Brancato L, Itescu S, Skovron ML et al. (1989) Aspects of the spectrum, prevalence and disease susceptibility determinants of Reiter's syndrome and related disorders associated with HIV infection. Rheumatol Int 9: 137

Martel W, Braunstein EM, Borloza G et al. (1979) Radiologic features of Reiter disease. Radiology 132: 1

Salomon G, Brancato LJ, Itescu S et al. (1988) Arthritis, psoriasis and related syndromes associated with HIV infection (Abstr). Arthritis Rheum 31 [Suppl. 4]: 12

3.6.5 Oligoarticular Juvenile Rheumatoid Arthritis (Type II)

This disease is also known as the "late type" of nonsystemic mono- or oligoarticular juvenile chronic arthritis. It affects males more than females, and patients are positive for HLA-B27. Children present clinically with sacroiliitis that later may progress to ankylosing spondylitis. The peak incidence is between 10 and 15 years of age. Usually the disease has an insidious onset, only occasionally marked by temperature elevation to about 38°C. Because the disease is essentially nonsystemic, extra-articular manifestations are not very common; lymphadenopathy occurs in about 36% of patients, leukocytosis in about one-third, and *iridocyclitis* in 11%. Stöber and Kölle (1984) list the following diagnostic criteria for nonsystemic juvenile rheumatoid arthritis:

Seronegative:
1. Polyarthritis occurring at onset or within 3 months of onset, and lasting or recurring over a 12-week period.
2. Monarthritis or oligoarthritis (affecting 1–4 joints) lasting or recurring over a 12-week period (watch for exclusions); "extended oligoarthritis."
3. Morning stiffness.
4. Typical radiographic changes.
5. Typical findings at synovial biopsy (especially with monarthritis or oligoarthritis!).
6. Rheumatic iridocyclitis or uveitis.
7. Subcutaneous rheumatoid nodules.
8. Family history of rheumatic disease.

References

Stöber E, Kölle G (1984) Juvenile chronische Arthritis. In: Mathies H (Hrsg) Handbuch der Inneren Medizin, Rheumatologie B. Spezieller Teil I. Springer, Berlin Heidelberg New York, S 265

3.6.6 Enterospondylarthritis (Crohn's Disease, Ulcerative Colitis, etc.)

Synonyms: enteropathic spondylarthritis, intestinal arthropathies, arthritis associated with inflammatory bowel disease

> Erythema nodosum, aphthous mouth ulcers, uveitis, pyoderma gangrenosum; occasional clubbing of the fingers and toes with watchglass nails.
> **Clinical and radiologic signs:** acute or subacute, usually erosive oligo- or polyarthritis predominantly affecting the lower extremities; "variegated" sacroiliitis; periosteal ossification in the hands and feet.

Definition

Enterospondylarthritis refers to a group of mono-, oligo- or polyarticular joint diseases, often associated with sacroiliitis, whose occurrence correlates with any of the following chronic bowel diseases:

– ulcerative colitis,
– Crohn's disease,
– Whipple's disease,
– celiac disease,
– previous intestinal bypass operation or surgical isolation of bowel loops,
– pseudomenbranous colitis following antibiotic therapy.

General Clinical Features

The etiology and pathogenesis of the intestinal arthropathies, especially those associated with *ulcerative colitis* and *Crohn's disease*, are not fully understood. It is very likely that patients have a genetic predisposition (HLA-B27, see Table 3.6.1, p. 88; familial incidence with other diseases of the seronegative spondyloarthropathy group) leading to faulty immune regulation and the spontaneous onset of an autoimmune type of disease. It is interesting to note that arthritis in the extremities may precede the onset of bowel disease in up to 50% of patients, while spondylarthritis with sacroiliitis may precede bowel disease in up to 75%.

Oligo- and polyarthritis predominantly involving the lower extremities may have an acute to subacute or even insidious onset but usually subside within 4 weeks. Only a small percentage of patients continue to have arthritis for longer than 1 year. Specific ocular and cutaneous manifestations are described below.

Arthritis rarely develops in ulcerative colitis patients who have undergone colectomy. But resection of inflamed small bowel segments or of the colon does not improve the arthritic changes in patients with Crohn's disease.

Intestinal lipodystrophy (Whipple's disease) is a rare disorder manifested clinically by abdominal pain, chronic diarrhea, grayish-brown pigmentation of the skin, lymph node enlargement, weight loss (due to malabsorption), anemia, fever, polyserositis, and oligo- or polyarticular arthritis. Males in the fourth to fifth decade of life are most commonly affected. The etiology of Whipple's disease is unclear, but the detection of rod-shaped bacterial structures in macrophages from the bowel wall and lymph nodes suggests a bacterial pathogen (e.g., *Corynebacterium specialis*). The resolution of the disease with antibiotic therapy further suggests a bacterial origin. The diagnosis is established by small-bowel or lymph-node biopsy demonstrating macrophages that contain PSA-positive material (glycoproteins) and perhaps demonstrating bacteria-like structures. Joint symptoms may predate diarrhea by a period of years and consist of a transient oligo- or polyarthritis similar to that occurring in Crohn's disease or ulcerative colitis.

Approximately 60% of patients with Whipple's disease develop frank joint inflammation (pain, warmth, effusion, etc.) predominantly affecting the knees and ankles. Arthralgia alone is probably a far more common manifestation. Progression to chronic arthritis is rare. About 5% of patients with Whipple's disease develop ankylosing spondylitis, and about 7% develop isolated sacroiliitis.

Arthritis following *intestinal bypass surgery* most commonly occurs after a jejunocolostomy or jejunoileostomy performed for the treatment of morbid obesity.

The pathogenesis of arthritis following intestinal bypass surgery certainly relates to the alteration of bacterial flora caused by isolating small bowel loops and creating a blind pouch. If the original anatomic situation is restored, the arthritis disappears. The prevalence of rheumatic conditions is approximately 30% after jejunocolostomy and 40% after jejunoileostomy. Arthritic symptoms may begin immediately after the surgery, or some years later. *The large and small joints of the upper extremity are most commonly affected.* Clinical episodes of joint pain, swelling, etc. last for 2–14 days and are separated by intervals of 2–12 weeks. The oligoarticular involvement of large joints usually takes a protracted course, although true erosive and destructive joint changes are rare. Patients generally are negative for HLA-B27, and effusions are sterile (in conventional microbiological tests).

Arthritis in the setting of an antibiotic-induced *pseudomembranous colitis* is rare. The joint symptoms subside following regression of the colitic symptoms.

Arthritic changes are also rare in patients with *untreated celiac disease*. They take the form of a seronegative arthritis predominantly involving the hips, knees, and shoulders. The arthritic symptoms are transient and are not accompanied by destructive changes. It is important to note that clinical joint symptoms may antedate bowel symptoms by years and that the joint symptoms subside after treatment with a gluten-free diet.

Dermatology

Erythema nodosum (see p. 112) may develop in all intestinal arthropathies but is particularly common in Crohn's disease and ulcerative colitis. Both diseases are very often associated with chronic recurring *aphthous mouth ulcers*, *uveitis*, and *pyoderma gangrenosum*. Cutaneous manifestations are most likely to occur in patients who develop arthritis.

1. *Chronic recurring aphthous mouth ulcers* are extremely painful, recurrent lesions involving the anterior third of the oral cavity and the tongue. Usually no more than two to four ulcers are present at any one time. Foci of immune-complex vasculitis have been postulated as the underlying lesion.
2. *Pyoderma gangrenosum* is a focal cutaneous gangrene, presumably based on a hyperergic reaction. Its pathogenesis has been related to

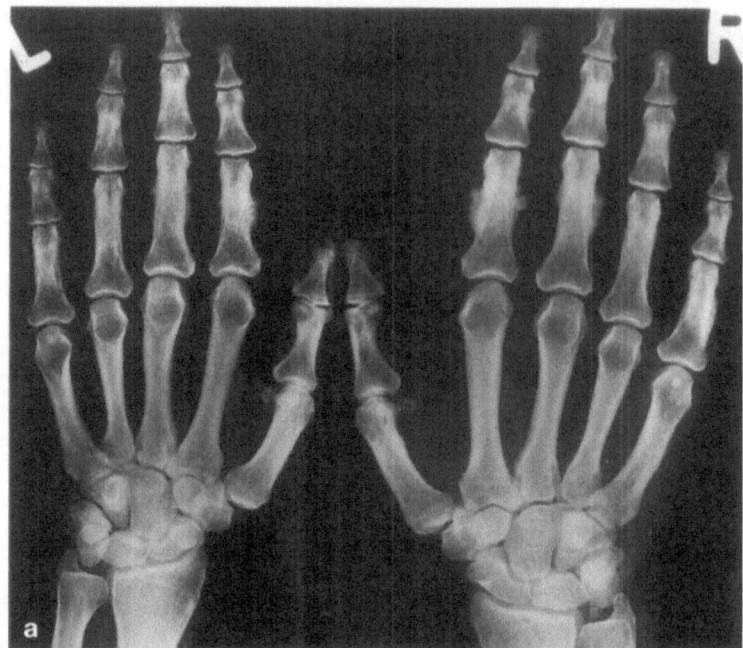

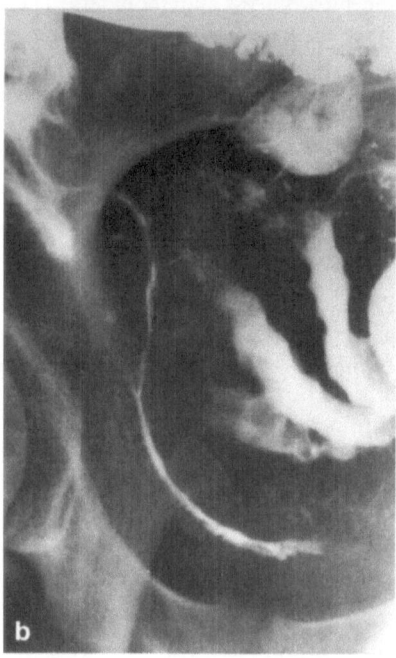

Fig.3.6.6a,b. Foci of periosteal ossification on the proximal and middle phalanges in Crohn's disease. The periosteal reaction shows an unusual brushlike pattern that is especially marked on the second and third proximal phalanges of each hand (**a**). When the film is viewed with magnification, finer sites of periosteal ossification are appreciated on the metacarpals. The patient presented clinically with watchglass nails and digital clubbing. These radiographs, obtained to investigate severe arthralgia in the hands and feet (where X-rays showed similar changes), prompted a search for pulmonary disease (see p. 185), but no evidence of such disease was found. But small bowel investigation revealed the classic features of advanced Crohn's disease (**b**) with severe narrowing of the terminal ileum and a cobblestone appearance of the more proximal loops. Fistulation from the bowel to other organs was also noted. The patient had no known history of Crohn's disease, although the radiographic findings are consistent with disease of long standing. As the inflammatory bowel changes responded to treatment, the periosteal ossifications also showed rapid and significant regression. Periosteal ossifications combined with clubbed fingers and watchglass nails constitute a form of hypertrophic osteoarthropathy (see p. 185)

a circumscribed necrotizing vasculitis. It should be noted that, despite its name, this condition is not a true "pyoderma." The single or multiple inflamed, reddish, pustular lesions most commonly occur on the lower extremities but may appear anywhere on the skin. They liquefy and coalesce to form extensive, spreading ulcerations. Typically the ulcers have a necrotic base surrounded by painful, dusky, undermined borders, some showing remnants of blister-like elevations of the epidermis.

Radiology

Because of its transient nature, the arthritis associated with Whipple's disease, intestinal bypass surgery, pseudomembranous colitis, or untreated celiac disease very rarely produces objective radiologic features of joint inflammation with erosion and destruction. By contrast, the typical chronic, recurring forms of Crohn's disease and ulcerative colitis are associated respectively with a 12% and 14% incidence of objective radiologic signs of inflammatory joint disease, which most commonly involves the small joints of the extremities. Both diseases also may be associated with *sacroiliitis* (about 10–18% of cases), especially in carriers of HLA-B27. Some 2–4% of cases may progress to the radiographic presentation of *ankylosing spondylitis* (see p. 89). A distinctive and not uncommon feature of Crohn's disease is the occurrence of *periosteal reactions* like those in hypertrophic osteoarthropathy (Marie-Bamberger disease). Patients present clinically with pain and swelling in the forearms, lower legs, metacarpals, and metatarsals; this may be accompanied by *clubbing of the fingers* and *watchglass nails* (see Fig. 7.3 a). Radiographs may show delicate layered, velvety, or occasional spiculated patterns of periosteal ossification about the metacarpal and metatarsal shafts (Fig. 3.6.6 a) and the shafts of the radius, ulna, tibia, and fibula. Radionuclide scans generally show a typical bandlike pattern of tracer uptake that encircles the affected cortex. A radiologist who encounters such changes in the absence of known bowel disease should first look for coexisting pulmonary disease (pleurisy, bronchiectasia, bronchial carcinoma). Only after eliminating these causes should the radiologist

proceed with a gastrointestinal examination to confirm Crohn's disease. We personally know of cases in which the periosteal ossifications and the joint symptoms, including sacroiliitis, clinically preceded the bowel disease (see Fig. 3.6.6 a), and a gastrointestinal contrast series had to be performed to establish the presence of ileocolitis (Fig. 3.6.6 b).

References

Freyschmidt J (1997) Skeletterkrankungen. Klinisch-radiologische Diagnose und Differentialdiagnose, 2. Aufl. Springer, Berlin Heidelberg New York

3.6.7 Undifferentiated Spondyloarthropathy

> Conjunctivitis, uveitis, keratoma blennor-
> rhagicum, circinate balanitis, onycholysis,
> chronic recurring mouth ulcers.
> **Clinical and radiologic signs:** asymmetric mono-
> or oligoarticular arthritis, predominantly in-
> volving the lower extremities; sacroiliitis,
> spondylitis.

Definition

Undifferentiated spondyloarthropathy is the
term applied to a disease with clinical and radiographic features suggestive of ankylosing spondylitis but not fulfilling the diagnostic criteria
for any of the established seronegative spondyloarthropathies (ankylosing spondylitis, psoriatic spondylarthritis, reactive arthritis including
Reiter's syndrome, enterospondylarthritis).

General Clinical Features

As the definition states, undifferentiated spondyloarthropathy is more of a provisional diagnosis than a subcategory in the group of seronegative spondyloarthropathies. "Undifferentiated" means that the spondyloarthropathy may
later evolve into one of the established seronegative spondyloarthropathies, it may be an abor-
tive form of a definite seronegative spondyloarthropathy, or it may represent an "overlap syndrome." Another possibility is that undifferentiated spondyloarthropathy is yet an unknown,
etiologically undefined subcategory of seronegative spondyloarthropathy that may be differen-
tiated in the future.

According to Zeidler et al. (1992), the following
manifestations *may* be present in undifferentiated spondyloarthropathies:

– arthritis with asymmetric joint involvement,
  predominantly mono- or oligoarticular and
  mainly involving the lower extremities;
– enthesopathy;
– sacroiliitis and other inflammatory axial involvement such as spondylitis or arthritis of
  the intervertebral, costovertebral, and cranio-
  cervical joints;

– characteristic systemic manifestations such
  as uveitis, conjunctivitis, and mucocutaneous
  lesions;
– rheumatoid factors negative;
– HLA-B27 associated.

In their survey work, Zeidler et al. (1992) report
the following clinical data on the frequency of
various signs and symptoms in patients with
undifferentiated spondyloarthropathies: male
preponderance of 62–88%; mean age of onset
16–23 years; low back pain 52–80%; peripheral
arthritis 60–100%; polyarthritis 40%; enthesopathy 56% (heel pain 20–28%); mucocutaneous
lesions 16%; conjunctivitis or iritis 33%; urogenital disease 28%; inflammatory bowel disease
4%; cardiac abnormalities 6%; elevated ESR
19–30%; HLA-B27 positive 80–84%; rheumatoid factor negative 100%; radiographic signs of
sacroiliitis 16–30%; spinal radiographic changes 20%.

These data reflect the broad and nonspecific
spectrum of clinical features in this disease. Patients may, for example, have unilateral sacroiliitis alone or combined with inflammatory eye
disease or peripheral arthritis, while other patients may have dactylitis alone or combined
with Achilles tendinitis, inflammatory eye
disease, or mucocutaneous involvement (see
above).

Dermatology

The dermatologic spectrum of undifferentiated
spondyloarthropathy is relatively broad and
includes keratoma blennorrhagicum, circinate
balanitis, onycholysis, onychodystrophy, and
chronic recurring mouth ulcers. One-third of
patients have conjunctivitis or iritis.

Radiology

The radiologic signs of sacroiliitis, spinal changes, and enthesopathies were reviewed in Sect.
3.6.1. Undifferentiated spondyloarthropathy has
identical radiographic features. Chronic forms
of peripheral arthritis are characterized radiographically by erosive and destructive changes.
Undifferentiated spondyloarthropathy has no
specific radiologic features, but the presence of
an undifferentiated seronegative spondyloar-

thropathy should be considered whenever a unilateral "variegated" type of sacroiliitis is discovered along with other atypical symptoms.

General Differential Diagnosis

The differential diagnosis is guided by the above definition and descriptions. The arthritis of undifferentiated spondyloarthropathy mainly requires differentiation from seronegative rheumatoid arthritis; sometimes this can be accomplished only by observing the course. As a general rule, rheumatoid arthritis without rheumatoid factors (seronegative polyarthritis) usually involves the joints of the hands and feet in a bilaterally symmetric pattern, while clinical and radiologic involvement of the spine and sacroiliac joints is less common and tends to occur late in the course of the disease.

References

Zeidler H, Mau W, Khan MA (1992) Undifferentiated spondyloarthropathies. Rheum Dis Clin North Am 18: 187

3.7 Other Forms of Reactive Arthritis

The diseases described in Sect. 3.6 constitute the largest group of reactive arthritides. Here we shall consider Lyme arthritis and rheumatic fever, which differ from the other reactive arthritides in that they are not associated with HLA-B27.

3.7.1 Lyme Arthritis

Synonyms: Borrelia-induced arthritis, erythema migrans borreliosis, erythema chronicum migrans disease

> *Early stage:* acute: erythema chronicum migrans, constitutional symptoms.
> *Subacute-chronic (untreated):* acrodermatitis chronica atrophicans, progressive encephalomyelitis, recurring oligo- or polyarthritis, possibly erosive.
> *Late stage:* myocarditis, pericarditis, meningitis, encephalitis, etc; lymphadenosis cutis benigna, juxta-articular nodules and ulnar striations.

Definition

Lyme arthritis is one of the main features of a multisystem infectious disease caused by the spirochete *Borrelia burgdorferi*. Other common manifestations are erythema chronicum migrans and meningopolyneuritis.

General Clinical Features

Lyme arthritis and Lyme disease are named for the town of Old Lyme, Connecticut, where the occurrence of arthritis in children bitten by ticks was first reported in 1975. Biting flies have also been implicated as a vector for *B. burgdorferi*. The disease can occur at any age following a tick bite, and no sex predilection is known.

It is interesting epidemiologically to note that approximately 10% of the German population has been infected with *B. burgdorferi* without contracting disease. The disease is most prevalent, of course, in persons who frequent wooded areas (lumberjacks, hunters, mushroom gatherers, etc.). It is estimated that approximately 30–40% of ticks are infected with *B. burgdorferi*, and that about 50% of persons bitten by an infected tick will contract the infection. The incidence of infection is highest during the summer and fall, but factors such as chronicity and asymptomatic intervals mean that physicians may encounter Lyme disease and Lyme arthritis at any time of the year.

The clinical presentation of Lyme disease is usually monosymptomatic or less commonly bisymptomatic, with cutaneous and neurologic symptoms predominating. Arthritis is less frequently observed.

The disease usually begins with the lesions of erythema chronicum migrans (see below), which appear from several days to several weeks after a tick bite. From days to several weeks or months into the illness, diverse symptoms appear that may include neurologic, cardiac, and articular manifestations. The *early stage of the disease* is marked by subjective complaints consisting of rapidly fluctuating and intermittent symptoms that may include general malaise, weakness, headache, fever, stiff neck, arthralgias, myalgias, and lymphadenopathy. The arthralgias and myalgias often last only a matter of hours and are migratory.

Unless the disease is diagnosed and controlled in its *early stage*, it will enter a *late stage* as much as 1 year after the original tick bite. This stage is characterized by myocarditis and pericarditis manifested by atrioventricular conduction defects that may include a complete AV block with atrial fibrillation and ventricular extrasystoles. Neurologic manifestations of Lyme disease at this stage are potentially severe and may take the form of meningitis, encephalitis, cranial neuritis, motor and sensory radiculoneuropathy, mononeuritis multiplex, or myelitis. These manifestations may occur intermittently for many months. They should be distinguished from spring-summer meningoencephalitis, another tick-borne disorder that is based on a viral disease. Allowed to run a spontaneous course, Lyme disease progresses to a *chronic stage* whose main features are acrodermatitis chronica atrophicans (see below), a progressive encephalomyelitis, relapsing oligo- and polyarticular arthritis, and chronic erosive arthritis.

The diagnosis of Lyme disease can be supported by detecting specific antibodies (IgG) in the immunofluorescence test and/or by PCR, but decisive are clinical data (Krause et al. 1998). The treatment of choice is antibiotic therapy (penicillin, tetracycline, or erythromycin). With prompt initiation of treatment, the disease has a favorable prognosis.

Dermatology

Erythema chronicum migrans (Fig. 3.7.1) starts as a small erythematous papule at the site of the tick bite. Usually this is on the lower extremity, but any area may be affected. Within a few weeks, the papule becomes surrounded by an erythematous macule that continues to spread peripherally with central livid regression. The lesions of erythema chronicum migrans may spread over large areas of skin 20–80 cm or more in diame-

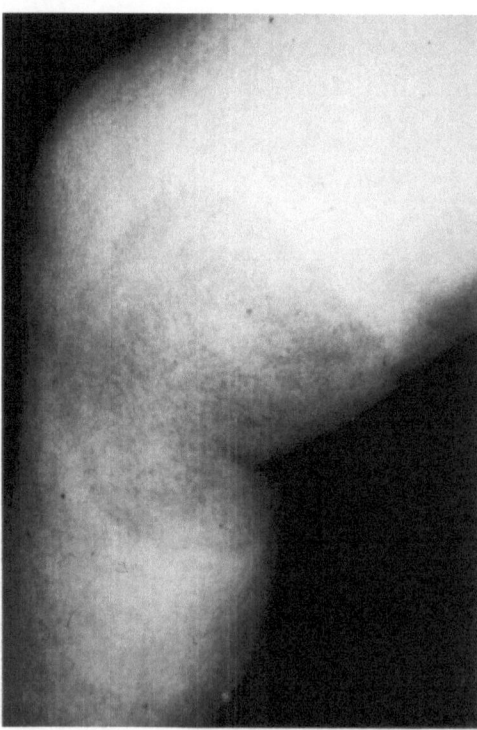

Fig. 3.7.1. Erythema chronicum migrans. The patient presented with headache, malaise, myalgias, arthralgias, and normal radiographic appearance of the symptomatic joints (as expected). Radiographs are not useful for the investigation of arthralgias in the early stage of Lyme disease

ter. Regional lymph node enlargement is not uncommon. Differentiation is primarily required from other figurate erythemas and, in the hand, from erysipeloid.

Acrodermatitis chronica atrophicans is distinguished by the thinned, "cigarette-paper" appearance of the affected skin combined with telangiectases and pigmentary changes. As subcutaneous fatty tissue is lost, cordlike venous markings appear. Red, inflamed margins separate the atrophic areas from normal skin. The above changes most commonly affect the extensor surfaces of the extremities and show a symmetric distribution. (Osteolytic changes at acral sites are discussed on p. 191.) The transition to the full presentation of acrodermatitis chronica atrophicans is of diagnostic importance; this is an inflammatory, edematous stage marked by a padlike edema of the skin with inflammatory redness followed by livid discoloration.

Another late cutaneous manifestation of Lyme disease is *lymphadenosis cutis benigna*, known also as borrelia lymphocytoma or Bäfverstedt's syndrome. The lesions consist of red to bluish-red dermal nodules about 1–2 cm in diameter with a smooth surface, occurring most commonly on the earlobes or other acral sites. They appear months to years after the onset of infection. Other late manifestations are *juxta-articular nodules* and *ulnar and/or tibial striations*. Appearing decades after the original infection, these lesions consist of rheumatoid nodule-like thickenings that occur over the elbow or knee, sometimes – in the case of elbow location – forming striations that pass across the ulna from the elbow.

Radiology

Arthritides usually occur in a late or chronic stage of Lyme disease, and only about 5–30% of patients recall the tick bite. Many patients have long forgotten an earlier bout of erythema chronicum migrans and do not relate it to the arthritis commencing weeks or months later. Lyme arthritis starts as an acute mono- or oligoarticular inflammation and runs an intermittent course, with attacks of several days' duration alternating with weeks of remission. The knees and other large joints are predominantly affected. Polyarticular involvement is less common,

and progression to chronic erosive arthritis is rare. Radiographs are of little value, as generally they do not show the obvious radiologic changes of arthritis (nondelineation of the subchondral plate, erosion, destruction). Periarticular soft-tissue swelling may be present but is an equivocal roentgen sign. Enthesopathy with heavy calcification or ossification may occur. Despite the minimal value of objective radiographic signs, we regard Lyme arthritis as a typical interdisciplinary disorder because we feel that radiographic evaluation is indicated in patients who present clinically with arthritic symptoms.

References

Ackermann R (1983) Erythema chronicum migrans und durch Zecken übertragene Meningopolyneuritis (Garin-Bojadoux-Bannwarth): Borrelien-Infektion? Dtsch Med Wochenschr 108: 577

Asch ES, Bujak DJ, Weiss M et al. (1994) Lyme disease: an infectious and postinfectious syndrome. J Rheumatol 21: 454

Krause A, Priem S, Burmester GR (1998) Borrelia – PCR: Diagnostic problems constantly remain? Why molecular biological diagnosis cannot be replaced by clinical examination (Editorial). Z Rheumatol 57: 79

Herzer T, Wilske B, Preac-Mursic V et al. (1986) Lyme-Arthritis: Clinical features, serological and radiographic findings of cases in Germany. Klin Wochenschr 64: 206

3.7.2 Rheumatic Fever

Synonyms: acute articular rheumatism, strepto-coccal rheumatism

> High fever, epistaxis, pungent sweat; erythema anulare, rheumatoid nodules; purpura; papular erythema; migratory polyarthritis with no radiographic changes; in the case of Jaccoud's arthritis deformities and occasional osteoporosis.

Definition

Rheumatic fever is a systemic febrile disease occurring 2–3 weeks after a pharyngeal infection with group A beta-hemolytic streptococci. It is associated with articular and/or visceral inflammatory changes and various cutaneous manifestations of variable degrees.

General Clinical Features

Rheumatic fever has become a rare disease. It most commonly affects children and adolescents, with a peak incidence around 10 years of age. Young and middle-aged adults are rarely affected. Malnutrition, heavy physical exertion, hypothermia, crowded living conditions (with opportunity for mass infections), and a moist climate are considered predisposing factors. It is believed that an infection with beta-hemolytic streptococci induces the formation of autoantibodies directed against host tissues such as the synovial membrane, the sarcolemma of myocardial cells, and the endocardium.

Between about 8 and 20 days following a tonsilar, pharyngeal, sinus, or laryngeal infection caused by beta-hemolytic streptococci, the disease starts with a fever as high as 41°C, accompanied by severe malaise and epistaxis. The patient secretes large amounts of watery sweat with a sharp, pungent odor. The arthritis is *migratory* and predominantly affects the large joints (especially the ankles), causing significant swelling, warmth, and extreme pain and tenderness. The disease in children is complicated by visceral inflammations in up to 80% of cases, and often this is the dominant feature. The most important of these complications are endocarditis with mitral

and aortic valve sequelae and pleurisy. Dermatologic manifestations are described below. A small percentage of children with rheumatic fever develop chorea minor after the inflammatory changes have subsided.

Laboratory tests demonstrate elevated antistreptolysin titers.

In most cases the symptoms resolve in about 3–6 weeks, but inadequate treatment carries a high risk of recurrence, which is particularly dangerous for the heart. Rarely, the arthritis of rheumatic fever may progress to a chronic, deforming *Jaccoud's arthritis* characterized by a reversible ulnar deviation and slight flexion of the metacarpophalangeal joints, variable hyperextension of the proximal and distal interphalangeal joints, and carpal and carpometacarpal deformities. The main clinical features of Jaccoud's arthritis are arthralgias, especially during weather changes and after infections, and mild periarticular soft-tissue swelling – features unlike those of rheumatoid arthritis.

Dermatology

The most typical skin lesion in children with acute rheumatic fever is *erythema anulare rheumaticum* (Fig. 3.7.2). This rapidly appearing and rapidly clearing erythema erupts on the chest, abdomen, flanks, back, and occasionally on the inside of the thighs. The multiple, blotchy, pale-pink macules of this subtle erythema rapidly develop into annular figures. The erythema is at skin level, blanches on compression, and is not infiltrated; there is no pruritus. These lesions signify cardiac involvement (endocarditis), and the examiner should make a diligent search for them owing to their prognostic importance.

The following types of erythema should be considered in the differential diagnosis:

Erythema infectiosum: butterfly facial rash with no constitutional symptoms.
Erythema anulare centrifugum: brownish-red erythema with fine scales, infiltrated; no malaise.
Recurring syphilitic exanthema: involves the palms and soles of the hands and feet.
All drug rashes.

Rheumatoid nodules are among the cardinal signs of rheumatic fever. They tend to occur at acral sites, and their appearance correlates with rheumatic episodes. Occasionally they appear

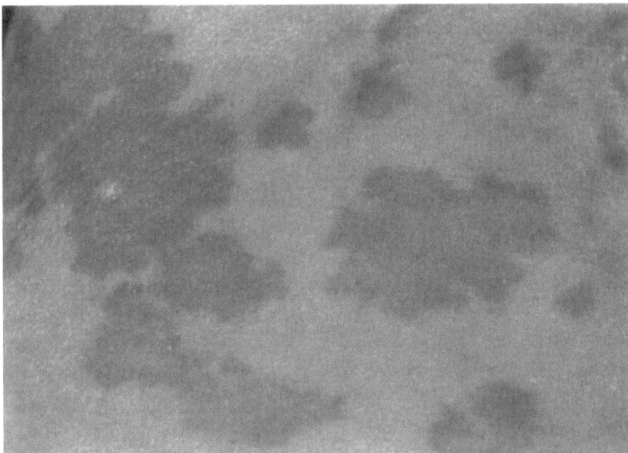

Fig. 3.7.2. Erythema anulare rheumaticum

between the initiating streptococcal infection and the onset of fever. Rheumatoid nodules tend to appear and disappear quickly, although some may persist for months while fluctuating in size. They may occur over the elbow joint, on the dorsal aspects of the hands and feet, over the knee, the malleolar region, the dorsal spinous processes, the scapular angle, or the iliac crest. They are palpable as firm, nontender nodules ranging from a few millimeters to several centimeters in size. As the rheumatic disease improves, the nodules regress.

Nonspecific dermatologic reactions that may accompany rheumatic fever:

1. *Urticaria rheumatica* is most common in the early stage, its course paralleling that of the systemic disease manifestations.
2. *Purpura* may result from toxic vessel wall damage caused by medications (salicylates) taken during the course of the disease.
3. *Papular erythema*, occurring in symmetrical groups on the extensor surfaces of the extremities, over the elbow joints, knees, and dorsal aspects of the hands and feet and consisting of red, lentil-sized nodules that correlate with the activity of the rheumatic fever.
4. *Erythema nodosum* (see p. 112).
5. *Erythema exudativum multiforme*, a variant of erythema nodosum.

Radiology

The radiologic features of rheumatic fever are usually sparse compared with its dramatic clinical features and consist mainly of a broadening of the soft-tissue shadow of joints due to synovitis and effusion. Erosions and significant demineralization are less common. Even in Jaccoud's arthritis there is little decalcification of the subchondral bone, little joint space narrowing, and only occasional, subtle erosive changes in the metacarpal heads. These subtle findings contrast with the significant ulnar deviation of the metacarpophalangeal joints and other potential deformities mentioned above. The diagnostic criteria for Jaccoud's arthritis are a prior history of rheumatic fever, an acquired mitral or aortic valve defect, and (occasionally) elevated antistreptolysin titers.

References

Behrend T, Lawrence JS (1977) Epidemiologie der rheumatischen Erkrankungen. In: Blohmke M et al. (Hrsg) Handbuch der Sozialmedizin. Enke, Stuttgart

Girgis FL, Popple AW, Bruckner FE (1978) Jaccoud's arthropathy. A case report and necropsy study. Ann Rheum Dis 37: 561

Hartmann F (1982) Entzündliche Gelenkserkrankungen. In: Gross R, Schölmerich P (Hrsg) Lehrbuch der Inneren Medizin. Schattauer, Stuttgart

3.8 Behçet's Syndrome

Iritis with hypopyon, keratitis, conjunctivitis; more than five aphthous ulcers in the
oral mucosa in the posterior part of the oral
cavity; shallow, elliptical genital aphthous ulcers; pustular acneiform and papulonecrotic skin lesions.

Clinical signs: symmetric nonerosive polyarthritis, less commonly mono- or oligoarthritis; positive pathergy test.

Definition

Behçet's syndrome is a multisystem disease,
probably a vasculitis, marked by a triad of iritis
(with hypopyon), aphthous stomatitis, and aphthous ulcerative lesions of the genital mucosae.
The syndrome is named for the Turkish physician Behçet, who first described it in 1937. For
many years it was counted among the seronegative spondyloarthropathies, but today this classification is outdated.

General Clinical Features

Various clinical and histologic findings suggest
that Behçet's syndrome is based on an immuno-
logic vasculitis most likely triggered by viral infections or environmental antigens in genetically predisposed individuals. A genetic predisposition is evidenced by the frequent presence of
HLA-B5 in Behçet patients – an antigen that is
highly prevalent along the historic "silk route"
extending from Japan through China to the Me-
diterranean. The syndrome itself is most prevalent in these regions and in northern Africa. The
geographic distribution suggests that the genetic predisposition started from an unknown lo-
cale and spread through mass migrations along
the eastern trade route. The condition predominantly affects males between 20 and 30 years of
age.

The main clinical symptoms of Behçet's syndrome are recurring mouth ulcers combined
with recurrent genital ulcerations, ocular inflammation, and various skin lesions in addition
to a positive pathergy test (see below). Less common manifestations are subcutaneous or deep

venous thrombosis, occlusions or aneurysms
that may involve major arteries (e.g., in the lung),
and CNS involvement with meningoencephalitis
and occlusive vascular disease.

Joint involvement is highly variable. The arthritis is symmetric and polyarticular, less commonly mono- or oligoarticular, and tends to be
fleeting. Some patients experience only joint
pain with no objective signs of inflammation.
The most common sites of involvement are the
knees, ankles, wrists, elbows, hands, and shoulders. The hips, toes, temporomandibular joints,
and sternoclavicular joints are less commonly
affected. Contrary to former beliefs, sacroiliitis
occurs in less than 1% of patients. A similar incidence is reported for the development of an ankylosing spondylitis.

A fairly specific sign for Behçet's syndrome is a
positive pathergy test, signifying an unusual hypersensitivity to needle pricks. In a positive test,
pustules form 24–48 h following a needle prick
or the injection of 0.1 ml physiologic saline so-
lution at the site of the injection.

Dermatology

The spectrum of *ophthalmologic changes* includes iritis with hypopyon (pus formation due
to the accumulation of sterile leukocytes) and
accompanying conjunctivitis, also keratitis,
uveitis, chorioretinitis, retinal phlebitis, retinal
vasculitis, and vitreous hemorrhage. Glaucoma
and cataract may develop in the wake of these
changes. A detailed description of these ophthalmologic conditions would exceed our scope.

The presence of *more than five aphthous mouth
ulcers* should raise suspicion of Behçet's syndrome, especially if the mucosal lesions involve
the posterior part of the oral cavity and the individual lesions are remarkably large and have
bizarre configurations. They require differentiation from the recurring aphthae in certain seronegative spondyloarthropathies (see pp. 97,
110), which tend to involve the front of the oral
cavity and usually number no more than two to
four. Coexisting aphthous genital ulcers that are
shallow and elliptical and have well-defined,
nonundermined margins with no obvious signs
of inflammation further support the diagnosis
of Behçet's syndrome. The genital ulcers are relatively nontender and may be found on the scro-

tal skin, at the base of the penis, or on the labia majora and minora.

Pustular (sterile) acneiform and papulonecrotic skin lesions most commonly arise on the face, neck, and trunk. Nodular lesions may take the form of erythema nodosum (see p. 112) on the extensor surfaces of the lower leg.

Radiology

Behçet's syndrome is associated with few radiographic skeletal changes, because most joint involvement is transient and does not produce objective signs such as erosion or destruction. This occurs only in the small minority of cases (<1%) that develop chronic erosive-destructive arthritis primarily involving the toes, ankles, hands, wrists, temporomandibular joints, sternomanubrial joints, and hips. Periarticular osteoporosis is reportedly more common than erosive and destructive changes. As mentioned, there was a former tendency to overstate the incidence of axial involvement with sacroiliitis and ankylosing spondylitis. Today it is thought that these conditions develop in less than 1% of cases. Their radiologic features are described on p. 90ff.

References

Jorizzo JL (1986) Behçet's disease: an update based on the 1985 international conference in London. Arch Dermatol 122: 556

Numan F, Islak C, Berkmen T (1994) Behçet Disease: Pulmonary arterial involvement in 15 cases. Radiology 192: 465

Rosenberger A, Adler O, Haim J (1982) Radiological aspects of Behçet's disease. Radiology 144: 261

3.9 Acne-Associated Skeletal Changes

Acne conglobata with papules, pustules, and painful nodules with hemorrhagic crusts; *acne fulminans* with patchy areas of necrosis and liquefaction, often with severe malaise.

Clinical and radiologic signs: Reiter-like features with sacroiliitis, spondylitis, erosive enthesopathy, erosive oligo- or polyarthritis of hands and feet with periosteal ossification; features of chronic recurrent multifocal osteitis with dense sclerosis and sternocostoclavicular involvement.

Definition

The skin lesions and skeletal abnormalities encompassed by the term "acne-associated skeletal changes" cannot be clearly defined at present. However, published reports and our own observations indicate that severe forms of acne may be associated with pathologic changes in the bones and joints. Authors in different countries use different nomenclature for these severe forms of acne. In Germany, the standard dermatology textbook by Braun-Falco et al. (1991) describes acne fulminans as a "rare but serious disease of unknown cause beginning acutely and found almost exclusively in young males, aged 13–16 years, with acne conglobata." Thus, acne fulminans is described as developing from acne conglobata. On the other hand, American authors such as Ellis et al. (1987) state that acne fulminans usually occurs in white male adolescents as an acute febrile illness with ulcerating skin lesions and joint symptoms, while acne conglobata typically occurs as a severe cicatricial acne in adult black men with chronic skin disease comprising the dermatologic *triad of acne, hidradenitis suppurativa, and dissecting cellulitis of the scalp* (the "follicular occlusion triad"). These two types of acne are described as differing in their skeletal manifestations: acne fulminans is associated more with polyarthralgias or arthritis, while the skeletal changes of acne conglobata closely resemble those in Reiter's syndrome (sacroiliitis, spondylitis, erosive oligo- and polyarthritis involving large and small joints).

In this chapter about acne-associated skeletal changes we follow the German dermatologic nomenclature, and we shall base our clinical and radiologic descriptions on personal observations and on general information already published on acne-associated skeletal changes.

General Clinical Features

The pathogenesis of acne fulminans and the associated bone and joint changes is poorly understood. It may relate to a bacterial infection (e.g., with *Propionibacterium acnes*) that triggers an immunopathologic process transforming acne conglobata into a fulminant form with severe systemic manifestations. Arthritis, spondylitis, and nonspecific inflammatory bone changes may be considered reactive phenomena as in Reiter's disease.

Patients with acne fulminans have an acute febrile illness with malaise, weight loss, high septic temperatures, and leukocytosis up to 40,000/mm^3. Infectious anemia and an elevated ESR may also be present. Endocarditis and glomerulonephritis may develop in rare cases. Patients complain of polyarthralgia and polyarthritis primarily affecting the large joints (shoulders, hips, knees, and ankles). Effusions may occur. Involvement of the axial skeleton is manifested by low back pain. There may be inflammatory enthesopathy (fibro-osteitis) with associated radiographic changes.

Dermatology

The face, chest, and back may exhibit all the features of acne conglobata such as comedones, papules, pustules with hemorrhagic crusts, and painful indurated nodules which become confluent and bleed (Fig. 3.9 a). It is not the scope of this book to describe in detail the consecutive changes of acne conglobata. Acne fulminans is additionally associated with patchy necrotizing liquefaction of the cutaneous nodules.

Radiology

Transient polyarthralgia and polyarthritis of the large joints produce no radiographic changes other than the expansion of periarticular soft-tissue shadows due to effusion. In other cases, as

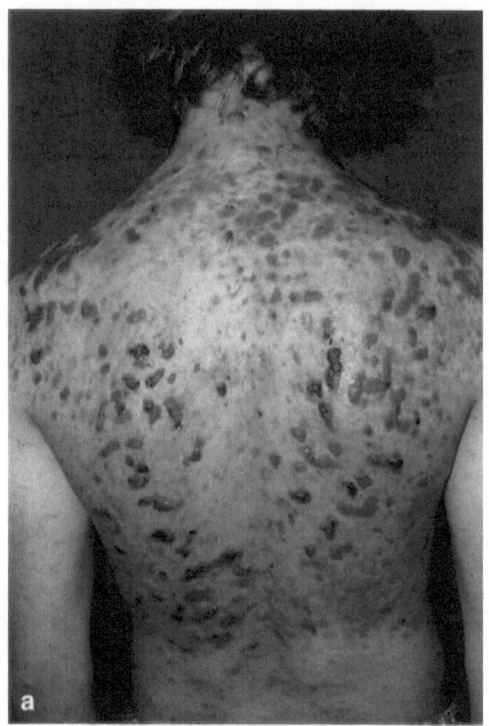

Fig. 3.9 a–g. Acne-associated skeletal changes. **a** Typical skin lesions of acne conglobata. Male 16 years of age with severe acne conglobata accompanied by extensive sclerotic skeletal changes (as in chronic multifocal recurrent osteomyelitis) combined with erosive polyarthritis of the large joints. Radionuclide bone scans (**b**) show intense tracer uptake in the right clavicle and manubrioclavicular joint, at the synchondrosis between the sternal body and manubrium, in the right proximal and distal femur, right proximal tibia, left proximal tibia, and about the ankle joints. Increased uptake was also observed in the right shoulder and left elbow (not shown). The sternocostoclavicular involvement is reminiscent of pustulotic arthroosteitis (PAO), but at presentation the patient did not have palmoplantar pustulosis. Radiographically, the positive areas on the bone scans displayed marked sclerosis with expansion of the right medial clavicle and destruction of the manubrioclavicular joint on the right side (**c**). Note the osteolytic defect in the lower part of the sclerotic area in the clavicle. Knee radiograph (**d**) shows marked erosive lesions of the medial femoral condyle and tibial margins and pronounced sclerosis of the subchondral bone, especially in the upper tibia. Similar changes were seen on the contralateral side. The left elbow joint also shows erosions and striking periosteal ossification on the radial neck (**e**, *asterisk*) **f, g** see p. 130

f, g see p. 130

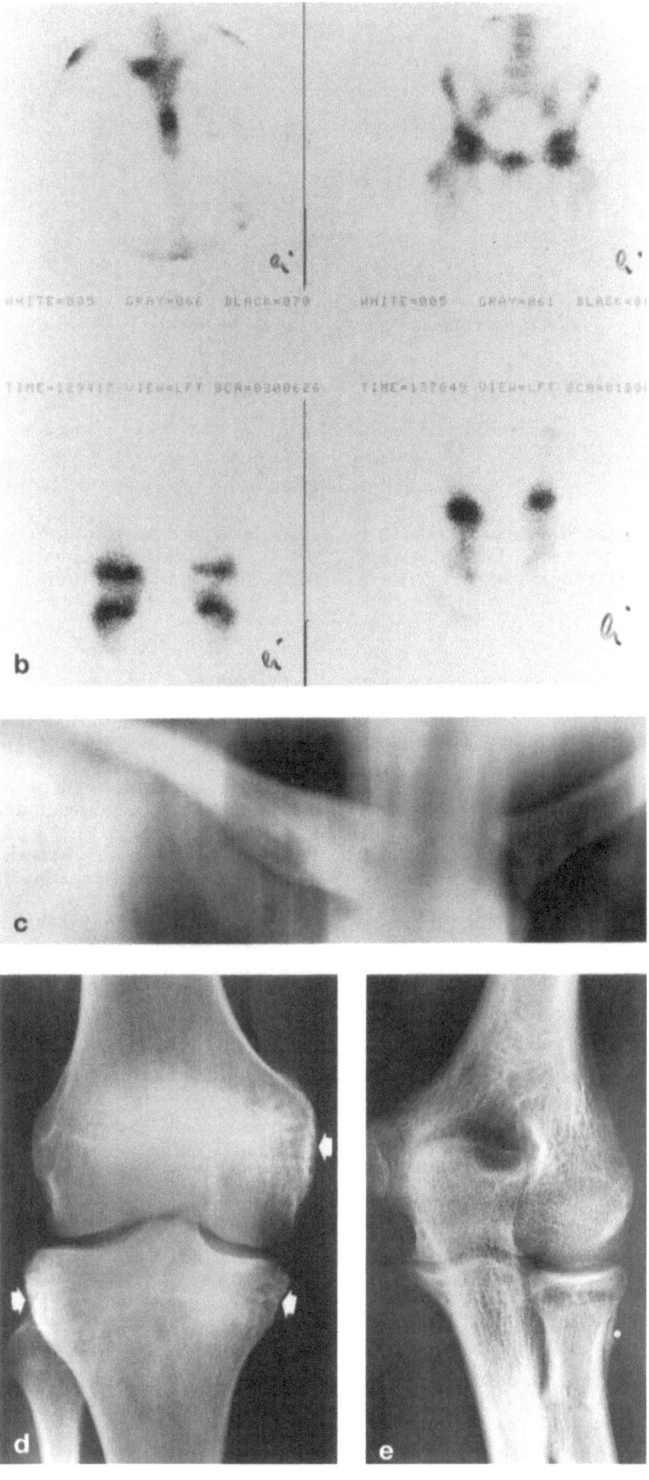

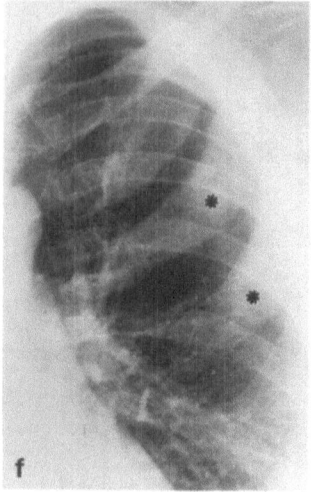 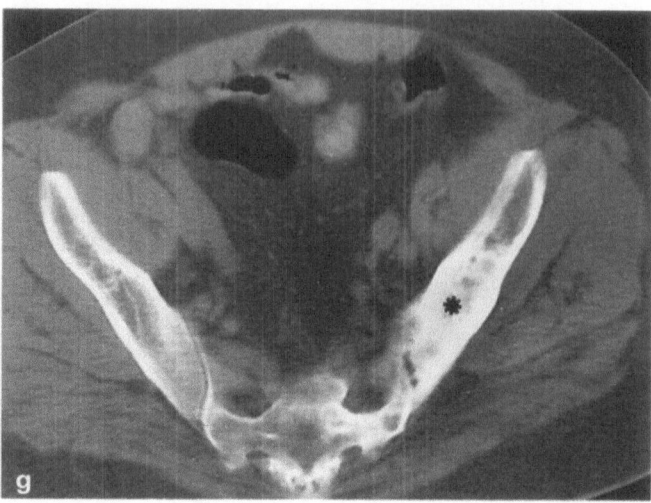

Fig. 3.9 (*continued*). **f, g** Man 32 years of age referred to us with a diagnosis of "severe acne," found to have extensive sclerotic changes in the left upper anterior rib segments (**f**) and pelvis (**g**) (*asterisks*). (Images courtesy of Dr. A. Wittenborg, Ruhrgebiet Rheumatology Center, St. Josef Hospital, Herne)

described for acne conglobata in the American literature, there may be conspicuous Reiter-like changes consisting of sacroiliitis (see p. 90), spondylitis with parasyndesmophyte formation (see p. 100), and enthesopathies. Ellis et al. (1987), Davis et al. (1981), and Rosner et al. (1982) described an erosive, often destructive oligo- and polyarthritis showing asymmetric involvement of the hands and feet and displaying all the features of erosive arthritis such as periarticular osteoporosis, erosions, and destructive changes, usually combined with foci of periosteal proliferation. Our own clinical material includes one case referred with "severe acne" showing the features of chronic multifocal recurrent osteomyelitis (CMRO) with extensive sclerotic changes in the pelvis and several ribs (Fig. 3.9 f, g) and a second case (acne conglobata) showing multifocal periarticular sclerosis combined with erosive arthritis mainly involving the knees, ankles, right manubrioclavicular joint, and the synchondrosis between the manubrium and body of the sternum (Fig. 3.9 b–e).

References

Braun-Falco O, Plewig G, Wolff HH, Winkelmann RK (1991) Dermatology, 3rd edn. Springer, Berlin Heidelberg New York

Davis DE, Viozzi FJ, Miller OF, Blodgett RC (1981) The musculoskeletal manifestations of acne fulminans. J Rheumatol 8: 317

Ellis BJ, Shier CRK, Leisen JJC et al. (1987) Acne-associated spondyloarthropathy: Radiographic features. Radiology 167: 541

Goldschmidt H, Leyden JJ, Stein KH (1977) Acne fulminans: investigation of acute febrile ulcerative acne. Arch Dermatol 113: 444

Kelly AP, Burns RE (1971) Acute febrile ulcerative conglobata acne with polyarthralgia. Arch Dermatol 104: 182

Lane JM, Leyden JJ, Spegel RJ (1976) Acne arthralgia. J Bone Joint Surg 58A: 673

Rosner IA, Richter DE, Huettner TL et al. (1982) Spondylarthropathy associated with hidradenitis suppurativa and acne conglobata. Ann Intern Med 97: 520

4 Infectious Diseases

4.1 Leprosy

Synonym: Hansen's disease

Nonspecific general symptoms with anesthetic, hypopigmented skin areas, muscular atrophy, and chronic nasal obstruction or epistaxis.
Tuberculoid leprosy: erythematous macules or plaques with anesthesia.
Borderline type: soft, raised, reddish skin lesions disseminated over the face and trunk.
Lepromatous leprosy: symmetric papular and nodular eruptions on the nose, ears, hands, and buttocks; diffuse facial involvement is marked by infiltrative swelling with loss of the eyebrows and eyelashes and subsequent depression of the nasal bridge.
Clinical signs: progressive mutilation of fingers and toes.
Roentgen signs: progressive bone resorption in the hands and feet, starting peripherally and extending proximally; granulomas in lepromatous form appear as cystlike lucencies, usually near joints (osteitis leprosa multiplex cystica); periosteal new bone formation.

Definition

Leprosy is a chronic multisystem infectious disease caused by *Mycobacterium leprae.*

General Clinical Features

Leprosy is mainly endemic to India, Africa, and South America. The WHO estimates that there are approximately 15 million cases throughout the world. About 130 cases were reported in the Federal Republic of Germany in 1985 (Mende et al. 1985). With the steady growth in tourism, the rising tide of immigration from endemic areas, and increases in international business travel, it is likely that greater numbers of leprosy cases will be seen in temperate regions. Nevertheless, our scope is too limited to explore all aspects of this complex disease, and we can do no more than outline its dermatologic features.

Two polar forms of leprosy are recognized based on clinical manifestations and the immune status of the host: *tuberculoid leprosy* (normal immune response) and *lepromatous leprosy* (impaired immune response). Intermediate between these extremes is a range of "borderline" or "dimorphous" forms.

Leprosy is usually acquired in childhood or adolescence due to transmission from "open cases," which consist mostly of borderline cases or the multibacillary lepromatous form. The mode of transmission is not precisely known. It is known that the bacilli are not transmitted via the airways and that prolonged, intimate contact and impaired host resistance are predisposing factors. Infection is also promoted by the presence of skin breaks, chronic ulcerations, and suppurative skin lesions caused by insect bites or stings. Sites of predilection for colonization by *M. leprae* are the skin, mucous membranes, upper respiratory tract, and peripheral nerves. The incubation period is extremely variable, ranging from 3 to 20 years. The *earliest symptoms* are usually nonspecific and include hypopigmented skin areas (Fig. 4.1a), anesthesia, muscular atrophy, chronic catarrh, or epistaxis. Lepromatous leprosy, known also as malignant leprosy, has a poor prognosis. Braun-Falco et al. (1991) note that patients with this malignant, anergic form of the disease may have a bacillary load of up to 1 kg in their bodies. Tuberculoid leprosy has a favorable prognosis and often resolves spontaneously due to effective host defenses. In other cases it may cause significant

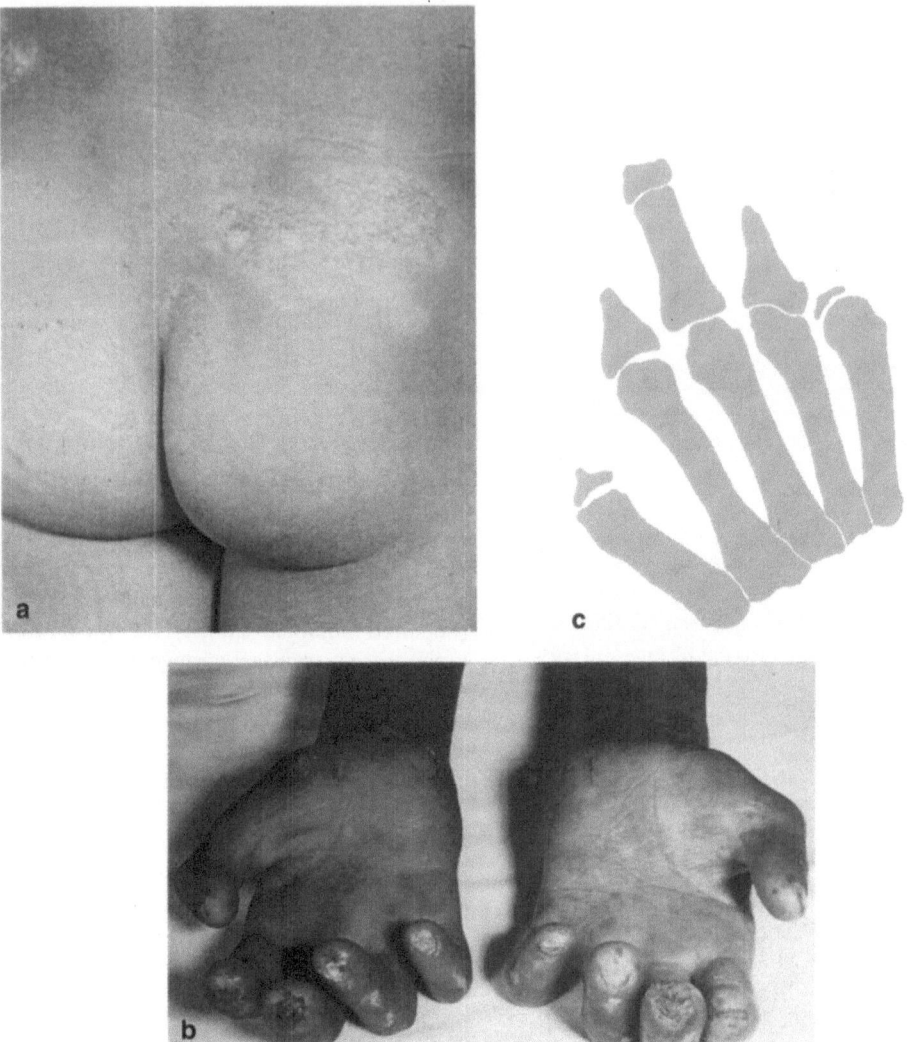

Fig. 4.1 a–e. Leprosy. **a** Early hypopigmented lesions over the buttock. **b** Gross clawhand deformity in tuberculoid leprosy with very severe trophic disturbances involving the distal phalanges of both hands. The distal phalanges of the third fingers are already resorbed, and the stumps are ulcerated. **c** Typical radiographic appearance of the hand in leprosy. Very severe but painless trophic disturbances have caused extensive "pencil-like" resorption of the distal and middle phalanges and incipient resorption of the proximal phalanges. Basically the same radiographic changes are seen in progressive scleroderma (see Fig. 2.1 d). **d, e** see p. 133

mutilation and disability due to involvement of the nervous system (Fig. 4.1 b). Few if any bacilli are recoverable from skin lesions. Tuberculoid or sarcoid granulomas are found on histologic examination. Lymph nodes are unaffected in the tuberculoid form.

Both polar forms, especially the tuberculoid, can cause severe nerve damage because of the ex-treme affinity of the bacilli to Schwann cells. Even external inspection of the peripheral nerves may reveal inflammatory granulomatous foci. Nerve destruction leads to palsies and muscular atrophy, with facial manifestations including facial nerve palsy, ptosis of the upper eyelids, and a masklike facies. Atrophy of the small hand muscles leads to contractures with

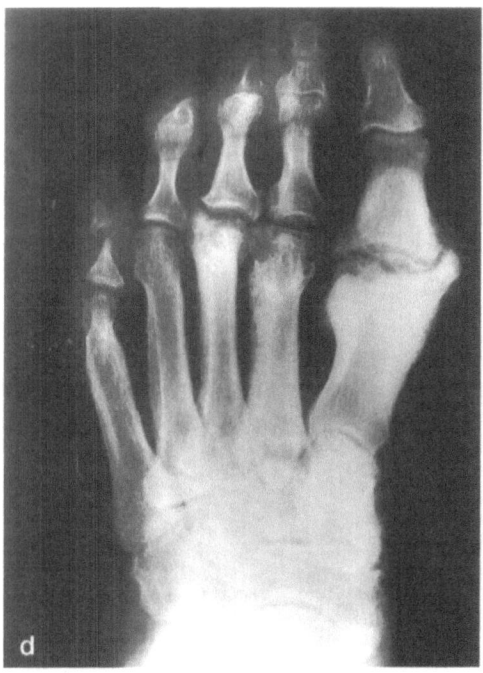
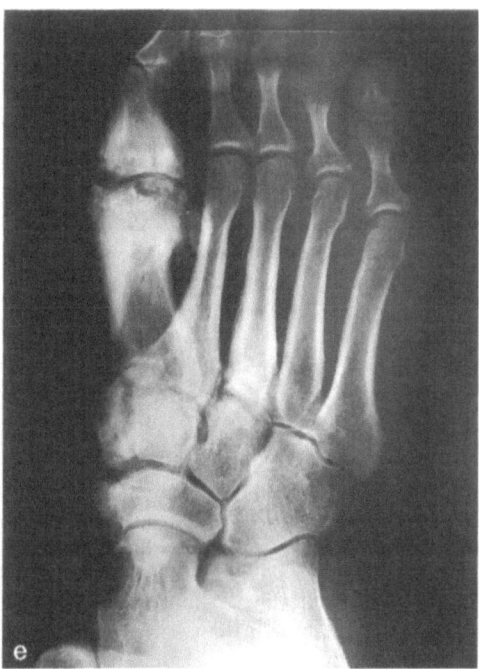
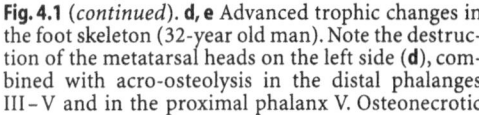

Fig. 4.1 (*continued*). **d, e** Advanced trophic changes in the foot skeleton (32-year old man). Note the destruction of the metatarsal heads on the left side (**d**), combined with acro-osteolysis in the distal phalanges III–V and in the proximal phalanx V. Osteonecrotic changes in both medial tarsal bones and periosteal new bone formation in most of the metatarsal bones, looking like diabetic osteoarthropathy. (X-rays courtesy of Prof. Dr. Dietrich, Bernhard-Nocht-Institute, Hamburg)

clawhand deformity, and a "steppage gait" may result from atrophy of the small muscles of the feet. Trophic ulcerations develop, leading to bone destruction. The "nonspecific skeletal changes" described below are also neurotrophic in nature.

Dermatology

As noted earlier, the full spectrum of dermatologic changes in leprosy cannot be covered in this monograph but may be found in numerous specialized textbooks. It is interesting to note that, from the standpoint of internal medicine, leprosy is a "primary domain of dermatology" (Classen et al. 1994).

Four types of leprosy are distinguished on the basis of dermatologic criteria:

1. *Indeterminate leprosy* (uncharacteristic leprosy) starts with macular lesions that are erythematous or, in pigmented individuals, hypopigmented. This type may resolve spontaneously or may evolve into one of the following forms:

2. *Tuberculoid leprosy* is characterized by multiple hypopigmented or erythematous macules or plaques that have well-defined borders and are anesthetic. There are no sites of predilection.

3. *Borderline leprosy* is characterized by soft, elevated, reddish, sometimes scaly skin lesions, usually widespread and typically showing an asymmetric distribution on the face and a symmetric distribution on the trunk.

4. *Lepromatous leprosy* presents with symmetric papular and nodular lesions that appear first on the nose and ears and later on the hands, arms, and gluteal region. Diffuse facial involvement is marked by infiltrative "padlike" swelling with loss of the eyebrows and eyelashes, glossitis, and eventual destruction of the nasal cartilages with collapse of the nasal bridge. Nasal secretions contain massive amounts of leprosy bacilli.

Lepra reaction refers to the phenomena that occur during antileprosy therapy. Two types are
recognized:

Type 1: Erythematous infiltration and thickening of skin lesions, lasting about 3–
8 months in tuberculoid leprosy.

Type 2: *Erythema nodosum leprosum* (ENL), appearing as erythematous nodules of varying size on the arms and legs, may occur
as a type-3 immune reaction during the
treatment of lepromatous leprosy.

Radiology

Skeletal changes are found in approximately
60–70% of leprosy patients. Two main types are
distinguished:

1. *Specific skeletal changes* (lepromatous bone
changes) result from the hematogenous seeding of bacilli into the bone. The resulting granulomatous lesions incite a regional bone destruction that appears radiographically as a
cystlike lucency, usually juxta-articular, and
is manifested clinically by joint swelling. The
phalanges of the hands and feet are sites of
predilection. "Osteitis leprosa multiplex cystica" refers to the presence of multiple cystlike lucencies that may create a honeycomb
pattern similar to that in sarcoidosis (granuloma formation; see Fig. 5.6 e). Bone destruction increases as the changes progress. Bacilli that enter the periosteum will incite reactive new bone formation, which is especially
common on the ulna and fibula. Granulomas
in the facial region may erode the nasal skeleton, even causing loss of the nasal spine, or
they may cause bone destruction in the alveolar processes of the maxilla (osteitis leprosa
faciei). External manifestations consist of
saddle-nose deformity and loss of the incisor
teeth.

2. *Nonspecific skeletal changes* are usually secondary to neurotrophic disturbances and primarily affect the hands and feet, which show
striking acro-osteolytic changes that start
distally and progress proximally (Fig. 4.1 c).
In severe cases all the phalanges of the hand
may be resorbed, leaving sharply tapered
metacarpal stumps. In the bones of the feet,
the destructive lesions usually start at the
metatarsophalangeal joints and proceed in
both directions. Spontaneous fractures are
not uncommon. The foot may also show neurogenic osteoarthropathy-like changes with
necrosis and disintegration, similar to that
seen in diabetes mellitus (Fig. 4.1 d, e). The
nerve destruction causes anesthesia, so most
patients do not experience pain. The trophic
disturbances may also be manifested by
osteoporosis, especially in the hands. The in-
sensitivity to pain allows soft-tissue injuries
to go untreated, leading to secondary infections that spread to adjacent bones and cause
nonspecific inflammatory bone lesions.

References

Braun-Falco O, Plewig G, Wolff HH, Winkelmann RK
(1991) Dermatology, 3rd edn. Springer, Berlin Heidelberg New York
Classen M, Diel V, Kochsiek K (1994) Innere Medizin,
3. Aufl. Urban & Schwarzenberg, München, S 321
Mende B, Stein G, Kreysel HW (1985) Knochenveränderungen bei Morbus Hansen. Röfo 142: 189
Schaller KF (ed) (1994) Colour atlas of tropical dermatology and venerology. Springer, Berlin Heidelberg New York

4.2 Syphilis

Dermatologic features. *Congenital syphilis:* scaling papules, perioral rhagades, radiating perioral scars (Parrot's fissures), bullous eruptions on the palms and soles (syphilitic pemphigus).
Acquired (tertiary) syphilis: nodular syphilids on the face and scalp, gummas anywhere on the integument. Serpiginous nodular syphilids and gummas in the mucosa of the upper lip; gummas in the nasal septum, paranasal sinuses, hard and soft palate, and tonsils. Lentil-sized nodules on the dorsum of the tongue, gummas of the tongue in the form of deeply rooted nodules, dorsal interstitial glossitis occurring as a granulomatous inflammation. Miliary ulcerative syphilis of mucous membranes with superficial ulcerations.
Roentgen signs: *Congenital syphilis:* coarse erosions of proximal medial tibial metaphysis, metaphyseal lucent bands, occasional fragmentation; calcifying periostitis; late stage: corticocancellous bone defects (syphilitic osteitis).
Acquired syphilis: syphilitic periostitis, sometimes resembling fibrous dysplasia. Osteolytic lesions due to gumma formation.

General Clinical Features

Syphilis, a chronic systemic infection caused by *Treponema pallidum*, can lead to skeletal involvement in either its acquired or congenital (transplacental) form. Tertiary lesions of acquired syphilis generally develop only in untreated cases and are relatively rare today. But it may be seen with increasing frequency due to the resurgence of the disease in its later stages in the past decade.
The very complex manifestations of syphilis are beyond our scope, but its dermatologic features will be outlined in a way that will allow the nondermatologist to include syphilis in the differential diagnosis of certain clinical and radiographic skeletal changes so that patients can be referred for specialized dermatologic evaluation and treatment.

Dermatology

Primary and secondary syphilis need not be discussed, as they are not associated with skeletal changes. The tertiary lesions of cutaneous syphilis fall into two main categories:

1. The cutaneous lesions of *nodular syphilis* (nodular syphilids).
2. The subcutaneous lesions of *gummatous syphilis*.

The lesions of nodular syphilis are firm, reddish-brown, solitary papules or nodules ranging from 2 mm to 1 cm in size. Occasionally covered with crusts or scales, the lesions heal by forming shallow hyperpigmented or depigmented scars. As the eruptions spread peripherally, they form curved or serpiginous patterns. The lesions may ulcerate to form noduloulcerative syphilids.
The face and scalp are sites of predilection for serpiginous nodular syphilids. The subcutaneous lesion of tertiary syphilis, the *gumma*, may occur anywhere. It starts as a bean-sized subcutaneous nodule that slowly enlarges and fuses with the skin and deeper tissues. The overlying skin assumes a violaceous red or reddish-brown color. The nodule has a firm, rubbery consistency. Eventually it erodes through the skin (Fig. 4.2 a) and discharges a stretchy, yellowish, turbid fluid. Gummas are tender to pressure and take months to heal, causing significant tissue destruction. They may occur in any tissue plane between the skin and bone. The lymph nodes are not enlarged.

Mucous Membrane Lesions of Tertiary Syphilis

Serpiginous nodular syphilids and gummas commonly involve the mucosal surface of the upper lip. Syphilitic macrochelia refers to severe swelling of the upper lip in late syphilis. Gummatous involvement of the nasal septum, paranasal sinuses, hard and soft palate, and tonsils may consist of soft-tissue gummas or periosteal or skeletal gummas. The nasal septum is most commonly involved. Liquefaction occurs, causing extensive destruction and perforation of the palate. Gummatous syphilis spreads from the tonsil to the uvula and from there to portions of the soft palate. A less common intraoral site of gummatous involvement is the gingiva, where gummas usually coexist with a skeletal gumma of the mandible.

The *tongue* is a very common site of mucous membrane involvement in tertiary syphilis:

1. Lentil-sized nodules on the dorsum of the tongue may liquefy and destroy the lingual papillae, giving the tongue a smooth, shiny, scarred surface ("smooth atrophy").
2. Gummas of the tongue may occur singly or in groups. They appear as painless, deeply rooted nodules that are prone to liquefaction and perforation. They heal by forming a deep, hard, indrawn scar with raised edges.
3. Superficial interstitial glossitis represents an interstitial granulomatous inflammation involving the dorsum of the tongue. Portions of the dorsum later undergo a superficial shrinkage and sclerosis with destruction of the papillae. Deep interstitial glossitis in tertiary syphilis is a deeply seated, specific granulomatous inflammation marked by shrinkage and sclerosis of the tongue with deep furrowing of its surface.
4. Ulcerative miliary syphilis of the mucosae is characterized by superficial ulcerations with bizarre "gnawed" borders occurring throughout the oral cavity.

Congenital Syphilis

Early congenital syphilis (lues connata praecox) refers to cases in which cutaneous manifestations are present in newborns and infants, *late congenital syphilis* to cases in which the skin lesions do not appear until adolescence or adulthood.

The mucocutaneous lesions of early congenital syphilis consist of macules, papules, and scaling papules accompanied by impetigo-like syphilids, flat condylomata, and specific alopecia. Mucous patches appear on the mucous membranes. Deep fissures radiate from the lips and oral commissures and, after healing, leave deep radiating scars (Parrot's fissures). Unlike the adult form, early congenital syphilis may feature a bullous eruption (syphilitic pemphigus) on the palms and soles that spreads to the forearms and lower legs. Briefly, the signs of late congenital syphilis are saddle nose, Parrot's fissures (see above), Hutchinson's teeth (malformed upper central incisors), and an interstitial keratitis involving the corneal parenchyma.

Radiology

Congenital Syphilis

A severe intrauterine spirochetal infection transmitted through the placenta often leads to fetal death and miscarriage or to very early postnatal death. Surviving infants usually exhibit a three-stage sequence of postnatal radiographic changes that continue into the second year of life. In the *first stage*, syphilitic granulation tissue infiltrates the growing metaphyses, especially about the knee, shoulder, and wrist, to produce multiple irregular erosions known also as *metaphysitis*. Coarse erosions of the medial corners of the proximal tibial metaphyses (*Wimberger's sign*, Fig. 4.2 c) are a very striking and characteristic feature. They may be accompanied or preceded by broad, horizontal lucent bands in the metaphyses similar to those seen in leukemia or metastatic neuroblastoma. There also may be fragmentation of the metaphysis simulating scurvy. These changes may resolve swiftly in response to penicillin therapy, or a more gradual spontaneous regression may occur.

Cases that are not adequately treated progress to a *second stage* of *syphilitic periostitis* caused by infiltration of the periosteum by syphilitic granulation tissue. This stage is usually marked by symmetric areas of periosteal new bone formation, especially on the long tubular bones (Fig. 4.2 b, c). These changes will resolve with or without antibiotic therapy, but more slowly than the changes in stage 1.

The *third stage* is characterized by a syphilitic osteitis with cortical and cancellous bone destruction predominantly affecting the long tubular bones (Fig. 4.2 b).

Late skeletal manifestations of congenital syphilis include periosteal and endosteal new bone formation that most commonly affects the proximal two-thirds of the tibia and is sometimes combined with osteolytic lesions in the diaphyses of the long tubular bones. Patients may also develop arthritic conditions with recurring metaphysitis and dental malformations (Hutchinson's teeth).

Acquired Syphilis

The two main radiographic presentations of acquired syphilis are syphilitic periostitis and

Fig. 4.2 a–d. Skin lesions and bone changes in syphilis. **a** Perforated gumma. **b,c** Typical radiographic features of congenital syphilis include erosion of the medial corners of the proximal tibial metaphyses (Wimberger's sign) and sclerotic changes. The marked osteolytic lesions in the proximal radial shaft are typical of syphilitic osteitis. Note the sites of periosteal new bone formation, especially on the medial tibial border (syphilitic periostitis). The X-ray findings in **b** and **c** include the third stage as well as remnants of the first and second stage of congenital syphilis. **d** Syphilitic periostitis in an adult. The anterior tibial margin is thickened due to periosteal new bone formation. This is probably a periosteal reaction to underlying gummas, which appear as lucencies in the thickened bone

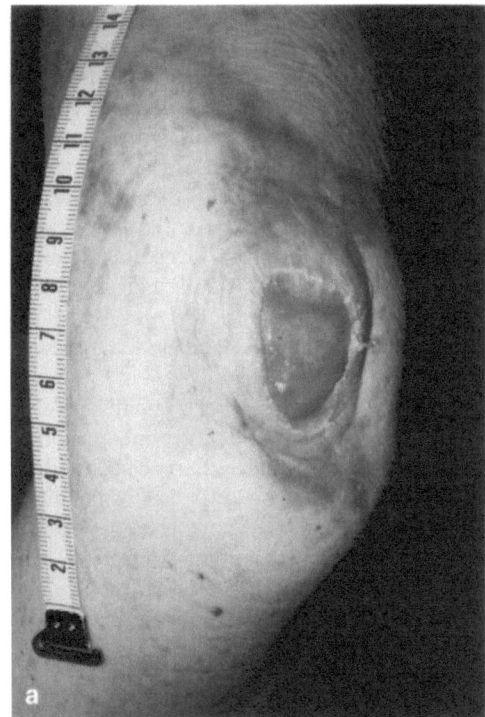

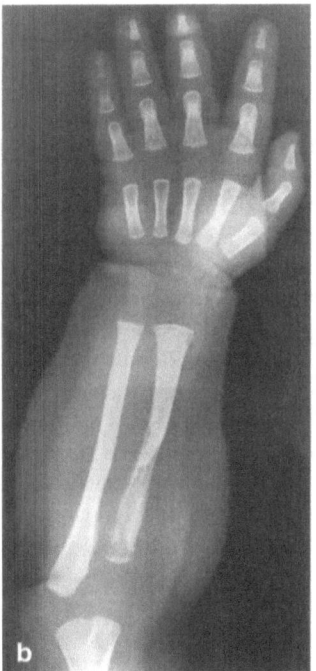

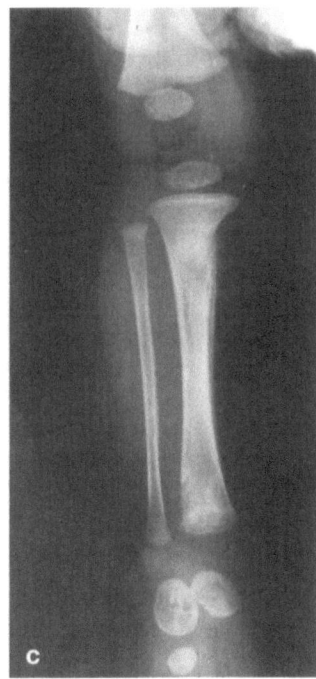

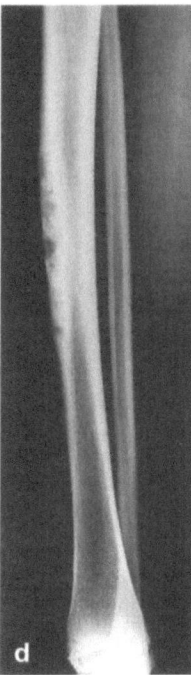

gumma formation. *Syphilitic periostitis* predominantly affects the anterior tibial margin and calvarium, which show solid periosteal new bone formation that may fuse with the subjacent cortex. The new bone may contain lucent areas representing gummatous cavities (Fig. 4.2 d). Differentiation is required from other periosteal reactions like those associated with varicose veins or the hypertrophic osteoarthropathy occurring in certain lung diseases. These changes are rarely as pronounced as those in syphilitic periostitis. The cranial and tibial changes may resemble fibrous dysplasia.

Gumma formation in acquired syphilis involves the development of circumscribed, rubbery nodules within the medullary canal and on superficial bone areas (e.g., the frontal bone, sternum, tibia, and clavicles). These lesions appear grossly as dry, gelatinous-appearing, caseating nodules that cause osteolysis predisposing to spontaneous fracture. Radiographs usually show a central lytic defect, occasionally combined with a sequestrum. Peripheral osteolytic lesions with an accompanying periosteal reaction are also seen.

References

Braun-Falco O, Plewig G, Wolff HH (1996) Dermatologie und Venerologie. Springer, Berlin Heidelberg New York

Murray RO, Jacobson HG (1977) The radiology of skeletal disorders, 2nd edn. Churchill Livingstone, Edinburgh

4.3 Actinomycosis

Firm, woody, bluish-red soft-tissue swelling (cervicofacial, thoracic, or abdominal) with small sinuses that exude pus on compression; "sulfur granules."
Roentgen signs: destruction of adjacent bones (i.e., the mandible).

Definition

Actinomycosis is an endogenous mixed infection caused by a gram-positive bacterium. The infection usually originates from the oropharynx and spreads hematogenously or, more commonly, by direct continuity to other tissues, where it produces a characteristic soft-tissue infiltration, usually with draining sinuses, that may destroy adjacent structures such as bone.

General Clinical Features, Dermatology, Radiology

Actinomycosis is an obligate endogenous mixed infection most commonly caused by *Actinomyces israelii* or *Actinomyces gerencseriae*. The pathogenic organisms are anaerobic or microaerophilic and grow in colonies composed of densely intertwined filaments. These colonies form the gritty, grayish-yellow or reddish "sulfur granules" that are found when the pus from actinomycotic lesions is spread beneath a coverslip on a microscope slide. Actinomycetes may occur on the skin and as a component of the normal intraoral flora. In the great majority of cases, trauma to the skin or mucous membranes allows the organisms to gain access to adjacent tissues, where an inflammatory granulation tissue forms and undergoes purulent liquefaction. This leads to multiple abscess formation and fibrous tissue proliferation with the formation of draining sinus tracts. The *areas of soft-tissue infiltration typically are indurated with bluish-red discoloration of the overlying skin and multiple small sinuses*, closely resembling neoplastic infiltration (Fig. 4.3).

Bone destruction in actinomycosis is generally a result of direct inflammatory infiltration. *Cervicofacial* actinomycosis is distinguished from the *thoracic* and *abdominal* forms and is of pri-

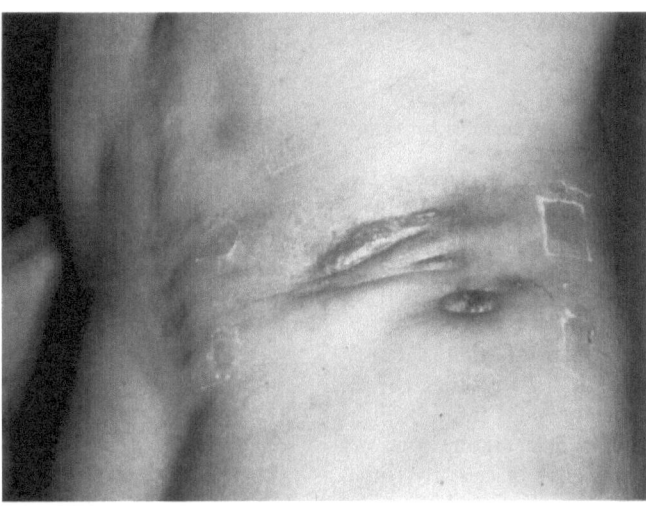

Fig. 4.3. Abdominal actinomycosis, marked by a typical woody swelling in the right lumbar region with at least four draining sinuses. The "sulfur granules" in the draining pus have a gritty feel when spread beneath a coverslip on a microscope slide

mary interest in this monograph, accounting for nearly 95% of all actinomycotic infections. Typically, cervicofacial actinomycosis is a mixed infection of mucous membranes that occurs following the extraction of a decayed tooth or a chronic, suppurative sinusitis. The initial manifestation consists of firm inflammatory nodules with associated buccal or submandibular swelling. This may give rise to a secondary cutaneous actinomycosis. The infection tends to spread along the side of the neck, producing a large, woody, infiltrative swelling over the angle of the jaw. The overlying skin is warm to the touch, shows bluish-red discoloration, and is riddled with sinuses that exude pus when compressed. The inflammatory process usually spreads to the mandible, causing extensive bone destruction. In rare untreated cases the process may infiltrate the muscles and spread to the cervical vertebrae. Hematogenous spread, especially to bone, is extremely rare. With prompt initiation of antibiotic treatment, the disease has a favorable prognosis.

References

Everts EC (1970) Cervicofacial actinomycosis. Arch Otolaryngol 92: 468

4.4 Mycetoma

Madura foot: tumefaction with livid skin discoloration, abscesses, and draining sinus tracts; little pain.
Roentgen signs: coarse, sometimes honeycomb-like pattern of bone destruction in the foot with reactive sclerosis; often a coarse, bristly periosteal reaction.

Mycetoma is a chronic infection acquired through a skin wound and characterized by abscess formation, draining sinus tracts, and the potential destruction of adjacent soft tissues and bone. Two different groups of causative organisms have been identified: the schizomycete group, including *Actinomyces israelii*, *Nocardia*, and *Streptomyces*; and true fungi (eumycetes), which include the *Madurella* species. Thus, the disease may be classified either as actinomycotic mycetoma or as eumycotic mycetoma (true maduromycosis). The latter was first observed in southern India and affected the foot almost exclusively, giving rise to the term "madura foot." Infections of the hand or other skeletal regions are relatively rare. Madura foot is not confined to southern India and may occur in any tropical region (Mexico, Africa, etc.) where hygienic conditions are poor and people often go barefoot. The soil-dwelling organisms enter the skin through small wounds (rhagades) or abrasions, usually in a hyperkeratotic sole. Once inside the tissue, the organisms form abscesses and sinus tracts, spreading through the plantar aponeurosis to attack the muscle and bone. This results in bone destruction with cavitary defects and reactive sclerosis.

Radiographs of the madura foot (Fig. 4.4 a) demonstrate multiple irregular bone erosions, honeycomb-like osteolytic defects, and thickened, irregular areas of periosteal and endosteal new bone formation. Anyone seeing an X-ray of the madura foot will not forget it. The *radiographic differential diagnosis* mainly includes tuberculous osteomyelitis of the foot, which generally is less proliferative, and advanced diabetic osteoarthropathy. Clinical inspection of the foot should quickly suggest the correct diagnosis (Fig. 4.4 b) by the massive tumefaction, livid skin discoloration, and multiple sinus tracts draining

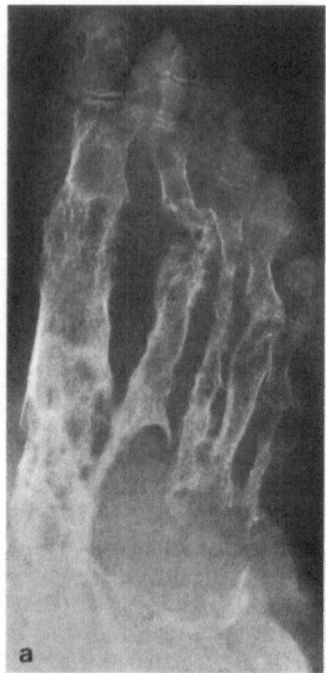

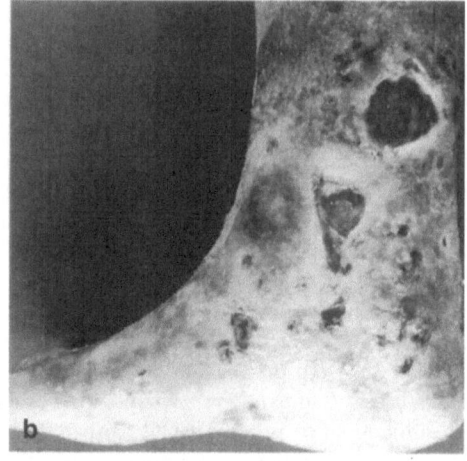

Fig. 4.4 a, b. Madura foot (from Gold and Mirra 1987). **a** Radiographic appearance. **b** Clinical appearance

blood and pus. The frequent absence of significant pain is noteworthy.

References

Gold RH, Mirra JM (1987) Case report 442: Madura foot (mycetoma pedis). Skeletal Radiol 16: 577
Reeder MM, Palmer PES (1981) The radiology of tropical disease. Williams & Wilkins, Baltimore, pp 364–378

4.5 Bacillary (Epitheloid) Angiomatosis in AIDS

Angiomatous papules; constitutional symptoms.

Roentgen signs: focal osteolytic bone lesions with periosteal reaction; positive radionuclide scans.

Definition

Bacillary angiomatosis is a multisystem infectious disease involving the reticuloendothelial system, mucous membranes, and especially the skin, which may show characteristic papular lesions consisting histologically of round vascular proliferations with prominent endothelial cells. The etiologic agents are the *Rickettsia*-like bacteria *Rochalimaea quintana*, *Rochalimaea henselae*, and *Bartonella bacilliformis*, which are similar to the causative bacterium of cat scratch disease.

General Clinical, Dermatologic, and Radiologic Features

HIV infections and AIDS may be associated with various musculoskeletal changes, most notably bacterial myositis (usually caused by *Staphylococcus aureus*), *HIV-associated seronegative disorders*, and acute *symmetric polyarthritis* (Freyschmidt 1993, 1997).

Non-Hodgkin lymphoma of the bone and osteomyelitis (septic, opportunistic) are relatively uncommon. We cannot discuss all these entities here, as most AIDS patients are referred to a specialist for dominant symptoms that are extracutaneous and extraskeletal (e.g., pulmonary or central nervous system involvement). The problem is different with bacillary angiomatosis, whose dominant features may be the cutaneous lesions and skeletal changes described below.

Bacillary angiomatosis is an opportunistic infection that presents clinically with fever, chills, night sweats, and weight loss. The liver, spleen, and lymph nodes may be enlarged. Mucosal involvement may lead to conjunctivitis and tracheobronchitis.

The dermatologic hallmark of bacillary angiomatosis is the *angiomatous papule*, which may be multiple and may occur on the upper trunk, face, and extremities. It appears as an erythematous, lentil-sized papule with well-defined borders that may be covered with hemorrhagic crusts. Hettmannsperger et al. (1993) note that the scaly collarette surrounding the papule (Fig. 4.5 a) serves to distinguish the lesion from Kaposi sarcoma (Fig. 4.5 b) and pyogenic granuloma (granuloma teleangiectaticum). Also, pyogenic granuloma is usually solitary. Histologic examination of cutaneous and visceral lesions shows *capillary proliferation* in an *edematous stroma* with myriad polymorphonuclear leukocytes. The bacterium can be identified in affected tissues by silver staining, electron microscopy, or antibody reaction. It is extremely difficult to culture, unlike the bacillus of cat scratch disease.

The *skeletal changes* in bacillary angiomatosis consist of destructive lesions in both tubular and flat bones, which may have a moth-eaten appearance with interrupted periosteal reactions and an overlying soft-tissue mass (Fig. 4.5 c, d). The ultimate radiographic picture is that of an aggressive osteomyelitis. Interestingly, the skeletal changes may precede the appearance of other symptoms, especially the cutaneous papules. Because osteolytic and osteomyelitic lesions due to other causes are extremely rare in AIDS, the presence of these radiographic changes in AIDS patients should raise immediate suspicion of bacillary angiomatosis. The *differential diagnosis* is aided by the fact that Kaposi sarcoma generally does not cause bone destruction. The radiographic differential diagnosis in AIDS patients also includes *non-Hodgkin lymphoma of bone*, but this lesion is also rare. In the series of Mitrou et al. (1991), only 3 of the 36 primary extranodal manifestations were located in bone. It is estimated that some 40% of patients with bacillary angiomatosis have skeletal involvement, suggesting a relatively high prevalence of osteolytic lesions in AIDS patients with bacillary angiomatosis.

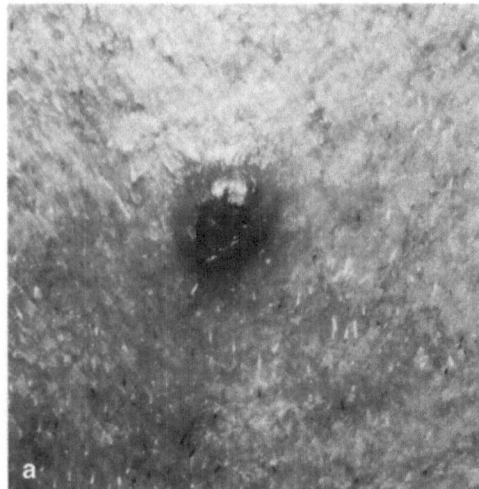

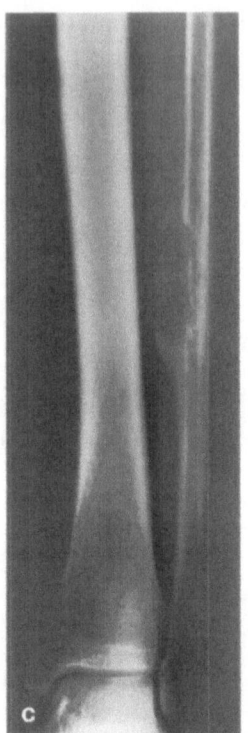

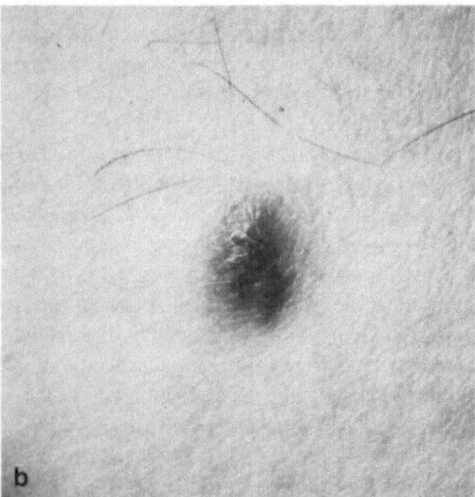

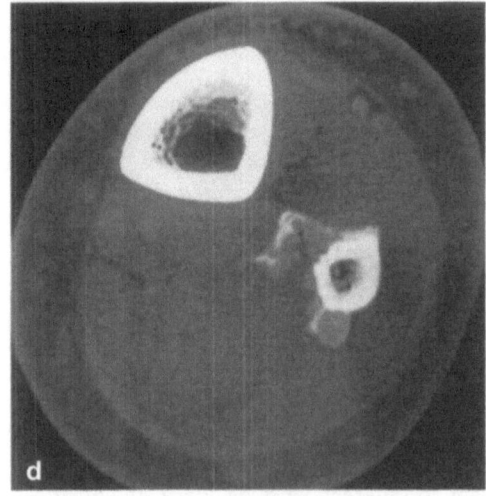

Fig. 4.5. a Angiomatous papule with central ulceration and a scaly collarette. **b** Typical Kaposi sarcoma. **c, d** Focus of bacillary angiomatosis in the fibula. Note the circumscribed "moth-eaten" lesions in the distal fibular shaft with partial destruction of the cortex on the tibial side. Spurs of periosteal new bone "encircle" the paraosseous soft tissues

References

Baron AL, Steinbach LS, Le Boit PE et al. (1990) Osteolytic lesions and bacillary angiomatosis in HIV infection: Radiologic differentiation from AIDS-related Kaposi sarcoma. Radiology 177: 77

Cockerell CJ (1992) The causative agent of bacillary angiomatosis. Int J Dermatol 31: 615

Freyschmidt J (1997) Skeletterkrankungen. Klinisch-radiologische Diagnose und Differentialdiagnose. 2. Aufl. Springer, Berlin Heidelberg New York Tokyo, S 699 ff.

Gomez-Jorge JT, Donabue F, Ganz W (1996) Osseous manifestation of bacillary angiomatosis. Skeletal Radiol 25: 505

Hettmannsperger U, Soehnchen R, Gollnick H et al. (1993) Bazilläre epitheloide Angiomatose bei fortgeschrittener HIV-Infektion. Hautarzt 44: 803

Mitrou PS, Serke M, Pohl C et al. (1991) Mit der HIV-Infektion assoziierte maligne Lymphome. Dtsch Med Wochenschr 116: 1217

5 Neoplastic and Granulomatous Diseases

5.1 Lymphoma

While primary extranodal lymphomas of the skin and bone do exist, they do not fall within our present scope. Only generalized (stage IV) lymphomas with cutaneous *and* skeletal manifestations fulfill the criteria of this monograph. As a rule, however, these patients have already been diagnosed and have been in the care of an oncologic specialist for some time, so the osseocutaneous signs of their disease are not a major diagnostic issue.

5.2 Mycosis Fungoides

Definition

Mycosis fungoides is a cutaneous T-helper-cell lymphoma (OKT-4+) whose various manifestations are initially limited to the skin and rarely spread to involve the internal organs and bone. From an oncologic standpoint, mycosis fungoides shows similarities to Sézary syndrome, which may progress from "erythroderma" to "plaques" and finally to a "tumor" stage with potential involvement of the bone marrow and lymph nodes.

General Clinical and Dermatologic Features

The estimated incidence of mycosis fungoides in Germany is approximately 0.1–1 case per 100,000 population per year. The etiology, genetics, and pathogenesis of this T-cell non-Hodgkin lymphoma, while certainly interesting, are beyond our present scope.

Mycosis fungoides is a *chronic disease* with variable and diverse manifestations. It is divided into three stages based on its dermatologic features (Alibert-Bazin classification). The cutaneous lesions that are typical of each stage may coincide.

1. The *premycotic stage* is marked by the gradual appearance of nonspecific cutaneous lesions that can mimic many other skin diseases such as nummular eczema, psoriasis vulgaris, and parapsoriasis en plaques. The lesions may appear as well-defined erythematous, scaly patches of variable size and shape (elliptical, round, arciform). Less commonly the lesions may be vesicular and bullous or covered with crusts. Sites of predilection are the trunk, extremities, and face. The lesions are pruritic.

2. The *infiltrative stage* (plaque stage) is marked by a plaquelike infiltration of lesions that either evolve from premycotic eruptions or develop on previously unaffected skin. The infiltrated areas have irregular but well-defined borders and may show scaling and crusting. Their color varies from red to reddish-brown or violaceous (Fig. 5.2). Peripheral extension and confluence occasionally lead to prominent raised areas (leonine facies). Larger lesions may encompass "islands" of normal skin. Pruritus that was present in the premycotic stage continues into the plaque stage.

3. *Tumor stage.* After the disease has been present for some years, tumors develop in existing plaquelike or erythematous lesions. The hemispheric tumors are relatively soft and sessile and have a tomato- or mushroom-like appearance. They are bluish-red or brownish-red in color and may ulcerate. It is common for tumors to regress spontaneously, leaving anular, crescent-shaped, or reniform remnants. Pruritus diminishes in this stage.

4. The *erythroderma form* has as its primary manifestation an initially nonspecific erythroderma followed by the development of a specific erythroderma with infiltration. The skin is reddened, thickened, and indurated.

Mucous Membrane Involvement

The oral mucosa, tongue, tonsils, and nasopharyngeal mucosa may be involved at any stage of the disease. Although mycosis fungoides is usually a cutaneous disease initially, it may eventually involve internal organs, lymph nodes, and the bone marrow, as in other forms of non-Hodgkin lymphoma.

Radiology

Very severe tumor growths can cause erosion of the underlying bone, especially in the facial skeleton and, as we have observed, in the calvarium. In patients with leukemic manifestations of mycosis fungoides and of Sézary syndrome, tumor cell proliferation can create a "moth-eaten" pattern of cancellous bone destruction (via osteoclasts). Rare cases may also show coarse areas of cortical bone destruction with involvement of adjacent soft tissues that resembles osseous involvement by malignant lymphoma.

References

Braun-Falco O, Plewig G, Wolff HH (1984) Dermatologie und Venerologie. Springer, Berlin Heidelberg New York, S 931 ff.

Classen M, Diehl V, Kochsiek K (1994) Innere Medizin, 3. Aufl. Urban & Schwarzenberg, München, S 187 f., 197

Edelson RL (1980) Cutaneous T cell lymphoma: Mycosis fungoides, Sézary syndrome, and other variants. J Am Acad Dermatol 2: 89

Kresbach H (1981) Mycosis fungoides. In: Korting GW (Hrsg) Dermatologie in Praxis und Klinik. Thieme, Stuttgart, 39.27 ff.

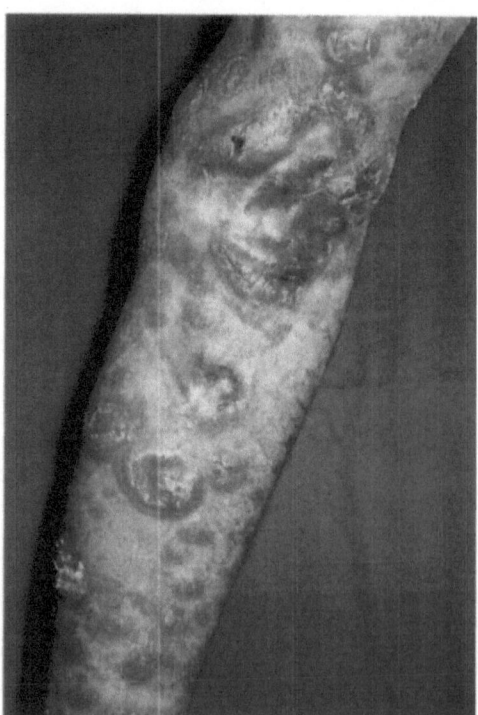

Fig. 5.2. Infiltrative-tumor stage of mycosis fungoides

5.3 POEMS Plasmacytoma

Diffuse grayish-brown to reddish-brown hyperpigmentation accompanied by edema of the trunk and lower extremities, also hypopigmented areas with scleroderma-like skin thickening involving the axillae, umbilical region, and trunk.

Roentgen signs: solitary or multiple areas of sclerosis.

Definition

POEMS plasmacytoma is a rare, special form of plasmacytoma whose overall features and prognosis differ from the more common plasma cell neoplasias such as multiple myeloma and disseminated non-osteolytic myelomatosis. POEMS is an acronym for the cardinal features of the syndrome: polyneuropathy, organomegaly, endocrinopathy, monoclonal protein, and skin changes.

General Clinical Features

In the majority of POEMS cases, lambda light-chain proteins are produced by the plasma cells. Fewer plasma cells are found in the bone marrow than in classic plasmacytoma. This finding has led some authors to classify POEMS syndrome as a plasma cell dysplasia rather than a true neoplasia. The syndrome responds swiftly and favorably to chemotherapy or radiation therapy (to affected skeletal segments).

Averaging 44 years of age, patients with POEMS syndrome are generally younger than plasmacytoma patients. Men are affected four times more often than women.

The organomegaly affects the liver, spleen, and lymph nodes. Endocrinopathic features include an elevated estrogen level with gynecomastia in men and amenorrhea in women. Glucose intolerance may also occur.

The polyneuropathy does not result from a secondary amyloidosis like that seen with long-standing plasma myeloma but is caused partly by anti-myelin-sheath autoantibodies that are formed by the plasma cells. These autoantibodies may also relate to the sclerotic, non-osteo-

lytic bone changes that are the radiographic hallmark of POEMS syndrome.

Lautenschlager and Itin (1993) described a case in which chronic urticaria, leukocytoclastic vasculitis, intermittent fever, bone pain with associated areas of sclerosis, and a monoclonal gammopathy developed in a 60-year-old man over a 10-year period. The authors ascribed these changes to **Schnitzler** syndrome, whose dominant features are a monoclonal IgM gammopathy with chronic urticaria, fever, and joint pain. The authors noted the difficulty of differentiating that condition from POEMS syndrome. Although the syndromes have different dermatologic symptoms and polyneuropathy was not present in the case described, it can be speculated that Schnitzler syndrome may be a variant or incomplete form of POEMS syndrome. It is known that the symptoms represented by the "POEMS" acronym may be metachronous: symptoms that have been absent for years may supervene on symptoms already present. In a recent paper (Lecompte et al. 1998) about Schnitzler's syndrome the authors deny explicitly a relationship to POEMS-Syndrome.

Dermatology

The dermatologic literature to date contains few reports on the cutaneous manifestations of POEMS. They consist of diffuse, grayish-brown to reddish-brown hyperpigmentation accompanied by edema, mainly affecting the trunk and lower extremities (Fig. 5.3 a). Interspersed hypopigmented areas with sclerodermiform skin thickening are found in the axillary and umbilical regions and may involve smaller areas on the trunk (Fig. 5.3 b).

It may be helpful in this context to review the classic cutaneous manifestations – both specific and nonspecific – of plasmacytoma. *Specific skin lesions* may occur in the setting of a primary extraosseous plasmacytoma and consist of multiple small red papules or nodules that grow and may metastasize in the skin. Other specific plasmacytoma lesions are cutaneous or subcutaneous nodules that have metastasized from a plasmacytoma of bone. More aggressive tumors may break through the cortex and infiltrate the overlying subcutaneous tissue and skin. Suggestive changes visible within the oral cavity include coarsening of the gingiva and/or polypous growths and tumors with a shiny red surface. The *nonspecific skin lesions* of plasmacytoma can result from *amyloid deposition* in the skin and tongue (macroglossia!). Additionally, cryo-

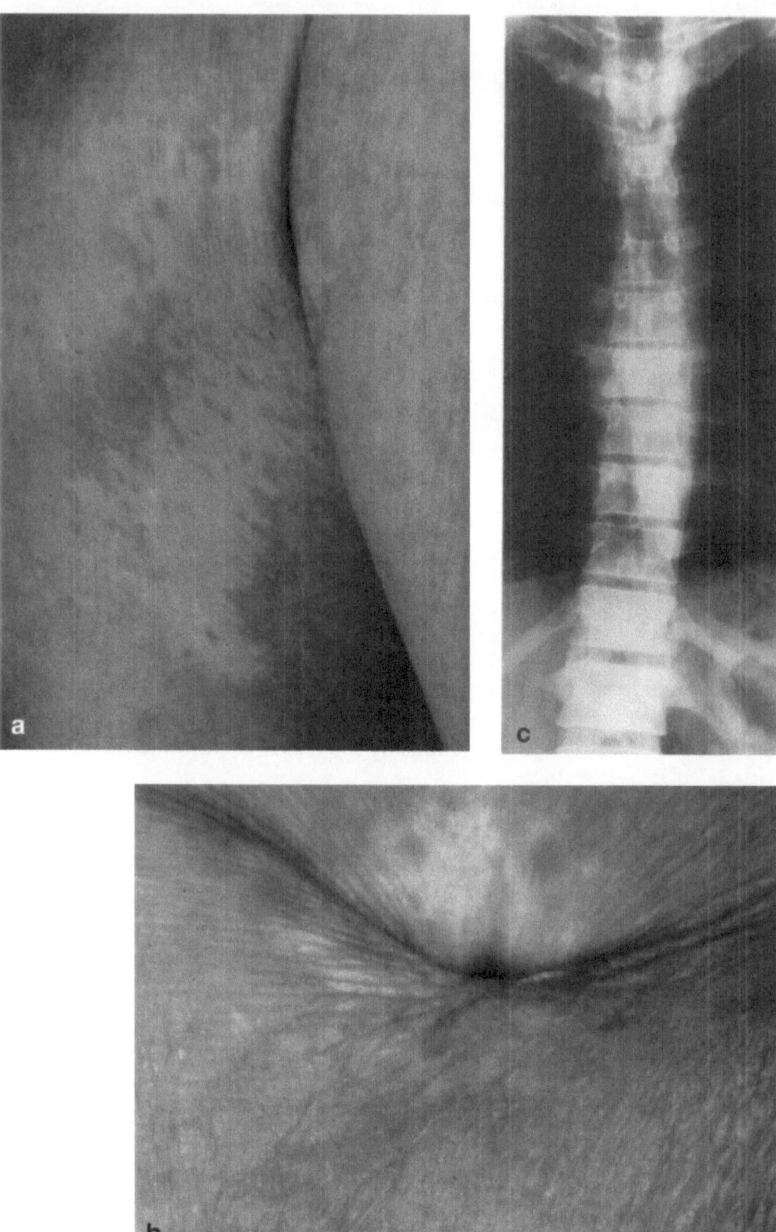

Fig. 5.3 a–e. POEMS syndrome. **a** Typical grayish-brown to reddish-brown hyperpigmentation alternating with hypopigmented areas. **b** Sclerodermiform skin thickening in the periumbilical region. (Photo from the collection of Prof. Dr. S. Borelli, Director, Department of Dermatology, Technical University of Munich) **c, d** Disseminated sclerotic bone changes in a 39-year-old man. The T10, T12 and L1 vertebral bodies are almost completely opaque, and patchy sclerosis is visible in the sacrum, the posterior portions of the left ilium, the right ischium, and the right proximal femur. **e** Unusual presentation of an initially solitary plasmacytoma in the humerus, showing extensive sclerotic areas in the shaft and proximal metaphysis with thinning of the cortex (different patient). Clinical symptoms included pain and signs of polyneuropathy. Years passed before cutaneous lesions appeared. **d, e** see p. 147

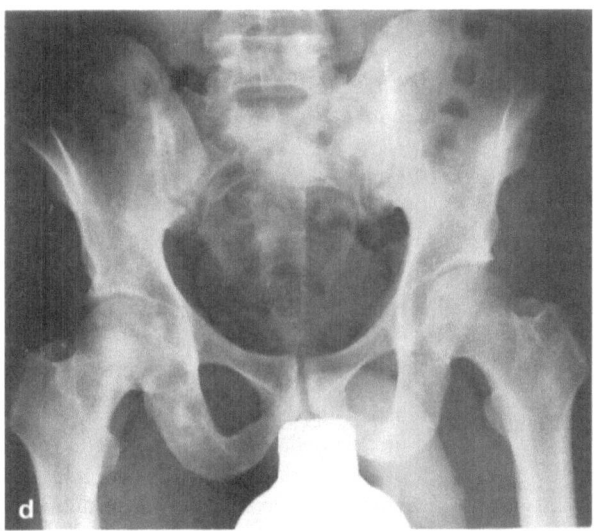

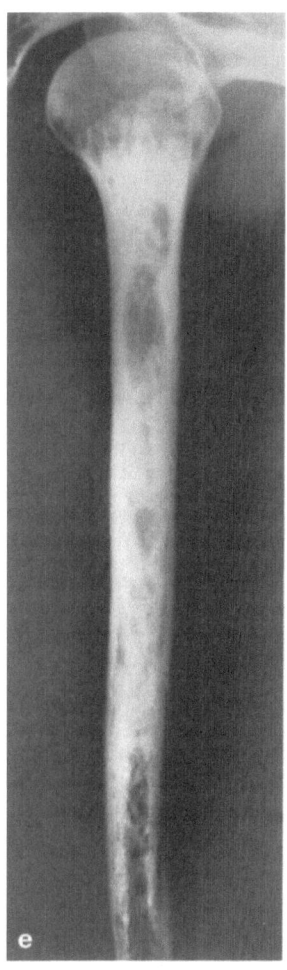

Fig. 5.3 d, e. See legend on p. 146

globulin formation and precipitation in the superficial cutaneous vessels can lead to *cold-induced purpura*, marble skin, Raynaud's phenomenon, and occasionally to urticaria, necrosis, and ulcerations of the skin. Other nonspecific dermatologic signs are scleromyxedema (elephant-like skin thickening, lichenoid nodules, hyperpigmentation, scleroderma-like features), pyoderma gangrenosum (chronic cutaneous gangrene based on a hyperergic reaction), planar xanthomas, and complicated infections (e.g., generalized herpes zoster).

Radiology

The very diverse radiologic features of plasmacytoma are beyond our scope. While classic plasmacytoma or multiple myeloma is marked chiefly by destructive bone changes in the form of severe osteoporosis and/or disseminated osteolytic lesions, POEMS syndrome is characterized by productive bone changes in the form of multiple or solitary *osteosclerotic foci* in the spine and pelvis (Fig. 5.3 c, d). Osteolytic lesions are infrequent and, when present, are surrounded by a sclerotic rim. The pathogenesis of the osteosclerosis is unclear but may relate to osteoblast-stimulating substances formed by plasma cells that are analogous to the osteoclast-stimulating factor (OSF,

OAF) produced in classic plasmacytoma. It has also been postulated that an autoantibody in POEMS syndrome completely inhibits the synthesis of osteoclast-stimulating factor, allowing reactive bone formation to occur around focies of plasmacell-infiltration.

It is interesting to note that the osteosclerotic areas may appear negative on radionuclide bone scans and may disappear in response to chemotherapy. The absence of radiotracer uptake indicates that the foci are no longer metabolically active when detected.

References

Brandon C, Martel W, Weatherbee L et al. (1989) Osteo-sclerotic myeloma (POEMS syndrome). Skeletal Radiol 18: 542

Freyschmidt J (1997) Skeletterkrankungen. Klinisch-radiologische Diagnose und Differentialdiagnose, 2. Aufl. Springer, Berlin Heidelberg New York

Hall FM, Gore SM (1988) Osteosclerotic myeloma variants. Skeletal Radiol 17: 101

Hermann G, Sherry H, Rabinowitz G (1981) Solitary plasmocytoma associated with peripheral neuropathy. Skeletal Radiol 6: 217

Kelly JJ, Kyle RA, Miles JM et al. (1983) Osteosclerotic myeloma and peripheral neuropathy. Neurology 33: 202

Lautenschlager ST, Itin PH (1993) Das Schnitzler-Syndrom. Hautarzt 44: 781

Lecompte M, Blais G, Bisson G et al. (1998) Schnitzler's syndrome. Skeletal Radiol 27: 294

Resnick D, Greenway GD, Bardwick PA (1981) Plasma-cell dyscrasia with polyneuropathy, organomegaly, POEMS-syndrome. Radiology 140: 17

Schnitzler L, Hurez D, Verret JL (1989) Urticaire chronique – ostéocondensation – macroglobulinémie. Cas princeps. Etude sur 20 ans. Ann Dermatol Venerol 116: 547

Tanaka O, Ohsawa T (1984) The POEMS-syndrome. Radiologe 24: 472

5.4 Langerhans Cell Histiocytosis

Synonyms: Histiocytosis X, Langerhans cell granulomatosis

Langerhans cell histiocytosis can lead to four clinical syndromes whose pathogenesis involves a proliferation of Langerhans cells:

1. Abt-Letterer-Siwe syndrome
2. Hand-Schüller-Christian syndrome
3. Eosinophilic granuloma
4. Erdheim-Chester lipoid granulomatosis.

While the first three disorders are definitely part of the Langerhans cell histiocytosis spectrum, the inclusion of Erdheim-Chester lipoid granulomatosis is still controversial. Lichtenstein added the designation "X" in 1953 to underscore the unknown etiology of this disease group, but today we can omit the X, because we know that the above mentioned clinical syndromes are based on a focal proliferation of Langerhans cells. This proliferation can lead to only one lesion (i.e., skin, bone), to multiple lesions restricted to one organ system (i.e., skeleton), or to a multisystem disease. The first three syndromes (see above) share a common pathoanatomic feature – a focal accumulation of proliferating Langerhans cells accompanied by scattered multinuclear giant cells and varying numbers of eosinophilic granulomas. Ultrastructural examination of the proliferating Langerhans cells reveals Bierbeck granules in the cytoplasm, which distinguish the cells from normal histiocytes. The granules also occur in epidermal Langerhans cells. Abt-Letterer-Siwe disease, Hand-Schüller-Christian syndrome, and eosinophilic granuloma exist along a continuum, and one of these diseases may give way to another. *An additional feature of Hand-Schüller-Christian syndrome is the storage of lipoid (cholesterol ester) in the Langerhans cells, transforming them into foam cells. This transformation probably represents the transition between eosinophilic granuloma and lipoid granuloma in Hand-Schüller-Christian syndrome.* Finally, both disorders may resolve by going through a fibrotic or cicatricial stage in which a dense network of collagen or reticulin fibers is formed.

Studies by Brower et al. (1984) indicate that Erdheim-Chester lipoid granulomatosis should be classified as a fourth form of "histiocytosis X". Examining a lytic area in the proximal tibia, the authors found the typical morphologic pattern of eosinophilic granuloma but also saw areas in which the bony trabeculae had been replaced by connective tissue mixed with foamy histiocytes. The authors also found storage histiocytes in distal portions of the tibia that showed only sclerotic changes. They believed that the fibrosis combined with foamy histiocytes represented a transitional stage to the pathognomonic sclerotic bone changes of lipoid granulomatosis. This justifies the recognition of Erdheim-Chester lipoid granulomatosis as a special form of histiocytosis – X today known as Langerhans cell histiocytosis. There is no need to discuss Erdheim-Chester lipoid granulomatosis further in this monograph, as it is not known to have any specific cutaneous manifestations.

A newer classification based on clinical and prognostic criteria subdivides the histiocytoses into a *chronic focal histiocytosis*, which is localized and multicentric, and an *acute disseminated histiocytosis* (Bergholz et al. 1979). This concept avoids the blurred distinctions between the three classic forms of Langerhans cell histiocytosis. Because this classification is not yet widely used in dermatology, we shall retain the classic nomenclature in our further discussion of the histiocytoses.

5.4.1 Abt-Letterer-Siwe Syndrome

Abt-Letterer-Siwe syndrome is an acute or subacute progressive disseminated form of Langerhans cell histiocytosis characterized by typical skin lesions and visceral involvement. Frequently the prognosis is poor, especially with an early childhood onset. The peak incidence is in the first and second decades of life.

Clinically, affected children are seriously ill with septic temperatures, hepatosplenomegaly, swollen lymph nodes, and anemia. Pulmonary infiltrates and cystic transformation can lead to respiratory difficulties. Histiocytic infiltration may also involve the central nervous system.

The *cutaneous lesions* consist initially of fine, yellowish-brown, lightly scaling papules that may become hemorrhagic and necrotic. Nodular and ulcerative lesions are also observed. If untreated, these primary eruptions develop into a widely disseminated pattern of small, flat, brownish, crusted and scaly papules along with papulovesicular and papulopustular lesions, moist erosive lesions, and petechial hemorrhages. Sites of predilection are the scalp, ears, face, and trunk. The only skeletal changes described to date are a diffuse bone marrow infiltration by histiocytic cellular elements with incipient granuloma formation (without xanthomatous transformation).

5.4.2 Eosinophilic Granuloma

Circumscribed, plaquelike areas of inflammatory infiltration along with yellowish-brown papules on the scalp, temples, and anogenital region; plaquelike or nodular infiltrates in the oral mucosa.
Roentgen signs: geographic osteolytic lesions, some with sequestra; sclerotic margins in the healing stage (skull, pelvis, large tubular bones); vertebra plana.

Eosinophilic granuloma of bone is defined as a tumorlike, osteolytic proliferation of histiocytes (Langerhans cells) that can involve virtually any organ but generally is confined to the skeleton, showing a mono-, oligo- or polyostotic pattern of involvement. Multisystem involvement of lymph nodes, bone marrow, lungs, and skin is relatively rare and may signal progression to Hand-Schüller-Christian syndrome or lipoid granulomatosis.

Eosinophilic granuloma is classified as chronic focal histiocytosis in the Bergholz classification. Its prognosis is generally good, because the granulomas have a tendency to regress spontaneously or in response to radiation or cortisone therapy. Only rare cases (usually multicentric) involving skeletal segments that bear large stresses, such as the spine and femur, will require cytostatic therapy.

The prevalence of eosinophilic granuloma is uncertain, because a large percentage of cases apparently takes an asymptomatic course in which lesions are detected incidentally, i.e. after trauma. In our own retrospective analysis of 18 cases spanning a 12-year period, two-thirds of the cases were incidental diagnoses (Berning and Freyschmidt 1985). We believe that eosinophilic granuloma of bone is the most frequent cause of clinically silent osteolysis in children and adolescents. The peak incidence is in the first two decades, but primary adult manifestations may occur.

Unifocal eosinophilic granuloma is more common than the multifocal form. Multiple eosinophilic granulomas may exceed 40 in number, but the average number is 7. Multiple lesions may develop synchronously or metachronously in the same or different bones. Favored sites of involvement are, in decreasing frequency, the calvarium, femur, spine, pelvis, ribs, mandible, clavicle, humerus, tibia, and scapula.

As noted earlier, the lesions generally do not cause clinical complaints. Painless nodular swellings are sometimes found on the calvarium that correlate with radiographic bone defects. Granulomas that grow aggressively can cause pain and soft-tissue swellings that are not associated with significant hyperemia or local warmth. Sphenoid involvement may lead to orbital infiltration and exophthalmos. With spinal involvement, neurologic complications may be absent despite extensive destructive lesions. Unlike cranial manifestations, lesions located in tubular bones cause definite pain and swelling, especially in the lower extremities.

Most patients with chronic focal Langerhans cell histiocytosis do not have significant systemic manifestations. Laboratory findings generally are nonspecific. Multifocal lesions involving the skin and internal organs, however, lead to severe systemic manifestations with intermittent fever, weight loss, anemia, and an elevated ESR. Peripheral eosinophilia may be present, and the liver, spleen, and lymph nodes are enlarged. Pulmonary involvement can cause interstitial lung disease with a fine honeycomb pattern (due to hyperexpanded areas) with dyspnea and risk of spontaneous pneumothorax.

The *cutaneous lesions* consist of yellowish to brownish papules and circumscribed, plaquelike areas of inflammatory infiltration that may undergo painful ulceration. The scalp (Fig. 5.4.2 a), temporal areas, and anogenital region are most commonly involved. Examination of the oral mucosa may disclose plaquelike or nodular infiltrates that are prone to ulceration.

Radiographs (Fig. 5.4.2 b, c) generally show well-defined geographic lesions (punched-out lesions) that may have sclerotic margins. It is rare to find moth-eaten lytic lesions with cortical bone destruction and soft-tissue infiltration. Osteolytic lesions in the skull are round to elliptical in shape and may be 3 cm or more in diameter. Individual lytic areas sometimes coalesce to form large, geographic defects that may contain sequestra. The combination of calvarial bone defects with diabetes insipidus due to destruction of the sella and exophthalmos due to

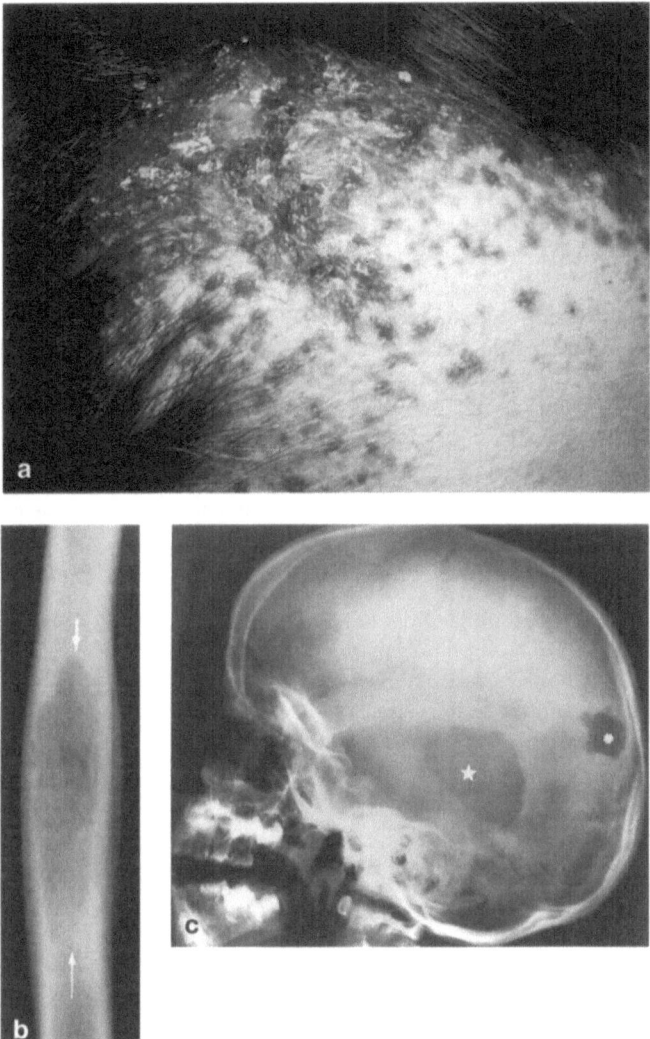

Fig. 5.4.2 a–c. Langerhans cell histiocytosis. **a** Scalp lesions consisting of plaquelike areas of inflammatory infiltration, some ulcerated, and brownish papules. Radiographs show typical foci of eosinophilic granuloma in the femur (**b**) and skull (**c**)

infiltration of the orbit is called the *Hand-Schüller-Christian triad.*

Lesions of the spine may involve the vertebral bodies, vertebral arches, or the transverse and spinous processes. Involvement of the vertebral bodies is most common and can rapidly lead to collapse of the affected vertebra (vertebra plana). Lesions in the pelvis resemble those in the calvarium. The small tubular bones of the hands and feet are almost always spared; lesions in oth-er long bones most commonly involve the diaphyses and diametaphyseal areas. More aggressive lesions may produce a moth-eaten pattern of cortical bone destruction accompanied by periosteal new bone formation. More slowly growing lesions tend to produce a well-defined lytic area. The periosteal reaction to diaphyseal lesions is usually of a solid or laminated type.

5.4.3 Hand-Schüller-Christian Syndrome

This disease is defined as a chronic form of Langerhans cell histiocytosis having the triad of features noted above. As mentioned in the introduction, the histiocytes in Hand-Schüller-Christian disease store lipoid; this transforms the histiocytes into foam cells and apparently differentiates the condition from eosinophilic granuloma. It is appropriate to ask whether Hand-Schüller-Christian "disease" might be more accurately described as the "chronic form of histiocytosis X" or merely as a special form of eosinophilic granuloma having the features of the Hand-Schüller-Christian triad.

As with multifocal eosinophilic granuloma, there may be involvement of the lungs, liver, spleen, and lymph nodes with corresponding systemic manifestations (see p. 150). The skin lesions are practically identical to those of eosinophilic granuloma and are described under that heading. The same applies to radiographic manifestations, especially in the calvarium. The prognosis is generally good, and the lesions spontaneously resolve in more than 50% of cases.

References

Bergholz M, Schauer A, Poppe H (1979) Diagnostic and differential diagnostic aspects in Histiocytosis X disease. Pathol Res Pract 166: 59

Berning W, Freyschmidt J (1985) Zur Klinik und Radiologie der Histiozytose X am Skelett – eine retrospektive Studie an 18 Patienten. Röntgenblätter 38: 400

Braun-Falco O, Plewig G, Wolff HH (1984) Dermatologie und Venerologie. Springer, Berlin Heidelberg New York

Brower AC, Worsham GF, Dudley AH (1984) Erdheim-Chester disease: a distinct lipoidosis or part of the spectrum of histiocytosis? Radiology 151: 35

Favara BE, Feller AC with members of the WHO committee on histiocytic/reticulum cell proliferation (1997) Contemporary classification of histiocytic disorders. Med Pediatr Oncol 29: 157

Freyschmidt J (1997) Skeletterkrankungen. Klinisch-radiologische Diagnose und Differentialdiagnose, 2. Aufl. Springer, Berlin Heidelberg New York

Freyschmidt J, Ostertag H, Lang W (1986) Erdheim-Chester disease. Case report 365. Skeletal Radiol 15: 316

Hefti F, Jundt G (1995) Langerhanszell Histiozytose. Orthopäde 24: 73

Lieberman PH, Jones CR, Steinman RM et al. (1996) Langerhans cell (eosinophilic) granulomatosis. A clinicopathologic study encompassing 50 years. Am J Surg Pathol 20: 519

McCullough (1980) Eosinophilic granuloma of bone. Acta Orthop Scand 51: 389

Resnick D (1981) Lipidosis histiocytosis and hyperlipoproteinemias. In: Resnick D, Niwayama G (eds) Diagnosis of bone and joint disorders. Saunders, Philadelphia, pp 1948–1991

Resnick D, Greenway G, Genant H et al. (1982) Erdheim-Chester disease. Radiology 142: 289

5.5 Multicentric Reticulohistiocytosis (MR)

Synonyms: lipoid dermatoarthritis, giant cell histiocytomatosis, reticulohistiocytic granuloma, giant cell reticulohistiocytosis, lipoid rheumatism

Firm, skin-colored to yellowish-red papules, sometimes with central molluscoid pitting, forming clusters mainly near joints and on oral and nasal mucosae.
Clinical signs: polyarthralgia, joint swelling.
Roentgen signs: any joint may be affected; marginal *and* central erosions and destructive lesions predominantly affecting the hands and feet; no osteoporosis or periosteal reactions.

Definition

Multicentric reticulohistiocytosis (MR) is a rare systemic granulomatous disease of the skin and synovial membranes whose joint manifestations consist of an erosive and destructive arthropathy.

General Clinical Features

The disease is based on the formation of granulomatous lesions composed of atypical, bizarre-shaped histiocytes with a finely granular cytoplasm and of multinucleated giant cells with a foamy-appearing, partially vacuolated cytoplasm. Apparently the different histologic components have contributed to the various names for the disorder. The granulomas occur mainly in the skin, subcutaneous tissue, and synovium and less commonly in the stomach, lungs, pleura, heart, bones, lymph nodes, muscles, liver, and kidneys.

Some 120 to 150 cases have been described in the previous literature. MR is probably far more common than these numbers would suggest, given the tendency for the disease to be *mistaken for a polyarthritis with negative rheumatoid factors*. MR is among the classic interdisciplinary disorders that are frequently and consistently misdiagnosed.

The disease seems to occur predominantly in women, and the average patient age is 40.

Joint complaints are usually polyarticular and consist of spontaneous arthralgias with pain on exertion. Clinical examination reveals swelling about the joints but no warmth or redness. Limitation of motion and instability can be demonstrated in affected joints.

Despite the sometimes extensive destructive bone lesions, especially in the hands and feet, MR has a favorable prognosis compared with rheumatoid arthritis, for example, as spontaneous remission may occur after the disease has run a course of about 6–8 years. However, residual joint damage will persist and culminate in a very severe degenerative arthritis. The involvement of parenchymal organs implies a poor prognosis.

Dermatology

The dominant cutaneous manifestation is a papular eruption consisting of firm, indolent, nonpruritic, smooth, skin-colored to yellowish- or brownish-red papules that are occasionally xanthoma-like and may show molluscoid central pitting. The lesions are disseminated over the skin and adjacent mucous membranes, especially the oral and nasal mucosae, and they tend to cluster around joints. In the case observed by the authors, the papules were irregularly distributed over the fingers, palms, and dorsal surfaces of both hands and formed sporadic clusters (Fig. 5.5 a). Only a few papules were visible on the lower legs.

Radiology

The radiographic manifestations of MR are produced by reticulohistiocytic granulomas, which occur within an edematous and highly vascularized stroma, especially on synovial surfaces. They produce the classic features of "synovial arthropathy," or joint disease originating from the synovium. The changes occur wherever there are articulations that have a synovial membrane. Most commonly affected are the joints of the fingers and toes, which are involved in some 70–80% of cases. Radiographs show well-defined defects or erosions at the joint margins and adjacent cortex and contour defects in the articular surface (Fig. 5.5 b, c, e). The joint space may be narrowed, although widening can result from coarse destruction of the articulating bone ends

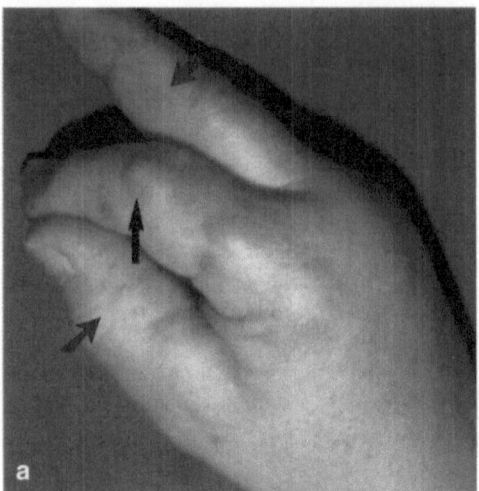

Fig. 5.5 a–e. Multicentric reticulohistiocytosis (37-year-old woman). **a** Disseminated papules on the fingers and distal dorsum of the hand (several clusters of lesions are marked with *arrows*). The radiographs in **b–e** show erosive and destructive lesions, some severe, involving the interphalangeal joints (**b**), carpal joints (**c**), hip joint (**d**), and metatarsophalangeal joints of the foot (**e**). Note the central location of the destructive changes in the interphalangeal joints and the complete absence of osteoporosis – a key differentiating criterion from rheumatoid arthritis. Note also the absence of periosteal reactions, differentiating this condition from psoriatic arthritis, for example. The changes had a bilaterally symmetric distribution. Destructive lesions were also found in the apophyseal joints of the cervical spine, the shoulder and elbow joints, and the knee and ankle joints

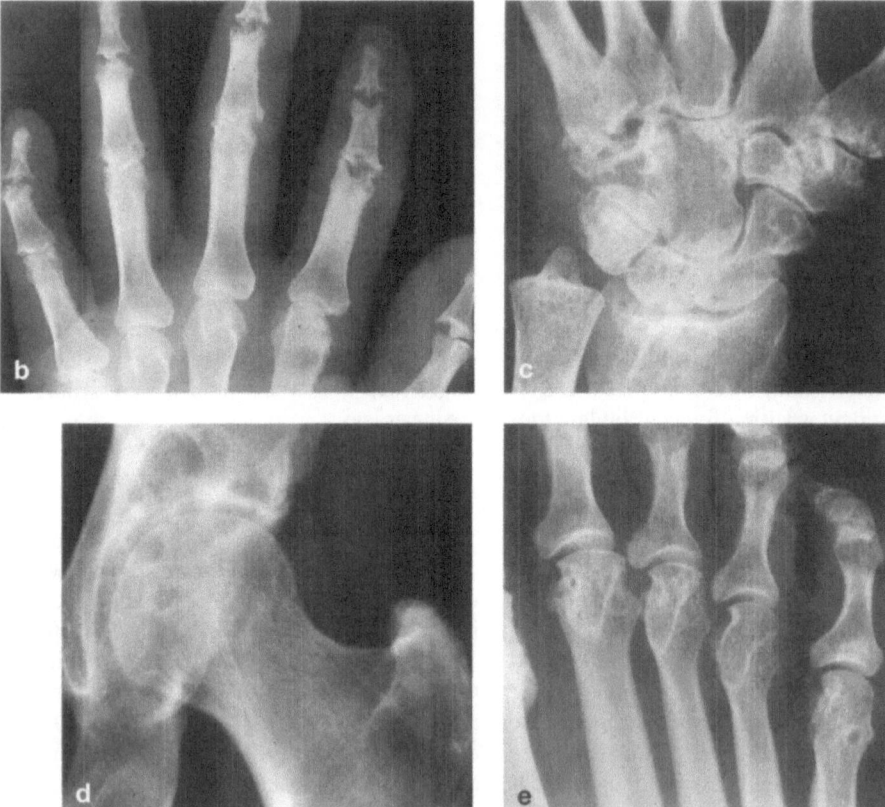

and edematous thickening of the synovium (Fig. 5.5 b). Various patterns are seen ranging to frank mutilation, but ankylosis apparently does not occur. In contrast to rheumatoid arthritis, peri-articular demineralization is not a feature. The absence of osteoproliferative changes aids in the differentiation from psoriatic arthritis. The overall differential diagnosis is challenging in cases where cutaneous lesions are absent or minimal at the time of initial presentation.

References

Erlich G, Young J, Nosheny SZ et al. (1972) Multi-centric reticulohistiocytosis (lipoid dermatoar-thritis), a multisystem disorder. Am J Med 52: 830

Freyschmidt J, Wilmowsky H von, Krmpotic L (1978) Multizentrische Retikulohistiozytose als Ursache einer „erosiv-destruktiven Arthropathie". Röfo 129: 605

Gold RH, Mezger AL, Mirra JM et al. (1975) Multicen-tric reticulohistiocytosis (lipoid dermato-ar-thritis). An erosive polyarthritis with distinctive clinical, roentgenographic and pathologic features. Am J Roentgenol 124: 610

Orkin M, Goltz RW, Good RA et al. (1964) A study of multicentric reticulohistiocytosis. Arch Dermatol 89: 610

5.6 Sarcoidosis

Synonym: Boeck's disease

Acute: erythema nodosum. *Chronic:* angio-lupoid (nose); disseminated papular form with purplish to brownish eruptions; circi-nate sarcoidosis (face, nuchal area); nodular-plaque form with violaceous plaques and lobulated nodules up to several centimeters in diameter (lupus pernio); mucous mem-brane involvement with glassy, padlike nod-ules or yellowish plaques.

Roentgen signs: lytic and sclerotic bone chang-es in the appendicular and axial skeleton with positive radionuclide scans; in the hand: polycystic, reticular-honeycomb pattern or larger bone defects, patchy cancellous osteo-sclerosis; characteristic chest radiograph.

Definition

Sarcoidosis is a noncaseating epitheloid cell granulomatosis with marked activation of the monocyte-macrophage system leading to multi-organ involvement with a predilection for the lung.

General Clinical Features

The prevalence of the disease in the German population is difficult to estimate, because a large percentage of cases are asymptomatic and undi-agnosed. Müller-Quernheim and Ferlinz (1988) report a prevalence of 43 cases per 100,000. The highest frequencies are found in Northern Europe, with a reported prevalence of 64 per 100,000 in Sweden versus only 0.04 in Spain. Women are affected slightly more often than men, and the peak incidence is at less than 40 years of age.

The etiology of the disease is unclear. Because the initial manifestations usually appear in the mediastinal and hilar lymph nodes and the lungs, the disease apparently is caused by an ex-ogenous agent that enters the body through the airways and incites a granulomatous tissue re-sponse. The granulomas are composed of epithe-loid cells, giant cells, activated macrophages, and predominantly activated T lymphocytes, which incite granuloma formation through the release of interleukin-2. During this process the epithe-loid cells and macrophages produce angiotensin converting enzyme (ACE), whose serum levels correlate with the total mass of granulomas in the various organ systems.

The disease may have an *acute* onset with severe constitutional symptoms, usually accompanied by erythema nodosum, uveitis, and/or *arthritis*. Cases with a subacute onset are generally asymp-tomatic and usually are detected incidentally on a chest radiograph. *Chronic* sarcoidosis is said to be present if the disease has lasted for more than 2 years. Most of these patients are over 30 years of age. Up to 20% of patients with lung involve-ment eventually develop pulmonary fibrosis, im-plying a less favorable prognosis. Almost half of these patients have extrathoracic manifestations. The general clinical aspects of sarcoidosis are be-yond our scope, but it may be noted that the di-agnosis is usually established by bronchoalveo-lar lavage demonstrating a characteristic shift in the ratio of T-helper cells to suppressor cells (to the range of 4:1 to 20:1) with a marked increase in total lymphocytes, combined with a positive chest radiograph and/or positive histology. The radiographic stages of thoracic involvement (stage 1: bilateral hilar adenopathy; stage 2: pul-monary parenchymal changes with granuloma formation; stage 3: interstitial fibrosis) have nothing to do with the clinical evolution of the disease. A full 80% of cases in stage 1 and stage 2 undergo complete resolution, while the chang-es in stage 3 are largely irreversible and tend to progress despite immunosuppressive therapy. Table 5.6 lists the frequencies of involvement of specific organ systems in sarcoidosis. Reports on the frequency of radiographic skeletal involve-ment range from 5.3% to 26% in the German-language literature. The Anglo-American litera-ture cites a 1% to 13% incidence of skeletal changes in patients with demonstrable pulmo-nary manifestations or involvement of other or-gan systems (Sartoris et al. 1985). This relatively large range of variation in the international lit-erature is due partly to the fact that skeletal in-volvement in sarcoidosis is often asymptomatic and that patients may or may not undergo radio-nuclide screening. A major reason is the lack of large-scale prospective studies based on the clin-ical stages of the disease.

Table 5.6. Frequency[a] of involvement of various or-gans in sarcoidosis. (According to Müller-Querheim and Ferlinz 1988)

Organ (system)	Involvement (frequency, %)
Lung	>95
Liver	25–70
Spleen	25–70
Prescalene lymph nodes	60–70
Skin	10–60
Erythema nodosum	30
Peripheral lymph nodes	30
Skeletal muscles	25
Eyes	10–25
Central nervous system	9
Myocardium	6
Bones	6
Lacrimal glands, salivary glands	4

[a] The frequencies vary greatly in different popula-tions, accounting for the large range of variation in published data.

The clinical manifestations of skeletal involve-ment are very diverse. As noted above, patients may be completely asymptomatic despite the presence of demonstrable lytic and sclerotic bone changes in the spine and appendicular skeleton. As a rule, destructive lesions of the spine must be extensive before neurologic symp-toms appear (Fig. 5.6 h, i). Up to 16% of patients with an acute disease onset complain of nonspe-cific arthralgias (Loefgren's syndrome) that mi-grate from joint to joint. Granulomatous syno-vitis generally is not present in these cases as an underlying lesion. Extensive involvement of the bone marrow can lead to a hypercalcemic syn-drome, with all its attendant complications, based on the ability of the sarcoid cells (macro-phages) to synthesize vitamin D and parathor-mone-like substances.

Dermatology

The typical dermatologic manifestation in the acute or subacute early stage of sarcoidosis is *erythema nodosum* (see p. 112, Fig. 3.6.4 a). It may appear as part of Loefgren's syndrome, which is characterized by erythema nodosum, bilateral mediastinal adenopathy, arthralgias, and a hy-poergic or anergic tuberculin skin test.

A rare, chronic facial manifestation of cutaneous sarcoidosis, most common in women, is *angio-*

lupoid, which chiefly involves the malar area and the bridge of the nose. It is characterized by soft, padlike lesions of a purplish brown color with telangiectases. On diascopic examination (glass-spatula pressure), the telangiectases disappear and a grayish-yellow "lupoid infiltrate" is seen. Angiolupoid shows little if any potential for spontaneous resolution and has a marked tendency to recur. The differential diagnosis should include pseudolymphoma, facial eosinophilic granuloma, lupus vulgaris, and acanthoma fissuratum.

The *disseminated papular form* of sarcoidosis (benign miliary sarcoid, Fig. 5.6 a) is characterized by purplish-brown maculopapular lesions ranging from the size of a pinhead to that of a small pea. Again, "lupoid infiltrate" is seen on diascopic examination. The probe sign is negative, in contrast to lupus vulgaris. Favored sites of occurrence are the face and the extensor surfaces of the extremities; the trunk and mucous membranes are less commonly involved. There may also be annular lesions with cleared atrophic centers.

Circinate sarcoidosis presents with bandlike, gyrate, slightly raised and scaly skin lesions that are yellowish-red in color (diascopic examination shows lupoid infiltrate). The typical pattern is one of centrifugal spread and central atrophy with depigmentation and central clearing. The *differential diagnosis* in patients with facial involvement should include necrobiosis lipoidica.

The *nodular-plaque form* of sarcoidosis consists of nodular or plaquelike lesions with a lobulated appearance that may reach several centimeters in diameter. They are purplish or brownish in color, have a firm consistency, and are associated with coarse telangiectases. The lesions most commonly involve the tip and bridge of the nose, the cheeks, and the earlobes; less common sites are the extremities and trunk. Larger sarcoid nodules on the face are often of a deep bluish-gray hue resembling pernio (chilblains), giving rise to the term *lupus pernio* (Fig. 5.6 c).

The *subcutaneous nodular type* of cutaneous sarcoidosis is associated with a palpable nodular infiltration. The overlying skin may appear normal or faintly violaceous. Sarcoid granulomas are present in the subcutaneous fat.

A notable feature of cutaneous sarcoidosis is its tendency to occur in scars. *Scar sarcoidosis* is attributed to a local inflammatory reaction leading to sarcoidal transformation of the scar tissue.

Mucous membrane manifestations of sarcoidosis may involve the conjunctiva, the nasal mucosa, the tonsillar and laryngeal mucosae, the buccal mucosa, or the palate. The lesions appear as padlike, glassy nodules or yellowish plaques that may ulcerate. Again, "lupoid infiltrate" is seen on diascopic examination.

The cutaneous lesions of sarcoidosis are rarely pruritic.

Radiology

The skeletal manifestations of sarcoidosis may consist of a diffuse infiltration of the medullary cavities by epithelioid cell granulomas with no visible effect on the surrounding bone. Once the granulomas interact with the surrounding bone, however, they can cause perigranulomatous destructive lesions in the cancellous bone or incite an early reactive sclerosis that shows increased uptake on bone scans and produces well-defined sclerotic densities on X-ray films.

The formation of epithelioid cell granulomas in the synovium can incite an acute, subacute, or chronic synovitis.

The pathoanatomic changes described above form the basis for the radiographic manifestations of sarcoidosis, which can be quite diverse. The skeletal manifestations include punched-out osteolytic lesions as well as permeative and "moth-eaten" areas of cortical bone destruction. The permeative pattern is caused by perivascular granuloma formation around vessels in the haversian canals. Osteosclerotic changes accompany the lytic destruction. There may be a disseminated skeletal involvement, which is rare, or the changes may be localized and perhaps limited to a single focus. We know from experience that sclerotic changes are more common in the axial skeleton (Fig. 5.6 h, j – m) while destructive lesions are more common in the appendicular skeleton.

The skeletal lesions in sarcoidosis primarily involve the small bones of the hands and feet (Fig. 5.6 e – g). Any of several forms may be encountered:

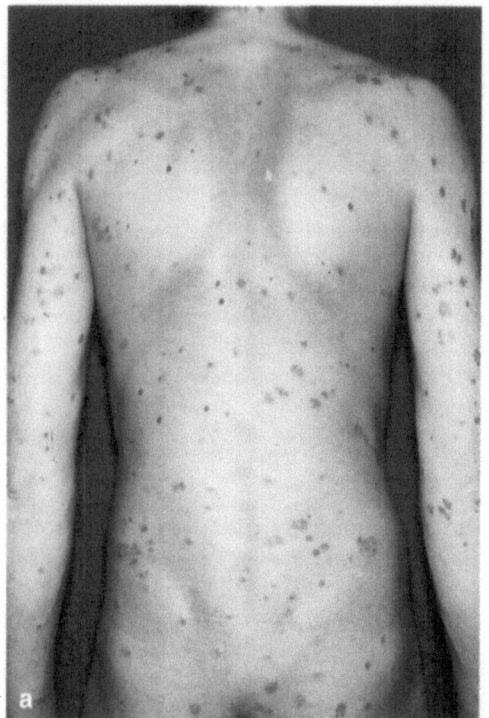

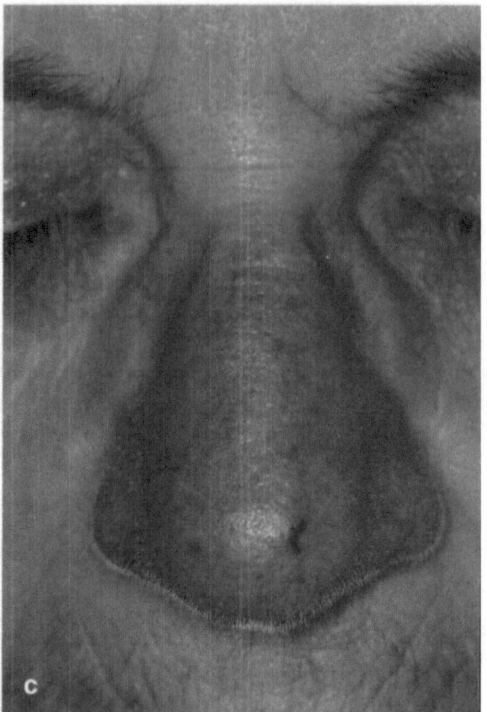

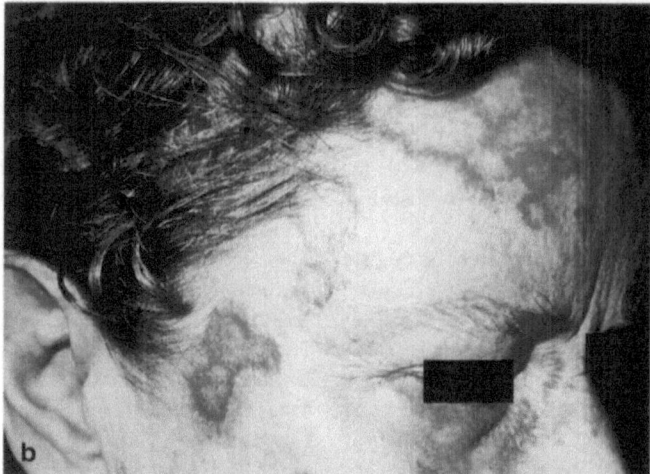

Fig. 5.6 a–m. Sarcoidosis. **a** Diffuse papular form with macropapular lesions ranging from the size of a pinhead to the size of a small pea. "Lupoid infiltrate" is seen on diascopic examination. **b** Circinate sarcoid lesions on the face. **c** Lupus pernio. **d** Typical radiographic appearance of sarcoidosis (radiographic stage 2) with bilateral hilar adenopathy and interstitial pulmonary infiltrates. **d–m** see pp. 159–161

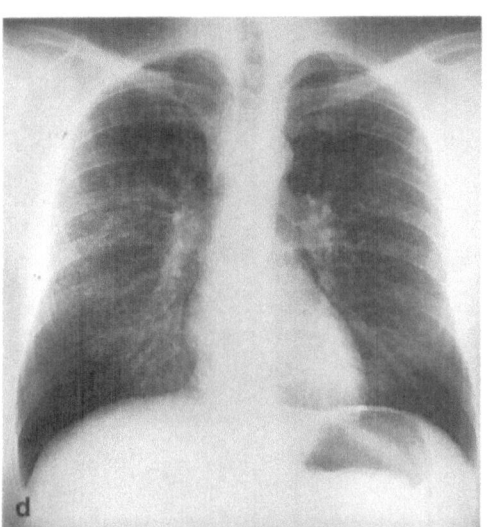

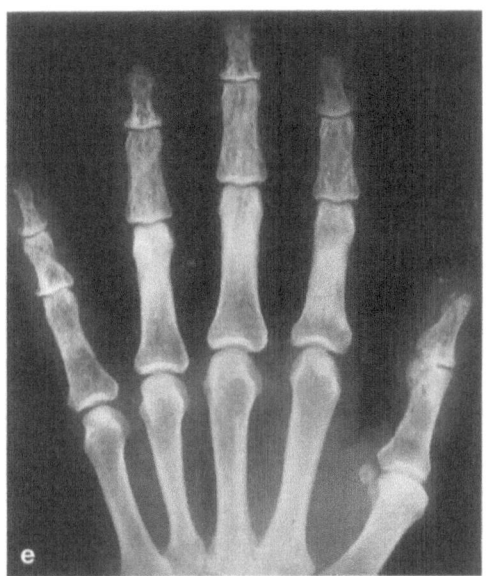

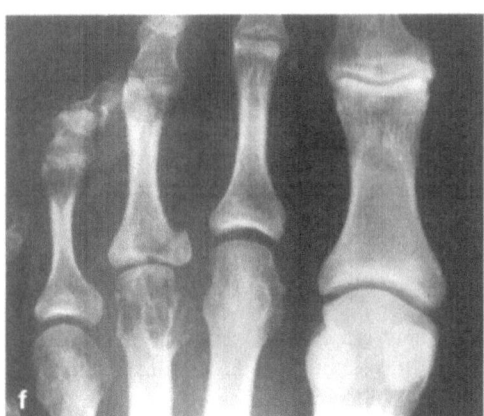

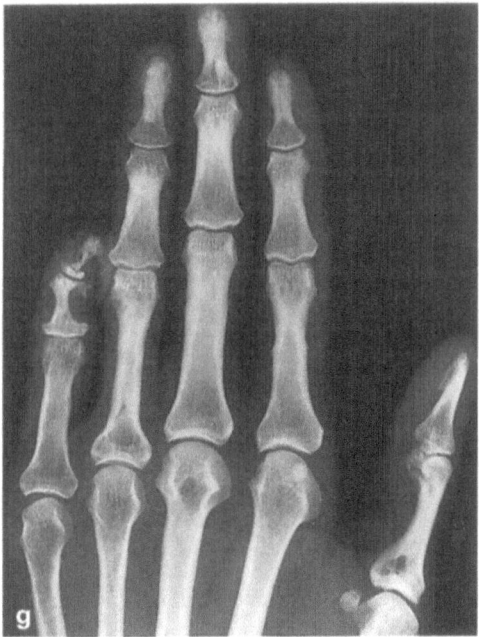

Fig. 5.6 (*continued*). **e–g** Skeletal sarcoidosis in the hands and feet showing a reticular-honeycomb pattern of structural changes in the middle and distal phalanges (**e**). Note the coarse destruction of the third metatarsal head and the osteolytic lesion at the base of the opposing proximal phalanx with a spontaneous fracture (**f**). Panel **g** shows the full radiographic presentation of Jüngling's multicystic osteitis. Note the osteolytic lesions at the bases of the first and fourth proximal phalanges, the pronounced mutilative changes in the middle and distal phalanges of the small finger, and the sclerotic foci in the second and third distal phalanges. Similar changes were seen in the opposite hand and in the feet. Radiographs **e–g** are from different patients. **h–m** see pp. 160, 161

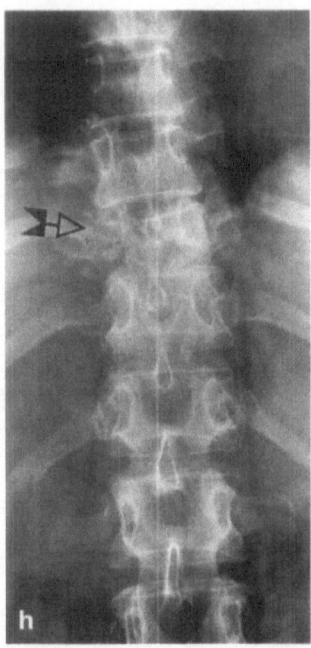

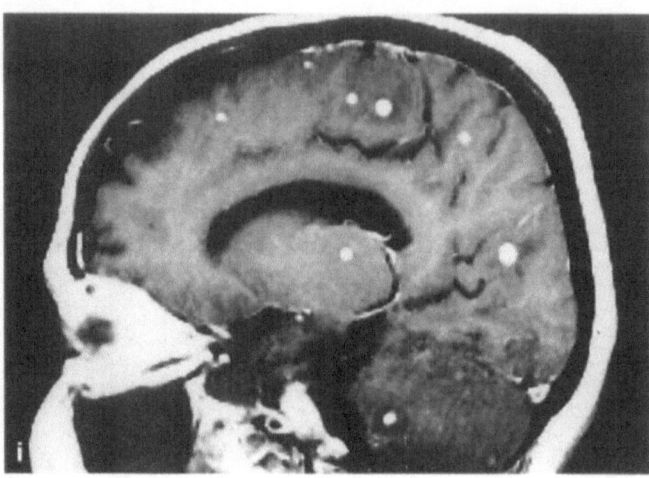

Fig. 5.6 (*continued*). **h, i** Woman 57 years of age with coarse destruction of T10 (**h**, *arrow*) and other predominantly sclerotic bone lesions in the pelvis (not shown). Later the patient developed disseminated infiltrates in the meninges and brain (**i**, coronal MRI showing scattered foci of high signal intensity). The patient also had coarse, atypical posterior mediastinal lymphadenopathy and relatively mild skin lesions. **j–m** see p. 161

– A *polycystic form* (Fig. 5.6 g) with round, punched-out defects mainly affecting the epimetaphyseal segments of the phalanges and occasionally the metacarpals and metatarsals (Jüngling's multicystic osteitis). The individual defects are rice-grain- to pea-sized and polygonal with very sharply defined borders.

– A *reticular-honeycomb pattern* (Fig. 5.6 e) initially involving the epimetaphyseal segments and later affecting the entire bone, with thinning of the cortex. New bone formation may cause thickening of residual cancellous bone trabeculae, accentuating the reticular pattern.

– *Relatively large, sharply marginated defects in the phalanges, metacarpals, and metatarsals*, occasionally with expansion of the bone and fine calcifications. These lesions sometimes resemble enchondromas.

– The *late mutilating form* is associated with relatively coarse destruction of the distal phalanges that may resemble neuropathic osteolysis (differential diagnosis: scleroderma, leprosy).

– *Patchy cancellous bone sclerosis* (Fig. 5.6 g) usually involving the terminal tufts of the distal phalanges.

– *Subperiosteal erosions* with frayed cortical outlines, similar to the findings in hyperparathyroidism.

– *Periosteal form* with spicules of new bone directed perpendicular to the shaft (very rare).

Given the diverse spectrum of skeletal changes in sarcoidosis, there are naturally cases in which the differential diagnosis is extremely difficult. A useful guide in these cases is the chest radiograph (Fig. 5.6 d), which will usually reveal stage 1 or stage 2 intrathoracic disease. Additionally, the radiologist should inspect the patient's integument, as the cutaneous manifestations (see above) are sometimes so characteristic that, when interpreted in the context of other findings, they can obviate the need for histologic evaluation of the skeletal lesions (e.g., by percutaneous biopsy).

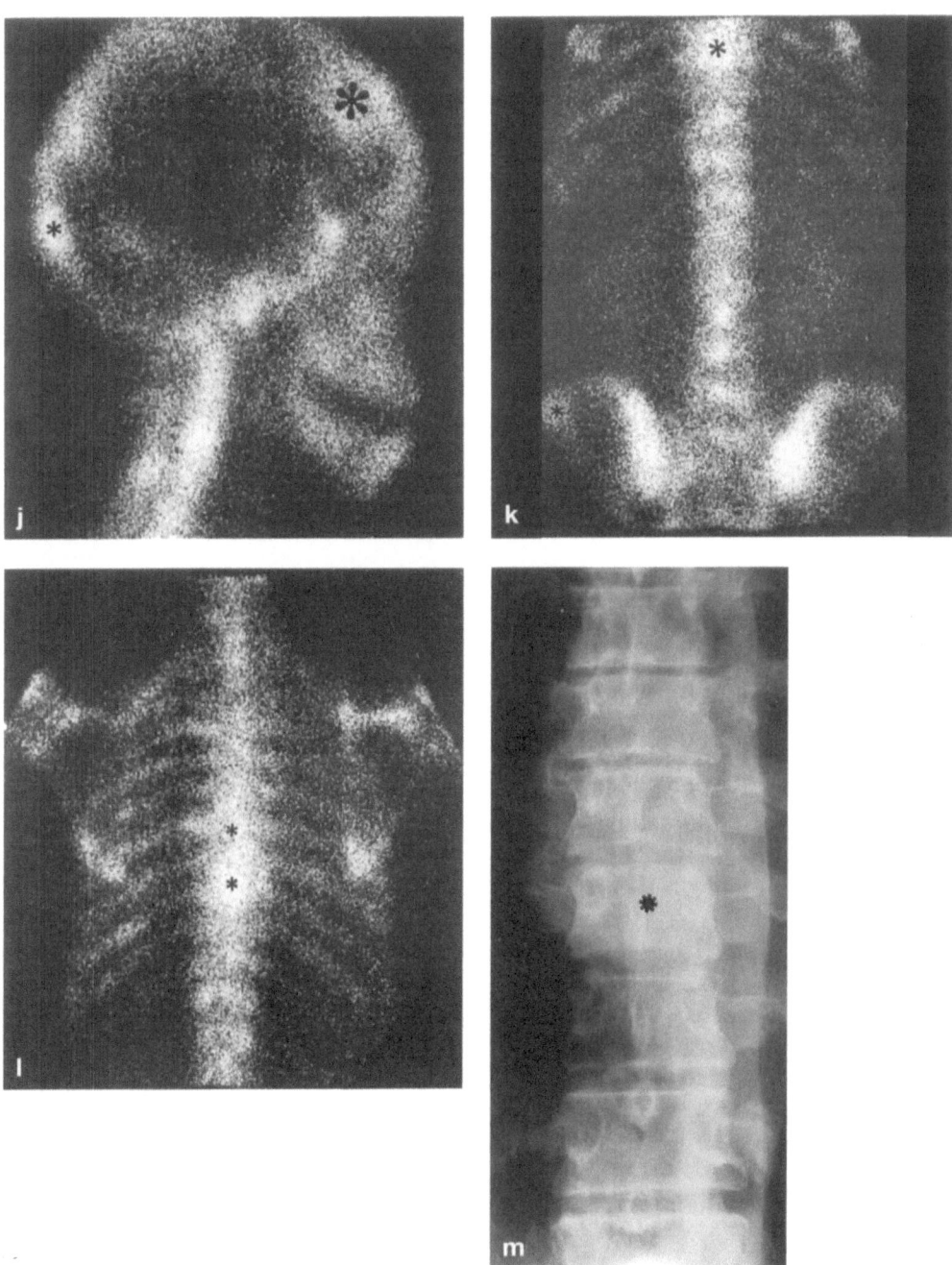

Fig. 5.6 (*continued*). **j–m** Sarcoidosis in a 39-year-old woman referred for radiologic evaluation of back pain. Radionuclide bone scans show areas of markedly increased uptake in the skull, T8 and T9, and the left side of the pelvis (**j–l**). These spots correlate with areas of nonspecific sclerosis on radiographs, as illustrated in T9 (**m**, *asterisk*). A chest film obtained as part of the differential diagnostic workup showed classic intrathoracic signs of sarcoidosis. All changes regressed completely with cortisone therapy. All the radiographs in **e–m** are from patients 40 years of age or older

References

Bonakdarpour A, Levy WM, Aegerter E (1971) Osteosclerotic changes in sarcoidosis. AJR Am J Roentgenol 113: 646

Braun-Falco O, Plewig G, Wolff HH, Winkelmann RK (1991) Dermatology, 3rd edn. Springer, Berlin Heidelberg New York

Fitzgerald P (1958) Sarcoidosis of hands. J Bone Joint Surg Br 40: 256

Müller-Quernheim J, Ferlinz R (1988) Sarkoidose, eine Immundysregulation. Dtsch Ärztbl 85: B-1179

Resnik CS, Young JWR, Aisner SC et al. (1990) Osseous sarcoidosis (osteolytic) of lumbar spine and pelvis. Case report 594. Skeletal Radiol 19: 79

Rodman T, Funderburk EE, Myerson RM (1959) Sarcoidosis with vertebral involvement. Ann Intern Med 50: 213

Sartoris DJ, Resnick D, Resnik C et al. (1985) Musculoskeletal manifestations of sarcoidosis. Semin Roentgenol 20: 376

Young DA, Lamann ML (1972) Radiodense skeletal lesions in Boeck's sarcoid. AJR Am J Roentgenol 114: 553

5.7 Mastocytosis

Synonyms: mastocytosis syndrome, urticaria pigmentosa with skeletal involvement

Numerous round to oval, reddish-brown, pruritic, lentil-sized lesions, mainly on the trunk, that urticate when rubbed; flushing, tachycardia, dyspnea, nausea, diarrhea.
Roentgen signs: irregular patches of osteoporosis (axial skeleton, pelvis), alone or combined with patchy osteosclerosis, *or* patchy osteosclerotic foci, *or* generalized "white bone." Circumscribed form is marked by tumorlike osteolytic lesions in the long tubular bones, skull, and pelvis. Positive radionuclide bone scans, showing either patchy areas of increased uptake or a "superscan" pattern.

Definition

Mastocytosis is a group of rare diseases characterized by mast (mastocyte) cell infiltration of the reticuloendothelial system of various organs, especially the skeleton, gastrointestinal tract, liver, spleen, lymph nodes, and skin. A benign form with urticaria pigmentosa, which may or may not show skeletal involvement, is distinguished from a malignant form (neoplastic mast cell reticulosis) that may progress to mast cell leukemia.

General Clinical Features

We cannot cover all the medical and dermatologic aspects of mastocytosis in this monograph and must limit our discussion to the forms that are associated with skeletal changes.

The proliferation of mast cells in the bone marrow is commonly associated with urticaria pigmentosa, as the cutaneous eruptions contain abundant subepithelial mast cells that release histamine in response to thermal and mechanical stimuli. This results in the well-known clinical picture of *urtication*, flushing, tachycardia, nausea, dyspnea, and intestinal symptoms in the form of diarrhea.

Laboratory tests show elevated histamine levels in the blood and urine, and alkaline phosphatase may be elevated in patients with skeletal changes. In 90% of patients with systemic mastocytosis, the diagnosis is established by aspiration biopsy of the bone marrow demonstrating mast cells. (The biopsy material should be sampled from osteoporotic areas.)

Urticaria pigmentosa with skeletal changes generally has a favorable prognosis, although sporadic cases may progress to mast cell leukemia, which is swiftly fatal. Generalized mastocytosis without urticaria pigmentosa usually pursues a malignant course with a rapidly fatal outcome. Systemic mastocytosis affects men about twice as often as women. Patients with radiographic skeletal changes are usually over 40 years of age.

Dermatology

Our discussion is limited to the *adult form of urticaria pigmentosa*, which features a combination of skin lesions *and* skeletal changes. The typical skin lesions consist of multiple, often disseminated, round-to-oval, reddish brown, lentil-sized macules and papules, occasionally with telangiectases (Fig. 5.7 a). The trunk is most commonly affected. Increasing pigmentation is apparent in older lesions. The dominant symptoms are pruritus and a urticarial skin reaction triggered by rubbing or thermal stimuli (e.g., hot and cold baths) due to histamine release from the mast cells. Drugs that cause histamine release should be strictly avoided due to the risk of shock, and patients should also avoid physical trauma and hot or cold stimuli.

Radiology

Mast cell proliferation can occur in any part of the skeleton that contains hematopoietic marrow (in adults: the skull, axial skeleton, and proximal long bones). Besides generalized mast cell hyperplasia of the bone marrow, there may be focal accumulations of mast cells with the size of miliary nodules. In time, these nodules may become obliterated and undergo metaplastic transformation to fiber bone, which has a denser, sclerotic appearance on radiographs. If the fiber bone formation occurs uniformly over the existing framework of cancellous bone, it will cause an initially irregular and later more *uniform thickening of the bony trabeculae*, with a re-

sultant "whitening" of skeletal areas that physiologically contain more cancellous bone (Fig. 5.7 b, c). This may be preceded or accompanied by resorptive changes near mast cell granulomas with the development of *irregular patchy osteoporosis* or a *mixed pattern of sclerosis and osteoporosis*. The heparin produced by mast cells very likely has a role in this process, as it appears to inhibit the formation of bony tissue through its effect on collagen synthesis.

Scrutinizing the radiologic manifestations of mastocytosis more closely, we are able to distinguish between a circumscribed and a diffuse form. In mastocytosis with urticaria pigmentosa, radiographic changes can be demonstrated in approximately 80% to 85% of cases.

In the *circumscribed form* of mastocytosis, the skeletal lesions may be lytic and sclerotic (Fig. 5.7 d) and can mimic tumors (i.e., osteoblastic metastasis) and bone marrow infarcts. This circumscribed form exclusively affects the long tubular bones, skull, and pelvis.

The *diffuse form* usually shows a mixed pattern of osteoporosis and sclerosis, with sclerotic changes predominating in most cases. The sclerosis may be dense enough to produce a "white bone" appearance. The ill-defined borders of the dense, thickened trabeculae help to distinguish this condition from other disorders such as marble bone disease and osteomyelosclerosis syndrome. Reticular densities may appear within the medullary cavities of the long tubular bones. This diffuse form most commonly affects the axial skeleton and femurs, usually in a symmetric distribution.

Radionuclide bone scans usually show increased uptake in affected skeletal areas, and occasionally this precedes the appearance of radiographic changes.

MRI studies of the bone marrow in patients with mastocytosis are very sensitive but nonspecific and are confined to special clinical questions (Avila et al. 1998).

The *differential diagnostic spectrum* includes metastases (from cancer of the breast or prostate), sarcoidosis, osteomyelosclerosis syndrome, and toxic exposures (e.g., fluorine).

Recent studies by Delling (personal communication, 1994) suggest that many cases of osteoporosis in males are attributable to mastocytosis, as indicated by histologic findings in iliac

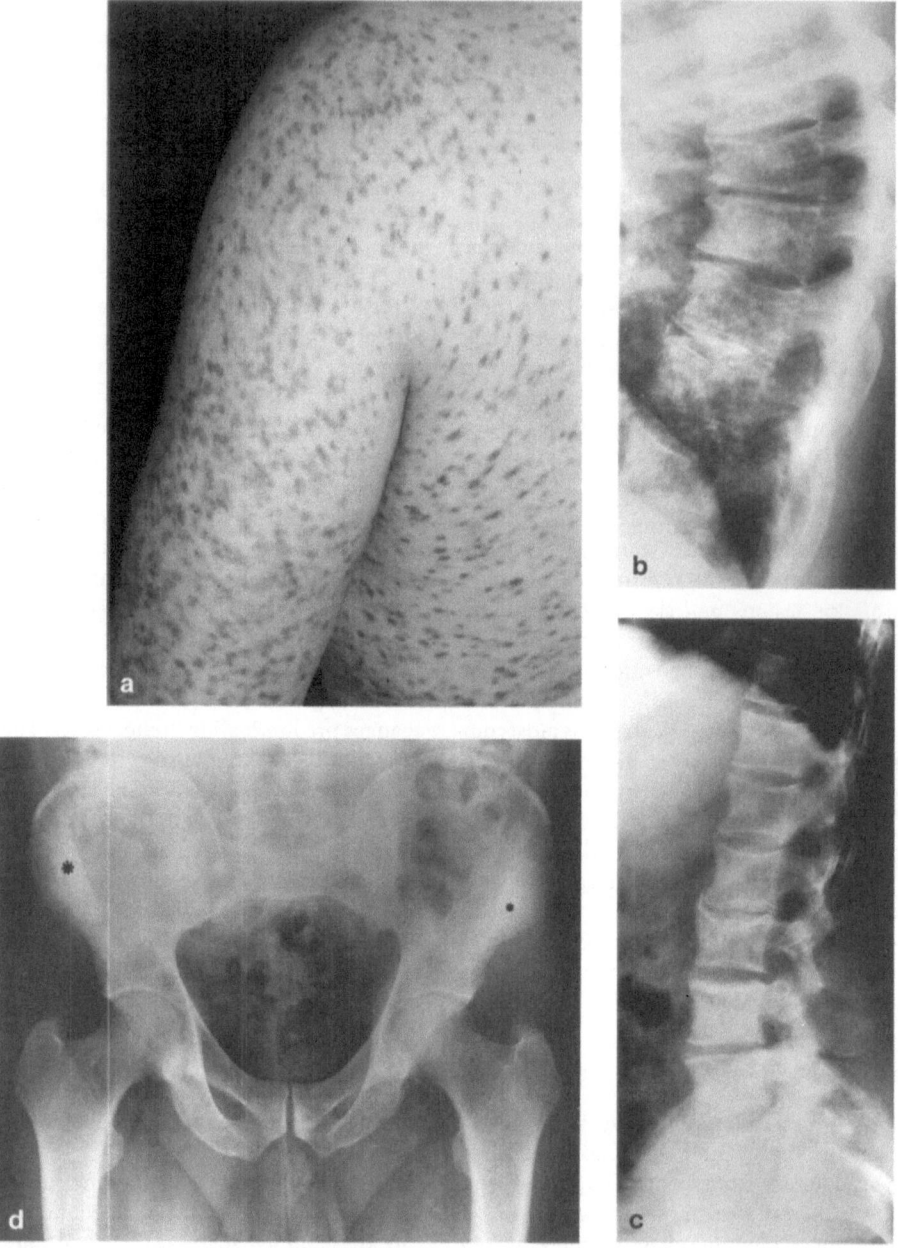

Fig. 5.7 a–d. Mastocytosis. **a** Disseminated round-to-oval, reddish-brown lesions that urticate when rubbed. Several older lesions already show hyperpigmentation. **b–d** Irregular reticular pattern of osteosclerosis in the thoracic and lumbar spine (**b, c**). The multiple collapsed vertebrae are suggestive of antecedent or concomitant osteoporosis. The pelvic radiograph (**d**) shows patchy sclerosis mainly involving the lateral portions of the iliac wings (*asterisks*) and the ischia

crest biopsies from osteoporosis patients. This possibility should be considered in evaluations of clinically overt osteoporosis, and a dermatologic examination should be performed.

References

Avila NA, Ling A, Metcalfe DD et al. (1998) Mastocytosis: MRI patterns of marrow disease. Skeletal Radiol 27: 119

Biehler EU, Wohlenberg H, Utech CH (1985) Die ossären Manifestationen bei der generalisierten Mastozytose im Skelettszintigramm im Vergleich zum Röntgenbefund. Röfo 142: 522

DiBacco RS, DeLoe VA (1982) Mastocytosis and the mast cell. J Am Acad Dermatol 7: 709

Horny HP, Parwaresch MR, Lennert K (1983) Klinisches Bild und Prognose generalisierter Mastozytosen. Klin Wochenschr 61: 785

Roberts II. LJ, Sweetman BJ, Lewis RA et al. (1980) Increased production of prostaglandin D_2 in patients with systemic mastocytosis. N Engl J Med 303: 1400

Rodenberg JC, Maegaard KK, Svanholm H (1986) Systemic mastocytosis. Case report 369. Skeletal Radiol 15: 334

Rohner HG, Bartl R, Klingmüller G et al. (1980) Die Mastozytose – eine Krankheit mit häufiger Systemisierung. Therapiewoche 30: 6773

Schweitzer ME, Irwin GAL (1989) Systemic mastocytosis. Skeletal Radiol 18: 411

Semerak M (1980) Urticaria pigmentosa mit Skelettbeteiligung – Mastozytosesyndrom. Röfo 133: 673

6 Angiodysplastic Skin Lesions and Skeletal Changes

Angiodysplastic skin lesions and skeletal changes present a broad clinical and radiologic spectrum ranging from small, trivial capillary nevi resp. hemangiomas to large, hemodynamically significant arteriovenous fistulas. Hemangiomas may occur on the skin, internal organs (e.g., liver), and bones. The great majority of these tumors are isolated and, unless they exceed a certain size, have no clinical importance. By definition, this chapter deals only with angiodysplastic lesions that are consistently associated with cutaneous and skeletal manifestations.

Congenital abnormalities of veins, arteries, and lymphatic vessels are commonly associated with an array of skeletal changes ranging from atrophy (dwarfism), hypertrophy (overgrowth), and sclerosis to osteolysis. The association with enchondromatosis (Maffucci's syndrome) was discussed on p. 15.

6.1 Congenital Angiodysplasias

Congenital angiodysplasias are classically subdivided into three types – Klippel-Trénaunay, Servelle-Martorell, and Weber – despite the fact that the dividing lines between the types (especially Weber and Klippel-Trénaunay) are not always clear. The symptoms of these disorders may overlap, and there are incomplete forms that are difficult to assign to a specific type. The essential features of the congenital angiodysplasias as defined by Langer and Langer (1982) are listed in Table 6.1. Today a fourth type, Stewart-Bluefarb syndrome, is also recognized owing to its dermatologic manifestations.

All four disorders may be associated with skeletal abnormalities whose pathogenesis is still poorly understood, as the manifestations may consist of atrophic or hypertrophic skeletal changes as well as extensive destructive lesions. Erosive bone lesions may be interpreted as a pressure-related phenomenon based on osteo-

Table 6.1. Findings associated with congenital angiodysplasias. (According to Langer and Langer 1982)

Finding	Weber type	Klippel-Trénaunay type	Servelle-Martorell type
Hypertrophy (overgrowth)	Proportional	Disproportional	–
Atrophy (dwarfism)	–	–	Disproportional
Hemangiomas	–	Frequent	Frequent
Arteriovenous fistulas	Consistently present	None (except for inactive microshunts)	None
Deep venous abnormalities	–	Occasional	Frequent
Corticocancellous bone lesions	Lacunar cancellous bone transformation and defects in cortical and cancellous bone	–	Destruction of cancellous bone structure, destruction and lamination of cortex, joint destruction
Prognosis	Uncertain	Favorable	Unfavorable

clast stimulation by dilated blood vessels, but this hypothesis cannot easily account for the hypertrophy of a whole extremity in Klippel-Trénaunay syndrome, for example. Formerly it was thought that venous stasis could stimulate growth zones. But this hypothesis is weakened by the fact that stasis is generally associated with hypoxia, which is not an effective mechanism for stimulating the proliferation of growth cartilage. On the other hand it is conceivable that venous stasis may trigger the production of certain growth agents that stimulate and sustain growth-cartilage proliferation. Meanwhile, the disproportionate skeletal shortening that occurs in the Servelle-Martorell type of angiodysplasia is easily understood when we consider that arteriovenous shunts deprive the growth plates of necessary oxygen, causing a quantitative reduction in growth. The presence of arteriovenous fistulas is the factor that distinguishes the Weber type of angiodysplasia from the Klippel-Trénaunay type. Some authors use the collective term Klippel-Trénaunay-Weber syndrome for both disorders.

6.1.1 Weber Type

In 1918, F. Parkes Weber described a condition in which arteriovenous fistulas were combined with the Klippel-Trénaunay syndrome. This description covers the essential features of the classic Weber type, in which the Klippel-Trénaunay triad is accompanied by arteriovenous shunting, especially in the lower extremity. If significant arteriovenous shunts exist in the bone as well as surrounding soft tissues, areas of lacunar resorption will form in the cancellous and cortical bone, appearing as serpiginous or bandlike lucencies on radiographs. These changes are usually accompanied by a proportionate hypertrophy (overgrowth) of the affected extremity or bone (Fig. 6.1.1 a), differentiating this condition from the disproportionate hypertrophy in Klippel-Trénaunay. If an arteriovenous fistula extends far enough into the subcutaneous tissue, it may be visible through the skin as a bluish-red mass with an associated doughy swelling that may have palpable pulsations. In contrast to Klippel-Trénaunay syndrome, there is no known association with cutaneous hemangiomas. The diagnosis and correct classification of the skeletal changes rely on arterial angiography, which typically shows an extensive mass of ectatic, convoluted veins that opacify in the early arterial phase (Fig. 6.1.1 b).

References are listed at the end of Chap. 6, p. 178.

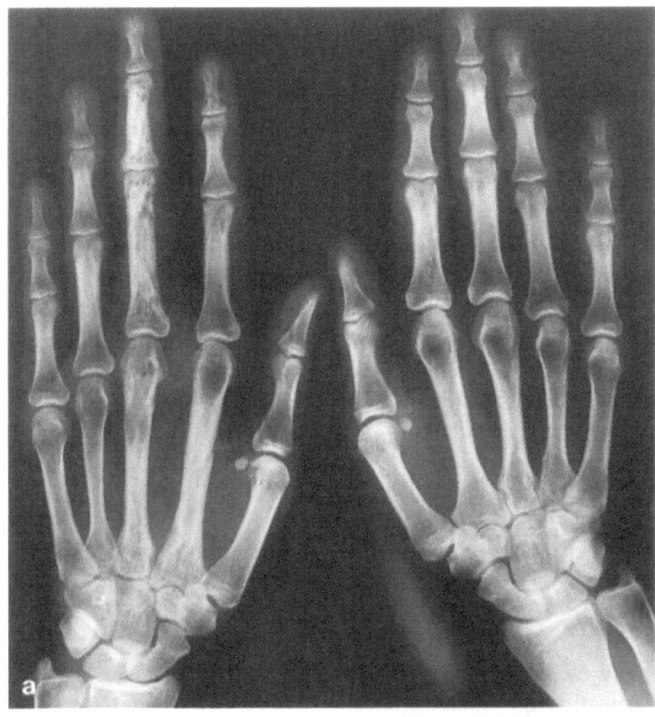

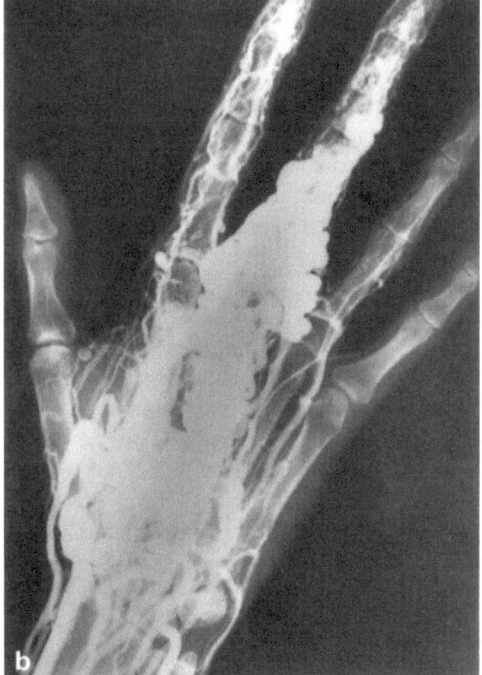

Fig. 6.1.1 a, b. Weber type of angiodysplasia in the left hand. **a** Radiograph shows proportionate hypertrophic elongation of the third ray. The bandlike lucencies in the metacarpal and proximal and middle phalanges represent broadened vascular beds and channels. Note the reactive sclerosis in the proximal and middle phalanges of the third ray and the subtle changes in the second ray. **b** The angiogram shows extensive vascular malformations with arteriovenous shunting (very early venous opacification in the early arterial phase). The blood supply to the thumb, ring finger, and small finger is markedly deficient due to a steal effect by the prodigious AV fistulas and varicosities in the third ray and carpus

6.1.2 Klippel-Trénaunay Type

Klippel-Trénaunay syndrome is characterized by the following triad of features:

1. Nevus flammeus (port-wine hemangioma), usually covering a large area of the affected extremity (Fig. 6.1.2 a, c).
2. Pronounced varicose veins.
3. Soft-tissue and bony hypertrophy appearing as partial gigantism of the affected extremity.

The lower extremities are predominantly affected (almost 80%). The hypertrophy may consist of an increase in length and circumference, the bone itself showing no structural changes besides elongation and occasional thickening. In cases where bone circumference is increased, lymphedema is usually present. The venous abnormalities mainly affect the deep venous system and include atresia, hypoplasia, ectasia, and the duplication of saphenous, popliteal, or ileofemoral veins (Fig. 6.1.2 b). A typical finding is persistent lateral marginal veins that drain into the internal iliac vein through dilated gluteal muscle veins and anastomoses, with absence of the external iliac vein and common femoral vein. The superficial veins may show true aneurysmatic transformation. Functionally, there may be significant impairment of drainage through the malformed, valveless deep venous system. The pronounced superficial varicosities handle most of the venous drainage. The global outflow obstruction leads to edema and trophic disturbances of the skin with increased susceptibility to microbial colonization.

Capillary and cavernous hemangiomas not only occur on the skin of the affected extremity but may also involve internal organs. Hemangiomas of the bowel are particularly common and may lead to bleeding and an exudative protein-losing enteropathy, especially when associated with arteriovenous malformations. Various other vascular lesions have been described including central nervous system aneurysms and renal vascular malformations with hematuria.

Klippel-Trénaunay syndrome shows a slight female preponderance. The hemangiomas may be present at birth or may appear shortly thereafter. The varicosities are noticed when the child begins to sit and stand. If pseudo-Kaposi-like skin lesions and painful ulcerations are also seen on the affected extremity, the condition is termed *Stewart-Bluefarb syndrome* (see below). A rare complication, seen most often in patients with extensive cutaneous hemangiomas, is *Kasabach-Merritt syndrome*, in which thrombocytopenia, decreased fibrinogen, and activation of the fibrinolytic system lead to a consumption coagulopathy with massive bleeding and/or purpura.

References are listed at the end of Chap. 6, p. 178.

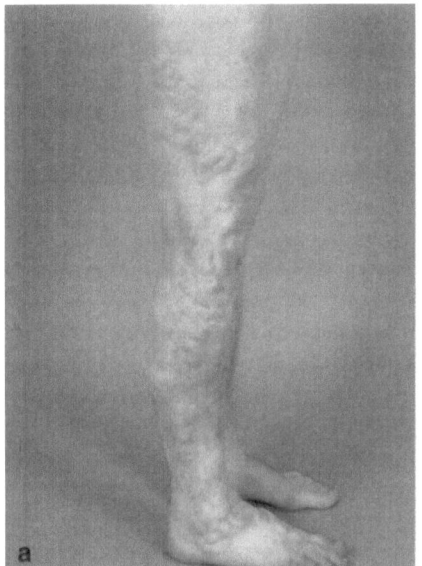

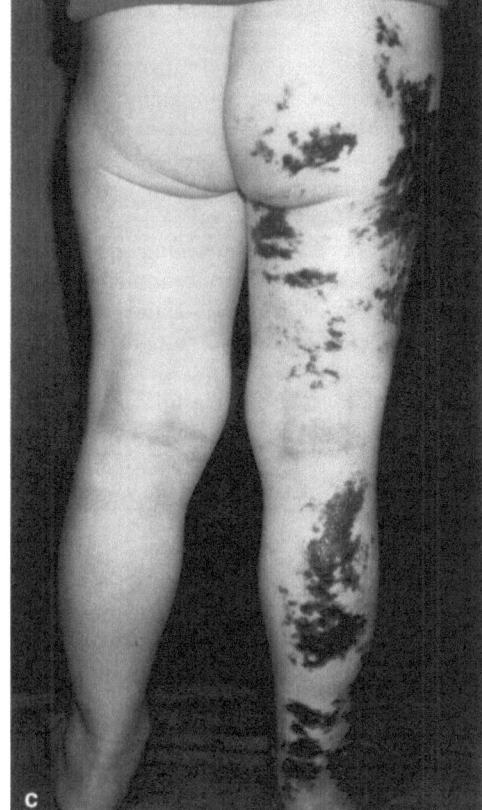

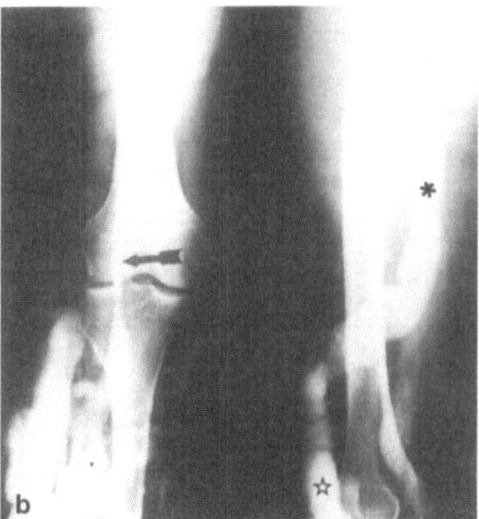

Fig. 6.1.2 a–c. Klippel-Trénaunay type of angiodysplasia. **a** Pronounced secondary varicosities, lateral marginal vein, and nevus flammeus on the right leg (which is 1.5 cm longer than the left leg). **b** Venograms in this 31-year-old woman demonstrate partial aplasia of the deep veins of the lower leg (not completely defined here) with segmental hypoplasia of the popliteal vein (*arrow*). The lateral marginal vein (*open star*) is cylindrically dilated; it ascends on the posterior aspect of the distal thigh and drains into the common femoral vein (*asterisk*). **c** Extensive angiomatous lesions ("port-wine hemangiomas") appear on the right lower extremity, which is hypertrophic. (Panels **a** and **b** courtesy of Prof. Dr. med. E. Paes, Aachen)

6.1.3 Servelle-Martorell Type

This syndrome is associated with arterial vascular malformations that are predominantly ectatic in nature. It is also associated with venous malformations in the form of pronounced varicosities, venous angiomas, and anomalous patterns of venous drainage. Affected skeletal segments show disproportionate shortening ranging from a few millimeters to several centimeters. Moreover, intraosseous hemangiomatous lesions are commonly associated with multiple cystlike lucencies in the cancellous bone with thinning and lamination of the cortex (Fig. 6.1.3 a, d). Periarticular spread of the angiomatous lesions can lead to massive joint destruction. In extreme cases the bone is so atrophic from the severe perfusion deficit that only vestiges of the original bone remain, accompanied by spontaneous fractures (Fig. 6.1.3 e–h).

Because of the pronounced venous malformations and hemangiomatous lesions, it is common for plain radiographs to show calcified phleboliths in the soft tissues of the affected extremity (Fig. 6.1.3 d–f).

References are listed at the end of Chap. 6, p. 178.

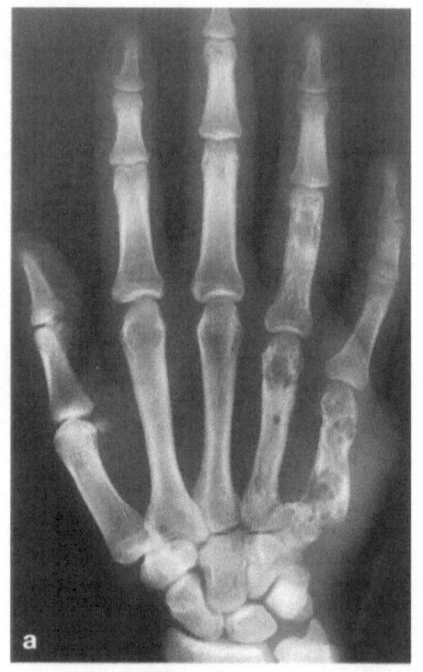

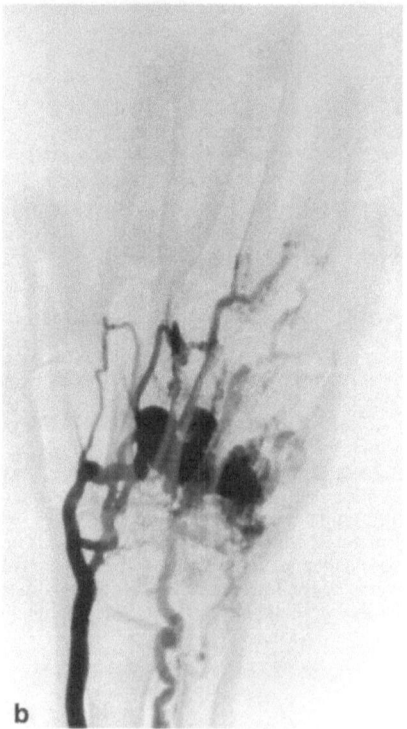

Fig. 6.1.3 a, b. See legend on p. 173

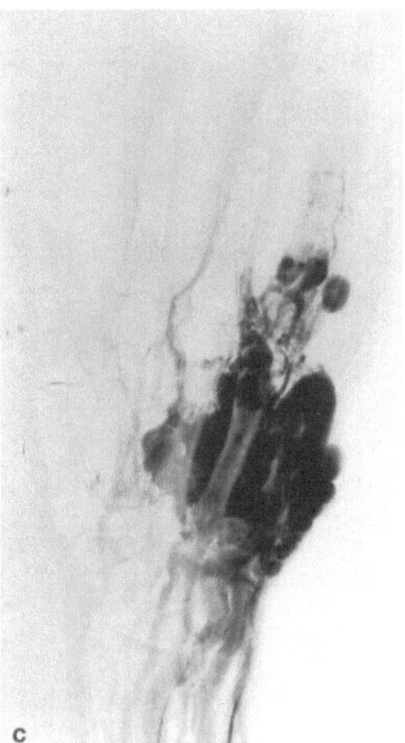

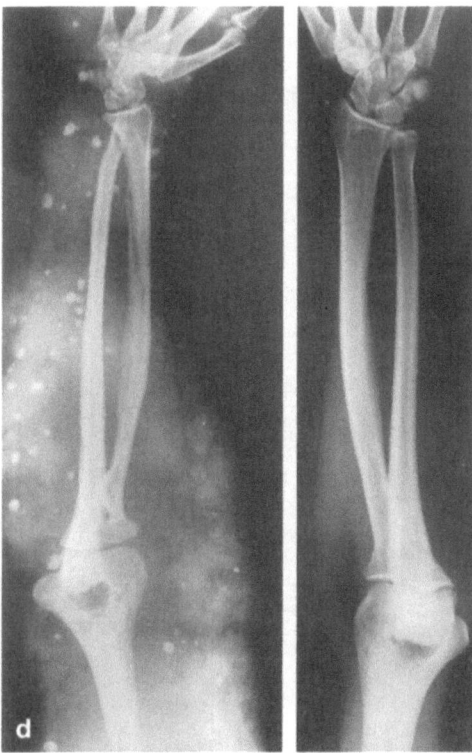

◁ **Fig.6.1.3a–h.** Servelle-Martorell type of angiodysplasia. **a–c** The fourth and fifth metacarpals show extensive structural changes with a spontaneous fracture near the base of the fifth metacarpal. Conspicuous lacunar and bandlike lucencies are seen in the fourth proximal phalanx. Marked soft-tissue swelling is visible about this phalanx and the lateral portion of the metacarpus. The angiograms show extensive arteriovenous shunting with early opacification of the severely ectatic, convoluted veins. Clinically, doughy swelling was found in the affected area with some bluish discoloration of the skin, and a bruit was noted on auscultation. Clubbing of the fourth and fifth fingers is apparently a result of the steal effect. **d** Another case showing disproportionate shortening of the right upper extremity with a general slenderness of the bones and structural changes in the radial shaft (the linear lucency represents a vascular bed with a deep groove on the inner aspect of the cortex). Coarse venous malformations appear as globular opacities throughout the soft tissues, and phleboliths appear as conspicuous nodular densities. **e–h** Grotesque mutilation due to bone resorption in the upper arm and forearm, with spontaneous fractures of the distal humerus and radius. These osseous changes are a result of very severe trophic disturbances secondary to extensive angiomatous lesions of the upper extremity. The structured soft-tissue densities are formed by coarse varicosities with numerous phleboliths. The patient presented clinically with extensive angiomatous lesions involving the left shoulder girdle, the left anterior pectoral region, and all of the grotesquely deformed left arm. The disease had started at age 2 with a cavernous hemangioma on the left forearm. When examined at age 70, the patient had been using her left arm only for simple tasks. Plastic surgery of the upper arm had been attempted when the patient was 10, and radiotherapy had been tried in the shoulder region, which shows typical postirradiation skin changes. This case could be interpreted as an unusual presentation of Klippel-Trénaunay syndrome with very severe secondary trophic changes. **e–h** see p. 174

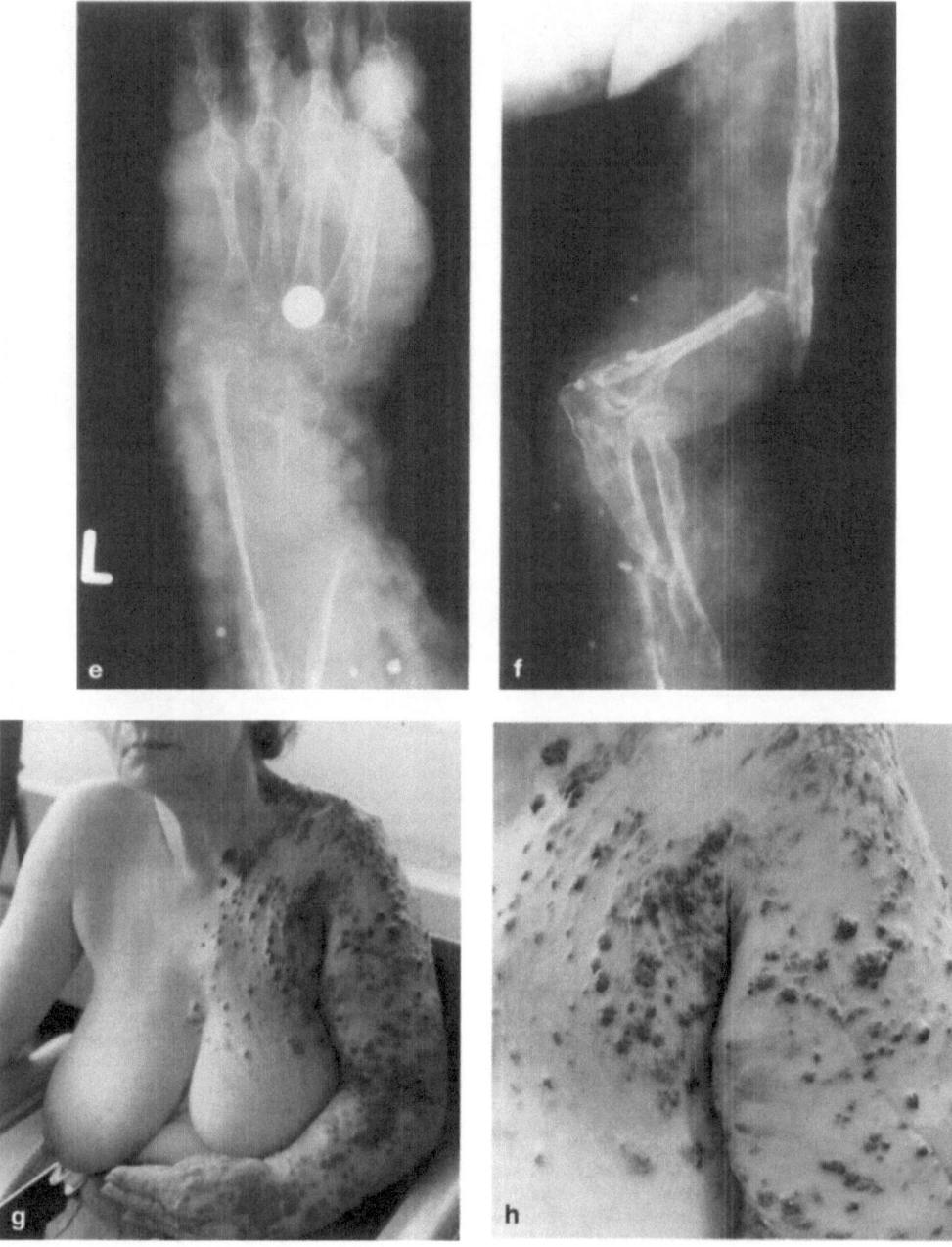

Fig. 6.1.3 e–h. See legend on p. 173

6.1.4 Stewart-Bluefarb Syndrome

As noted earlier, patients with Stewart-Bluefarb syndrome have pseudo-Kaposi-like skin lesions and painful ulcerations in addition to arteriovenous fistulas and hypertrophy of the affected extremity. Reportedly, Stewart-Bluefarb syndrome differs from other arteriovenous malformations in that there is a massive increase in thick-walled capillaries similar to capillary hemangioma.

The dermatologic lesions are described as "sharply marginated bluish-brown plaques" on the affected extremity, some of which are hyperkeratotic and papillomatous with interspersed pinhead-sized ulcerations. The surrounding area usually shows swelling, hyperhidrosis, and varicosities. These kaposiform skin lesions resemble not only Kaposi's sarcoma but also the pseudo-Kaposi lesions of *acroangiodermatitis mali*, which form on the dorsal surfaces of the feet due to chronic venous stasis but are most common in the fourth to sixth decade of life. Stewart-Bluefarb syndrome, on the other hand, is most common in adolescence. Similar hemangiomatous eruptions may be seen in the area of arteriovenous hemodialysis fistulas and following trauma. Apparently the AV fistulas, stasis varicosities, and ulcerations can lead to bone changes consisting not only of atrophic and destructive lesions as in Servelle-Martorell syndrome but also periosteal proliferation on the tibia, fibula, and other bones (Ueki et al. 1986).

References are listed at the end of Chap. 6, p. 178.

6.2 Acquired Angiodysplasias

A large percentage of acquired angiodysplasias have a traumatic etiology. Examples are synovial angiodysplasias following knee operations and cutaneous hemangiomas after trauma. In any given case, it cannot be determined with certainty whether hemangiomas of the skin *and* bone or glomus tumors are purely acquired lesions as opposed to congenital abnormalities (Fig. 6.2 a–c). Below we shall briefly describe hemangiomas with osteomalacia and glomus tumors as examples of acquired angiodysplasias that usually are first encountered in adults.

Brief mention should also be made of the "vanishing bone disease" of Gorham and Stout, which is characterized by massive bone resorption, chiefly in the shoulder girdle or pelvis, and very rarely is associated with cutaneous cavernous hemangiomas. A discussion of this disease would exceed our scope, however, as we are primarily dealing with purely osteologic problems.

References are listed at the end of Chap. 6, p. 178.

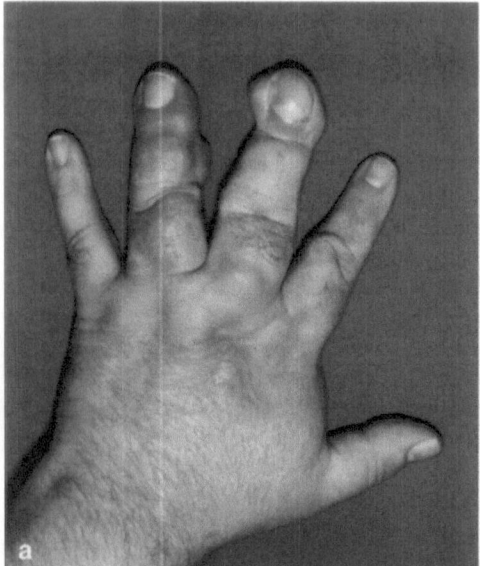
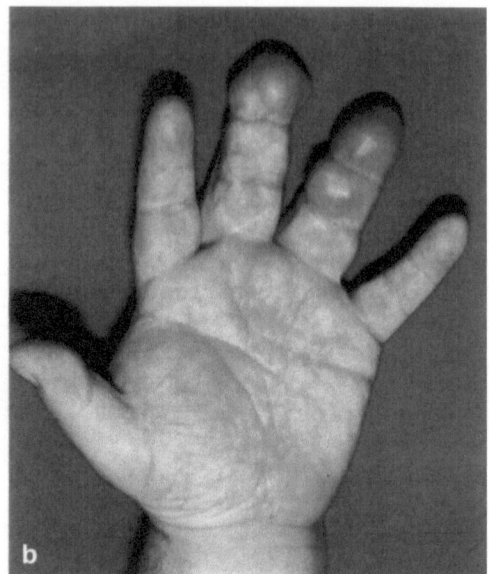
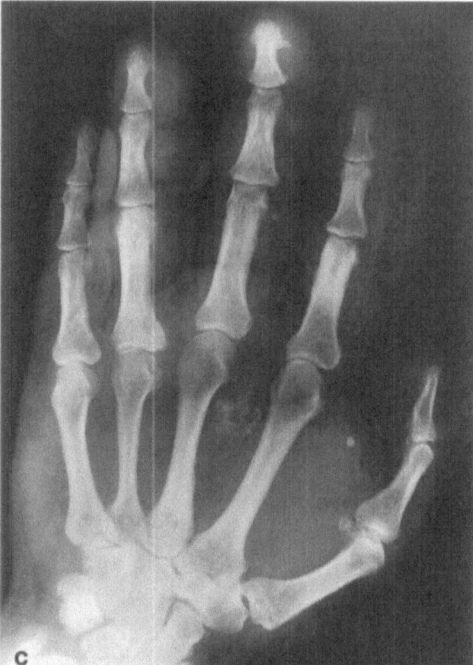

Fig. 6.2 a–c. Indeterminate angiomatous lesions involving the second through fourth fingers and distal metacarpal region. The patient stated that his hand seemed normal during childhood and adolescence but began to show increasing deformity, mainly of the third and fourth fingers, during the past few years. Previous vascular ligation surgery had been attempted elsewhere. The patient refused angiography, which might have clarified the nature of the angiodysplastic lesions. Clinical inspection (**a,b**) reveals massive swelling of the third and fourth fingers of the left hand caused by large cavernous hemangiomas and ectatic veins. The watchglass deformity of the third fingernail is probably the result of hypoxia (see Sect. 7.3). The radiograph (**c**) shows reactive sclerotic changes in the second and fourth proximal phalanges, the fourth middle phalanx, and the third distal phalanx. Several subtle lacunar defects represent pressure erosions from the dilated vessels. Irregular ossification between the second and third metacarpals is probably a metaplastic sequel to previous surgery (see scar in **a**). But its differential diagnosis would also include a cartilaginous tumor in the soft tissues, suggesting that the case may involve a late presentation of Marffucci's syndrome

6.2.1 Hemangioma with Osteomalacia

Various tumors of the bones and soft tissues, most notably hemangiomas, can induce hypophosphatemic osteomalacia (Nuovo and Dorfman 1989). It is likely that hemangiomas of the skin, internal organs, or bone synthesize a hormone-like substance that acts on the bone or bowel or affects phosphate reabsorption in the renal tubules. Renal phosphate clearance is always elevated, producing a hypophosphatemic state that apparently results in osteomalacia. It has also been suggested that the tumors may produce a substance that acts as a vitamin D antagonist, leading to the deficient dihydroxylation of vitamin D in the kidneys.

Whenever unexplained osteomalacia is found in a hypophosphatemic patient, the physician should look carefully for a hemangioma of the skin or internal organs or for some other tumor of the bone or soft tissues. Usually these tumors are richly vascularized and contain giant cells and primitive stromal cells. When the tumor is removed, the phosphate level and bone metabolism will return to normal. If the tumor cannot be surgically removed or irradiated (e.g., due to spinal involvement), the osteomalacia can be satisfactorily controlled with oral phosphate therapy.

Radiographs of large cutaneous and subcutaneous hemangiomas (Fig. 6.2.1) show broadening of the soft-tissue shadow along with rounded opacities representing phleboliths. Soft-tissue hemagiomas are better visualized by magnetic resonance imaging.

References are listed at the end of Chap. 6, p. 178.

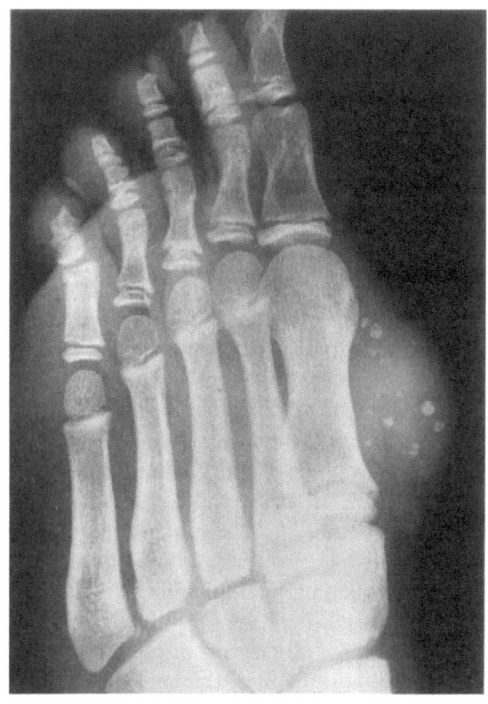

Fig. 6.2.1. Relatively large hemangioma medial to the first metatarsal in a child with extensive phleboliths. The lesion may be a cavernous hemangioma. This type of hemangioma, which is visible externally, may well be associated with hypophosphatemic osteomalacia

6.2.2 Glomus Tumors

Glomus tumors arise from nonchromaffin paraganglia, e.g., from the glomus jugulare (in the adventitia). Some authors classify glomus tumors as neurogenic tumors arising at paraosseous sites. Generally these tumors are richly vascularized and show marked abnormalities of vascular anatomy (ectasia, etc.). The great majority of glomus tumors is solitary. Multiple tumors may be confined to one region or may be widespread.

The most common site of occurrence is the area between the distal phalanx and nail. Pressure from the tumor gradually erodes a bony defect into the nail side of the distal phalanx (Fig. 6.2.2 b). Angiography defines the glomus tumor as a highly vascularized mass. Subungual tumors appear clinically as small, firm, exquisitely tender purplish or bluish-red nodules no larger than pea-size and sometimes forming a small hemispheric mound (Fig. 6.2.2 a).

A more detailed discussion of glomus tumors, especially those of the head and neck region (e.g., glomus jugulare, glomus tympanicum), would exceed the scope of this monograph.

References

Bluefarb SM, Adams LA (1967) Arteriovenous malformation with angiodermatitis. Stasis dermatitis simulating Kaposi's disease. Arch Dermatol 96: 176

Helmbold P, Pönitzsch I, Haustein U-F (1994) Klippel-Trénaunay-Syndrom mit intestinaler Beteiligung und Mammakarzinom bei einem Mann. Arch Dermatol 20: 288

Langer M, Langer R (1982) Radiologisch erfaßbare Veränderungen der Angiodysplasien Typ Klippel-Trénaunay und Typ Servelle-Martorell. Röfo 136: 577

Leipner N, Lackner K, Franzen M (1985) Röntgenbefunde bei einer angiomatösen Dysplasie (Typ Weber). Röfo 142: 571

Nuovo M, Dorfman HD, Sun C-C et al. (1989) Tumor induced osteomalacia and rickets. Am J Surg Pathol 13: 588

Paes E, Vollmar J, Echtler B (1992) Diagnostik und chirurgische Aspekte bei venösen Angiodysplasien der Gliedmaßen. Vasomed 4: 435

Phillips GN, Gordon DH, Martin EC et al. (1978) The Klippel-Trénaunay syndrome: clinical and radiological aspects. Radiology 128: 429

Schönlein KM, Worret W-J (1992) Das Stewart-Bluefarb-Syndrom. Hautarzt 43: 40

Stewart WM (1967) Fausse angiosarcomatose de Kaposi par fistules arterioveinulaires multiples. Bull Soc Fr Derm Syph 74: 664

Ueki H, Inagaki Y, Kohda M et al. (1986) Stewart-Bluefarb-Syndrom (kaposiforme arterio-venöse Kurzschlußverbindung mit Knochenveränderungen). Hautarzt 37: 673

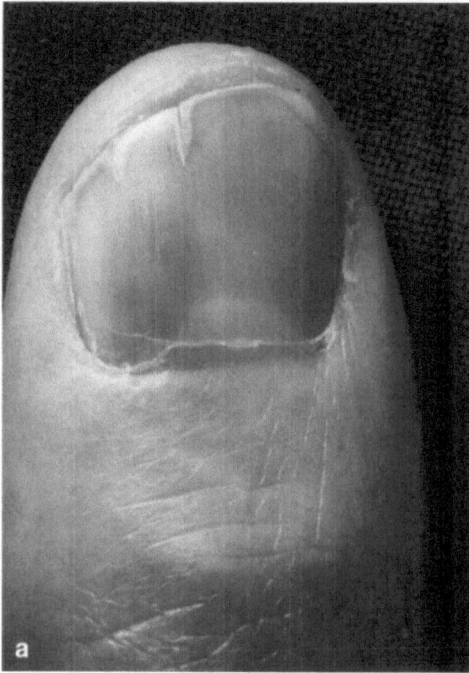
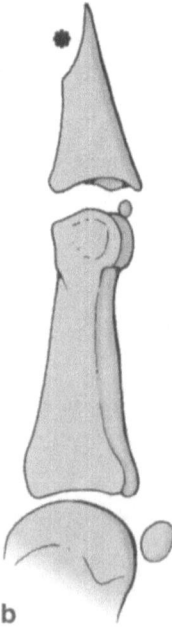

Fig. 6.2.2 a, b. Glomus tumor. **a** A bluish-red nodule is visible through the nail plate, where the lesion has formed a slight bulge. **b** Schematic drawing of terminal tuft erosion caused by a glomus tumor

7 Periostoses

There are a variety of pathologic periosteal reactions[1] in which mucocutaneous lesions or other external abnormalities (e.g., exophthalmos) occur as associated features, and a synoptic evaluation of *all* symptoms is needed in order to make a correct diagnosis. The congenital or acquired disorders discussed in this chapter are invariably associated with both periosteal and external changes, which constitute the major symptoms. These criteria are met by several other disorders which, though listed in Tables 7.1 and 7.2, are covered elsewhere in the book because of the way in which the chapters are organized. These tables also include entities in which periosteal reactions may or may not occur, such as certain collagen diseases and sarcoidosis.

In understanding pathologic periosteal reactions, it will be helpful to review some basic aspects of the anatomy and pathophysiology of the periosteum:

The periosteum forms the boundary between the osseous compartment and the surrounding soft tissues. The periosteum is composed of an external fibrous layer and an internal cellular layer, known also as the germinative layer or cambium. The germinative layer contains osteoblasts that may be activated at any time by various external and internal stimuli to synthesize new bone. Sharpey's fibers anchor the fibrous layer to the cortex. The periosteum is traversed by numerous vessels that enter the cortex through Volkmann's canals and then ramify in the haversian canals before entering the medullary cavity. These vessels play a major role in the initiation and spread of various diseases of the periosteum and bone (e.g., pathways for the spread of osteomyelitis, intra- and subperiosteal bleeding due to vascular tears, seeding of tumor cells, etc.). Any process that activates the osteo-

Table 7.1. Oligo- or polyostotic periosteal new bone formation, congenital or appearing in childhood, that may be associated with mucocutaneous lesions or other external abnormalities

---

Melorheostosis
Pachydermoperiostosis
Hereditary palmoplantar keratosis (Bureau-Barriére)
Rubella, infectious mononucleosis
Congenital syphilis
Scurvy
Inflammatory bowel disease (e.g., ulcerative colitis, Crohn's disease)
Leukemia
Pulmonary hypertrophic osteoarthropathy (e.g., in honeycomb lung)
"Diaphysitis" (see p. 202)
Congenital copper deficiency

Table 7.2. Adult forms of oligo- or polyostotic periosteal new bone formation that may be associated with mucocutaneous lesions or other external abnormalities (pattern of new bone formation is usually continued straight or undulating, rarely laminated or onionskin-like)

Pulmonary hypertrophic osteoarthropathy
Gastrointestinal hypertrophic osteoarthropathy (ulcerative colitis, Crohn's disease)
Pachydermoperiostosis
EMO syndrome
Collagen diseases (especially polyarteritis, progressive scleroderma, and lupus erythematosus)
Rheumatoid arthritis
Reiter's syndrome, psoriasis (periarticular)
Infectious mononucleosis
Sarcoidosis (hands, feet)
Multi-infarct disease (e.g., in pancreatitis)
Diabetes mellitus
Acromegaly
Arterial and venous blood flow disturbances (varicose symptom complex)
Lymphedema
Retinoid-induced
Syphilitic periostitis

---

[1] Some diseases, such as infectious mononucleosis and rubella, are not covered in this monograph because periosteal changes do not consistently occur and the general clinical features and organic disease symptoms are usually sufficient to make a diagnosis.

blasts will stimulate the formation of new bone. Activating stimuli include mechanical elevation of the periosteum by tumors, granulation tissue, pus, blood, edema, etc. In some cases the osteoblasts may be activated, and periosteal new bone formed, for no discernible cause. There may be substances that can directly stimulate the periosteal osteoblasts such as fluorine or tumor-synthesized factors. In systemic diseases that are associated with vasculitis (e.g., collagen diseases), the alteration in blood flow appears to have pathogenic significance. If venous drainage from the periosteum is impaired as a result of varicose disease or arteriovenous malformations, for example, edema can develop and stimulate osteoblastic activity. Similarly, the edema that accompanies inflammatory joint disorders is apparently able to stimulate periosteal new bone formation. The pathogenesis of systemic periosteal new bone formation like that occurring in hypertrophic osteoarthropathy is poorly understood. Changes in periosteal blood flow due to neural or other causes have been suggested as a possible mechanism (see Sect. 7.3 for further details).

Periosteal reactions become visible on X-ray films when the matrix formed by the osteoblasts of the germinative layer becomes mineralized. Depending on the underlying disease, it takes about 5–7 days in children and up to 4 weeks in adults for periosteal new bone to become visible on properly exposed radiographs. The radiographic appearance of periosteal new bone is shaped by various factors, and for the experienced radiologist it can provide important clues to the intensity, duration, and aggressiveness of the underlying disease. A thin, continuous strip of periosteal new bone that is demarcated from the underlying cortex signifies a fresh process, whereas a thicker, denser layer that is directly apposed to the cortex signifies a process of longer standing. A laminated, onionskin pattern of new bone deposition signifies an intermittent or episodic process. Discontinuous or interrupted periosteal reactions may indicate a more aggressive process that has disrupted preexisting solid periosteal new bone.

In interpreting new bone formation as the manifestation of a pathologic periosteal reaction, it is important not only to evaluate the pattern of bone formation itself and the underlying cortex but also to determine whether the process is circumscribed or systemic. In all cases the soft tissues surrounding the bone should be examined clinically for abnormalities (vascular changes? inflammatory induration?) along with the adjacent joints. If there is the slightest suspicion of a systemic periosteal process, radionuclide bone scans should be obtained. A single whole-body scan can accurately define the extent of the changes.

7.1 Pachydermoperiostosis

Synonyms: generalized hyperostosis with pachy-derma, Uehlinger's syndrome, Touraine-So-lente-Golé syndrome

Bulging cerebriform folds on scalp and fore-head; enlargement of the hands and feet; watchglass nails, digital clubbing; rheuma-toid complaints.
Roentgen signs: periosteal new bone formation on the epiphyses, metaphyses, and diaphyses of the bones of the hands and feet and long tubular bones. Acro-osteolysis.

Definition

Pachydermoperiostosis is a rare disease, prob-ably inherited as an autosomal dominant trait, that is characterized by circumscribed visible and palpable skin changes (pachyderma), club-bing of the fingers and toes, and hyperostotic skeletal changes.

General Clinical and Dermatologic Features

More common in males than females, pachyder-moperiostosis takes an insidious onset during or after puberty and rarely begins after age 30. Periosteal new bone formation is accompanied by rheumatoid complaints involving the affect-ed portions of the tubular bones. Pachyderma-tous changes affect the scalp, forehead, eyelids, and the palms and soles of the hands and feet. One of our patients was a 35-year-old man (Fig. 7.1 c) who presented with thickening and trans-verse furrowing of the forehead skin (cutis fron-tis gyrata) and occipital scalp (cutis verticis gy-rata). Thickening and transverse furrowing were reminiscent of the "bulging folds" of brain gyri. The upper eyelids were thickened and ptotic, and there was marked seborrhea associated with hy-perplastic sebaceous glands. The hands were en-larged with watchglass nails and clubbing of the fingers. The palms also showed marked pachy-dermatous changes with hyperhidrosis. Addi-tionally, the patient displayed an unusual, some-what feminine pattern of hair growth.
Pachydermoperiostosis is a self-limiting condi-tion with a favorable prognosis.

Radiology

The radiographic hallmark of pachydermoperi-ostosis is thick, solid *periosteal new bone forma-tion that involves all segments of the bone (diaph-yses, metaphyses, epiphyses); this distinguishes it from hypertrophic osteoarthropathy, which spares the bone ends* (Fig. 7.1 a, b, d–f). The peri-osteal new bone is directly applied to the cortex and is not visibly demarcated from it, so it can mimic cortical thickening. The new bone may have an undulating, bristled, or irregular contour and is most prominent at the midshaft level. Sites of predilection are the radius and ulna, the tibia and fibula, and the tubular bones of the hand. Thickening of the calvarium is rare, but we did observe thickening of the outer table in the case described. The facial bones and mandible are rarely affected. Acro-osteolysis may occur and most commonly involves the hands and feet (Fig. 7.1 f).

References are listed at the end of Chap. 7, p. 190.

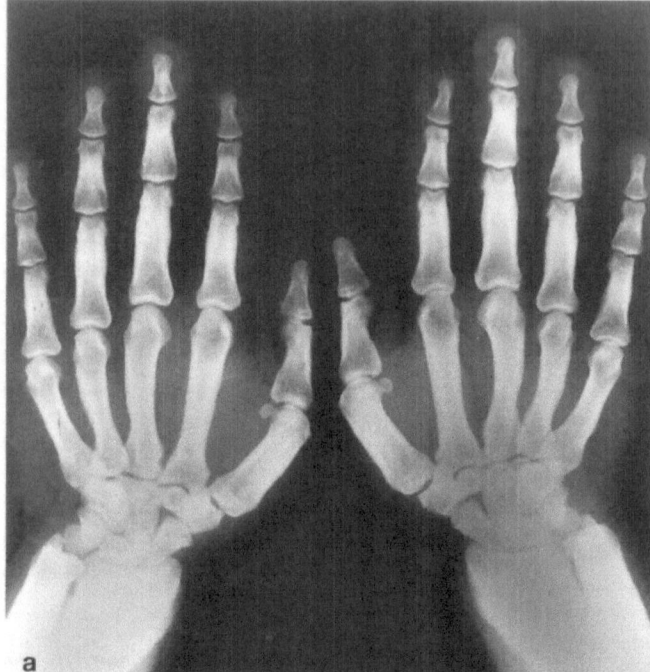

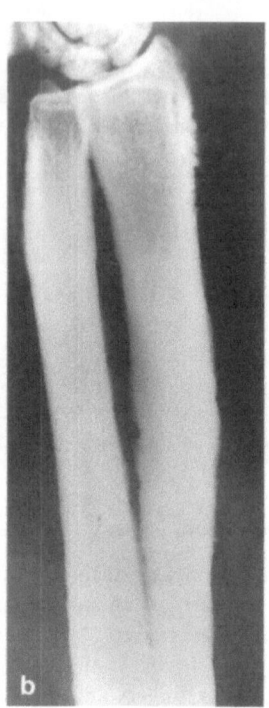

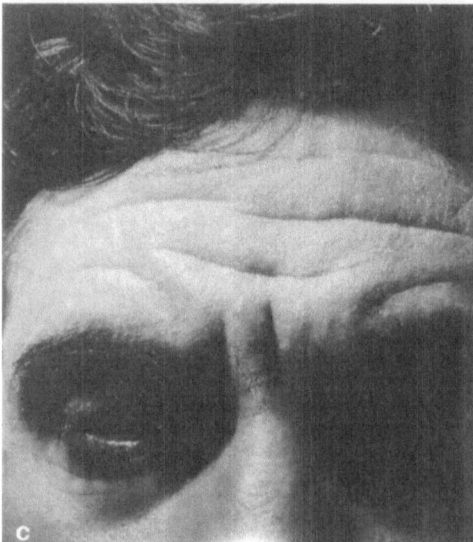

Fig. 7.1 a–f. Pachydermoperiostosis. **a–c** Man 35 years ▷ of age presented with marked thickening and bulging folds of the forehead skin (and occipital scalp, not shown) and thickened, ptotic upper eyelids (**c**). Clinically there was a marked overgrowth of the hands and feet with slight watchglass nail deformity and clubbing of the fingers. The changes in the hands and feet had commenced at age 15. When admitted, the patient suffered from increasing back pain and muscle pains in the arms and legs. Radiographs showed extensive periosteal new bone formation on the tubular bones of the hands (**a**) and on the radius and ulna (**b**). Similar changes were found in the feet. The periosteal reactions involved all bone segments including the diaphyses, metaphyses and epiphyses – a pattern consistent with pachydermoperiostosis. **d–f** Woman 58 years of age with extensive periosteal new bone formation, again including the metaphyses and epiphyses. The periosteal new bone is directly apposed to the subjacent cortex, which is slightly atrophic. The pronounced acro-osteolytic lesions with pencil-like tapering of the distal phalanges are apparently the result of a severe trophic disturbance. The soft-tissue swelling of the distal phalanges (clubbing) is clearly visible (**f**). The same changes were noted in the feet and were bilaterally symmetric. The classic clinical presentation and the involvement of the epiphyses by periosteal new bone formation were not consistent with a diagnosis of hypertrophic osteoarthropathy. **d–f** see p. 183

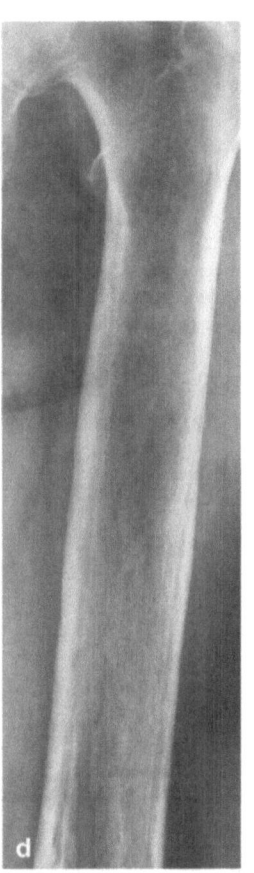

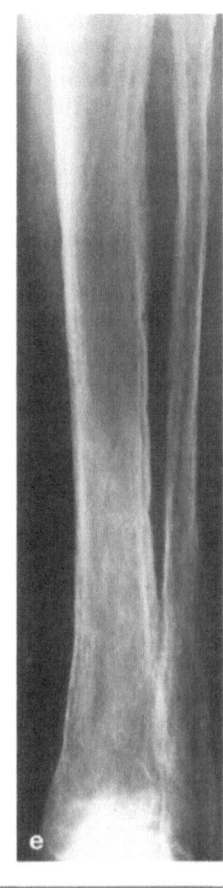

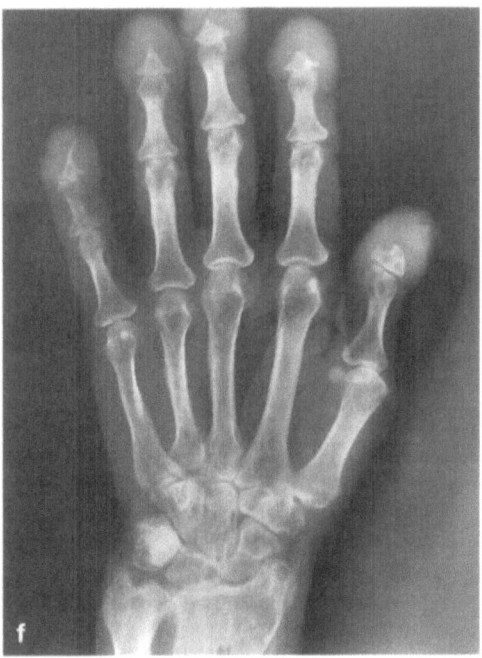

7.2 EMO Syndrome

Synonym: pituitary-thyroid acropachy

Prior treatment of hyperthyroidism.
Progressive exophthalmos, pretibial myxedema with orange-peel appearance of skin;
swelling of hands and feet.
Roentgen signs: periosteal new bone formation
on diaphyses of radius, ulna, tibia, fibula, and
tubular bones of hands and feet.

Definition

EMO syndrome is a sequela to anti-hyperthy-
roid therapy characterized by the triad of progressive exophthalmos, pretibial myxedema, and
periosteal new bone formation.

General Clinical and Dermatologic Features

The acronym EMO expresses the cardinal features of the disease: exophthalmos, (pretibial)
myxedema, and hypertrophic osteoarthropathy.
Braun-Falco and Petzhold introduced the term
"EMO syndrome" in 1967. Usually the disease
appears in patients who have been treated for hyperthyroidism from several weeks to several
years previously. The treatment modality seems
unimportant, as the syndrome may follow partial thyroidectomy, radioiodine therapy, or drug
therapy.

Most patients are hypothyroid or even euthy-
roid when the cutaneous and skeletal changes
develop. Important mediators of the disease are
the pathologic immunoglobulin LATS (long-act-
ing thyroid stimulator), EPS (exophthalmos-
producing substance), and TSH (thyroid-stimu-
lating hormone). LATS has been detected in
some 80% of reported cases with pretibial myxedema. The syndrome is estimated to affect approximately 1% of all hyperthyroid patients that
have been treated. There is no apparent predilection for a particular gender or age group.

The main clinical manifestations are pretibial
myxedema, characterized by a firm, plaquelike
infiltration on the anterior surface of the leg (Fig.
7.2 a), and swelling of the hands and feet with a
potentially painful clubbing of the fingers. The
symptoms are probably caused by the periosteal

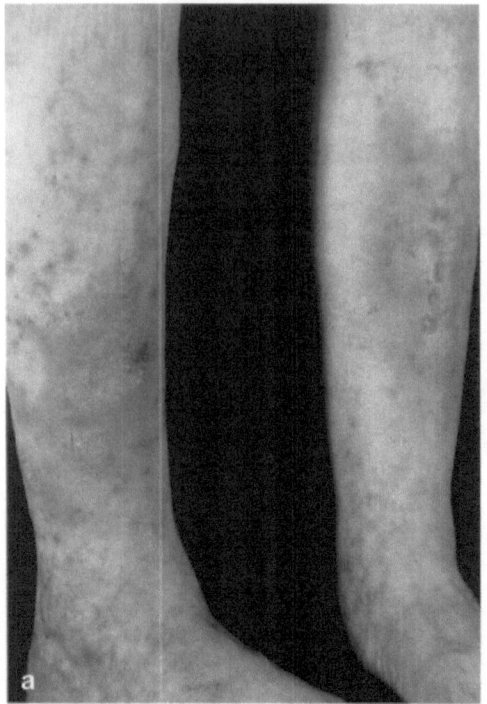

changes, which progress from an edematous stage to new bone formation. Accompanying features are rheumatoid complaints and a progressive exophthalmos. One case that we observed was unusual in that rheumatoid pain symptoms were the dominant feature.

Radiology

Periosteal new bone formation predominantly involves the diaphyses of tubular bones, especially the long bones of the forearm and lower leg and the small tubular bones of the hands and feet (Fig. 7.2 b, c). The sites most commonly affected in the hand are the radial aspects of the first and second metacarpals and the ulnar aspect of the fifth metacarpal. The new bone formation may have an irregular, frayed appearance or it may be bullous or spiculated, especially at the midshaft level. This radiographic pattern differs markedly from that seen in hypertrophic osteoarthropathy. The soft tissues show increased density on properly exposed films due to the presence of mucopolysaccharide deposits.

References are listed at the end of Chap. 7, p. 190.

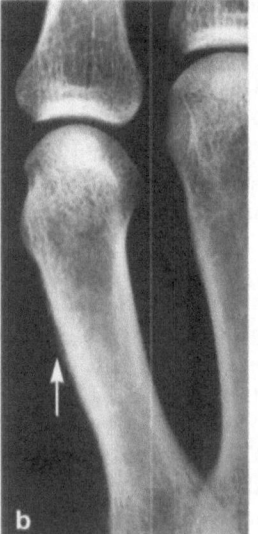

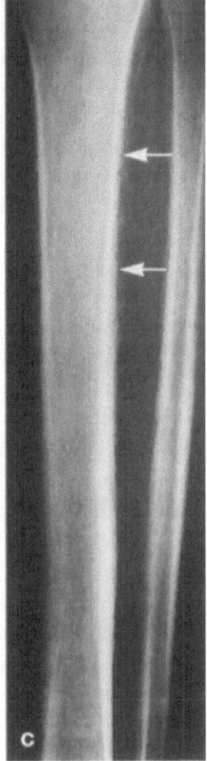

◁

Fig. 7.2 a–c. EMO syndrome. **a** Clinical appearance of pretibial myxedema. The dilated follicular orifices impart an orange-peel appearance to the affected skin. **b, c** Radiographs illustrate fine, irregular, frayed periosteal new bone formation (*arrows*), which may appear bullous or bristly when the film is viewed with magnification. The midshaft area is predominantly affected

7.3 Hypertrophic Osteoarthropathy

Synonym: Marie-Bamberger hypertrophic osteoarthropathy

Main clinical signs: clubbing of fingers and toes, rheumatic complaints.
Roentgen signs: solid, laminated, or bristled periosteal new bone formation on the diaphyses of tubular bones (especially the radius, ulna, tibia, fibula, metacarpals, and phalanges), usually showing a bilaterally symmetric distribution.

Definition

Hypertrophic osteoarthropathy is a condition of periosteal new bone formation that may accompany numerous inflammatory, suppurative, fibrotic, neoplastic (paraneoplastic syndrome), pulmonary, pleural, mediastinal, and occasionally gastrointestinal diseases.

General Clinical and Dermatologic Features

The pathogenesis of the periosteal new bone formation in hypertrophic osteoarthropathy is poorly understood. It is most common in patients with primary bronchogenic carcinoma (Fig. 7.3 f), but pulmonary metastases can also trigger the periosteal reaction. Von Bhate et al. (1980) describe a case of hypertrophic osteoarthropathy that was associated with liquefying pulmonary metastases from a squamous cell cancer of the cervix. It has been postulated that tumors may produce agents that stimulate periosteal osteoblasts, or that vagal nerve dysfunction may cause a "circulatory overload" of acral regions in which the increased blood flow is diverted and rerouted through the periosteal and capsular vessels. The latter hypothesis is supported by the finding that periosteal new bone formation and clinical symptoms regress following unilateral vagotomy. The periosteal new bone formation is also reversible following removal of the causative bronchogenic carcinoma. Other diseases that can incite hypertrophic osteoarthropathy include nonneoplastic pulmonary lesions (e.g., bronchiectasis) and chronic hypoxemic states. All forms of hypertrophic osteoarthropathy that are induced by intrathoracic processes are collectively referred to as the "pulmonary" form.

Somewhat less common is the "intestinal" form of hypertrophic osteoarthropathy, which occurs in the setting of inflammatory bowel diseases such as ulcerative colitis and Crohn's disease (see Fig. 3.6.6).

A characteristic feature of hypertrophic osteoarthropathy is progressive clubbing of the fingers and toes (Fig. 7.3 a) often combined with watchglass nails. Accompanying synovitis and periosteal new bone formation can cause significant pain resembling a systemic rheumatic disease. It is common to find periarticular warmth and edema with smooth, tense skin and other rheumatoid features. The clinical manifestations may precede the diagnosis of a pulmonary or intestinal disorder (see also Fig. 3.6.6). In cases caused by an intrathoracic neoplasm, digital clubbing is accompanied by an erythematous rim around the nail bed. It is interesting to note that digital clubbing in a setting of chronic pulmonary insufficiency does not cause significant pain.

Radiology

The most common radiographic manifestation of hypertrophic osteoarthropathy is periosteal new bone formation that symmetrically involves the diaphyses and diminishes toward the metaphyses, usually sparing the epiphyses (Fig. 7.3 b – e). The outer surface of the periosteal new bone is rough and grossly resembles tree bark. With passage of time, the periosteal new bone may be transformed into normal lamellar bone, virtually creating a new cortex while the original cortex undergoes cancellous transformation. This can cause a net increase in bone diameter. The most commonly affected bones (in decreasing order of frequency) are the radius, ulna, tibia, fibula, femur, humerus, metacarpals and metatarsals, proximal phalanges, and middle phalanges. Five radiographic patterns of periosteal new bone formation can be distinguished in hypertrophic osteoarthropathy:

1. Solid new bone with a smooth outer contour that is clearly demarcated from the subjacent cortex by a thin lucent line.

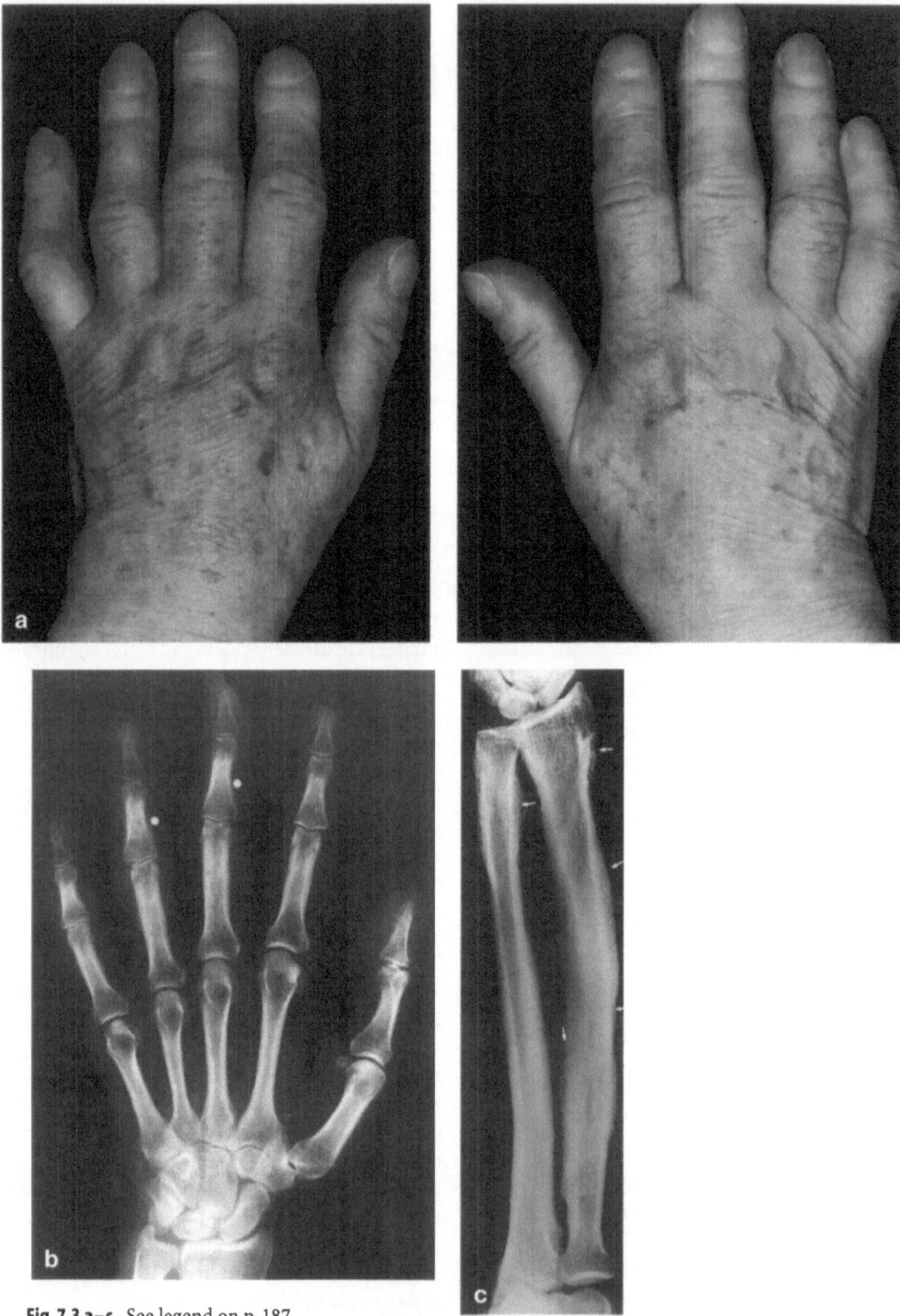

Fig. 7.3 a–c. See legend on p. 187

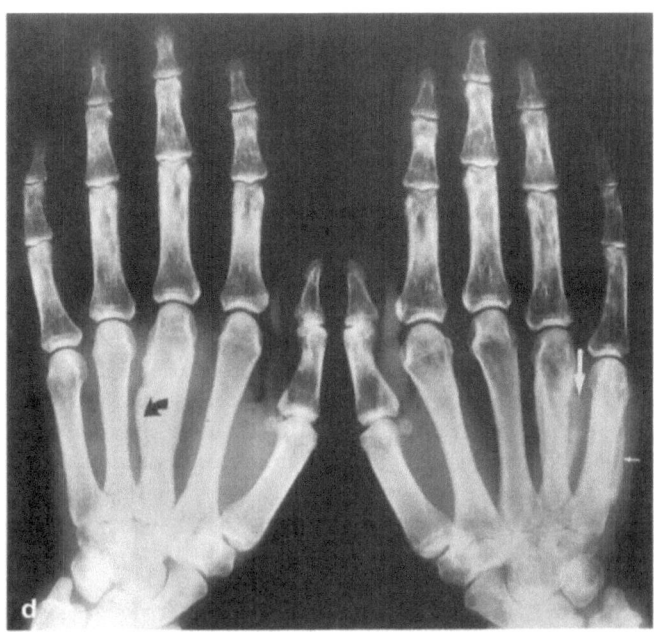

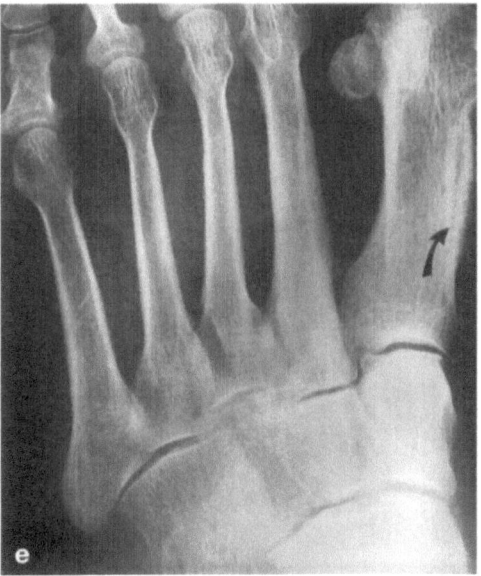

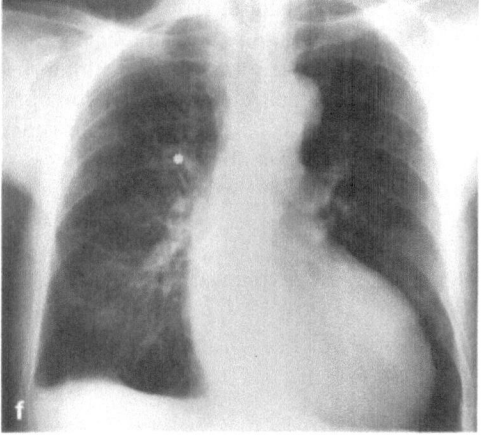

Fig. 7.3 a–f. Hypertrophic osteoarthropathy (in patients with bronchogenic carcinoma). **a** Watchglass nails and clubbing of the fingers with moderate dorsal and digital swelling in a patient with significant polyarthralgia. **b** Very subtle, bilaterally symmetric sites of periosteal new bone formation (also on the feet) accompanied by marked periarticular (Sudeck-like) osteoporosis reflecting a severe trophic disturbance and indicating the acuteness of the process. There are incipient acro-osteolytic changes. Clinically, the patient had severe pain and marked swelling of the fingers. **c** Solid periosteal new bone, some of which has already fused with the cortex. **d** Unusually prominent sites of periosteal new bone formation on the third metacarpal of the left hand and the fourth and fifth metacarpals of the right hand, showing both laminated and bristled configurations (*arrows*). Again, there is moderate periarticular osteoporosis, especially in the right hand. **e** Bristled pattern of periosteal bone formation along the medial side of the diaphysis of the first metatarsal. **f** Chest film reveals a typical bronchogenic carcinoma (*asterisk*) in the right upper hilum. **f** belongs to **e**

2. Laminar or onion-skin pattern of new bone formation.
3. Radial or bristled pattern of sporadic new bone formation (Fig. 7.3 e).
4. Predominantly solid mantle of new bone with a wavy outer contour (Fig. 7.3 c).
5. Mixed forms incorporating 1–3 (Fig. 7.3 d).
6. Cortical thickening due to fusion of the periosteal new bone with the original cortex (Fig. 7.3 c).

Besides occasional soft-tissue swelling, the synovitis causes no radiographic changes in the articulating bones. Clubbing of the fingers or toes appears as soft-tissue swelling of the distal phalanges without associated changes in the bone or periosteum.

Trophic acro-osteolysis is an uncommon finding that, when present, is usually accompanied by marked *Sudeck-like osteoporosis* (Fig. 7.3 b).

Differentiation is required from *acromegaly*, which may resemble hypertrophic osteoarthropathy in its very painful arthralgias and other clinical features. But the radiographic manifestations of acromegaly are readily distinguished by the anchor or spadelike configuration of the enlarged acral parts. The history alone is generally sufficient to differentiate hypertrophic osteoarthropathy from pachydermoperiostosis and EMO syndrome.

References are listed at the end of Chap. 7, p. 190.

7.4 Periosteal Ossification in Varicose Symptom Complex

Typical features of varicose symptom complex including venous stasis ulcers. Solid, laminated, or bristled periosteal new bone formation on the tibia and occasionally the fibula, often blending with the cortex.

Patients with varicose symptom complex have a chronic venous stasis that also affects the veins of the periosteum. The resulting edema stimulates the osteoblasts of the cambium layer to produce osteoid, which is transformed into radiographically visible periosteal new bone. Most periosteal new bone is solid, very dense, and very broad with a wavy outer contour (Fig. 7.4 c). If the venous stasis is intermittent, a laminated or bristled pattern of periosteal bone formation can occur (Fig. 7.4b). The new bone forms almost exclusively along the tibial shaft and less commonly on the fibula. Periosteal new bone formation is consistently found in patients with severe saphenous varicosity.

Fig. 7.4 a–c. Typical periosteal new bone formation in ▷ patients with varicose symptom complex and lower leg ulcers. **a** Massive stasis dermatitis with a typical leg ulcer (lateral view of the lower leg and ankle region). **b** Combination of solid and laminar periosteal new bone formation along the medial border of the tibia. **c** Predominantly solid, undulating periosteal new bone formation, most prominent on the tibial midshaft

7.5 Scurvy

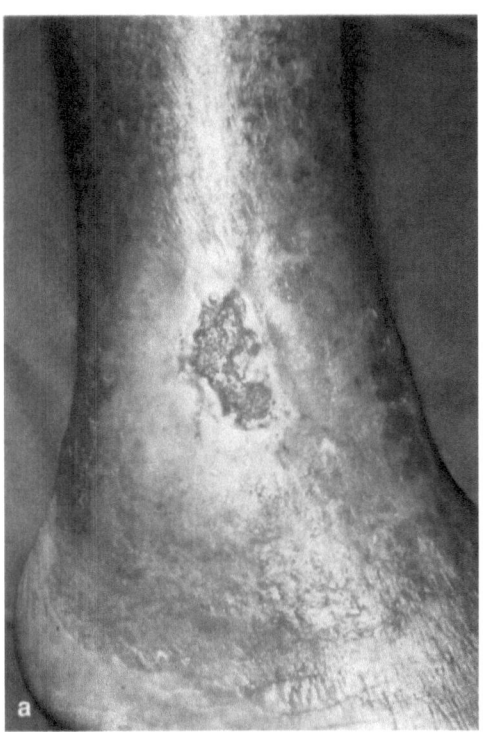

Children age 2 and under: bluish-red discoloration of the oral mucosa, purpura; pain in extremities.
Roentgen signs: periosteal new bone formation, metaphyseal white line, scurvy zone, Pelken's spurs, pseudo-double epiphysis.
In adults: rasp-like skin on the upper arms, also tibial and gluteal skin areas. Hemorrhagic papules with hyperkeratosis.
Roentgen signs: osteoporosis.

Definition

Scurvy is a vitamin C deficiency syndrome marked by characteristic changes mainly involving the oral mucosa, integument, and periosteum. A secondary impairment of collagen synthesis leads to osteoporosis in adults and growth disturbances in children.

General Clinical and Dermatologic Features

The *cardinal feature* of scurvy is tissue hemorrhages caused by a lack of proline hydroxylase activation, leading to a qualitative and quantitative connective tissue deficiency in blood vessels that is manifested by a *vascular purpura*.

In *children*, scurvy is known also as *Moeller-Barlow disease*. This disease has become rare in industrialized countries, where it is caused mainly by the vitamin C-deficient bottle feeding of infants with sterile milk during the first and second years of life. Rarely, the disease is seen in children with a severe malabsorption syndrome. The oral mucosa is swollen and shows areas of bluish-red discoloration that bleed easily. The teeth may become loosened. The skin shows *petechial hemorrhages* (purpura) typically located on the neck and shoulders and occasionally on the conjunctiva. Gastrointestinal and urinary tract bleeding are not uncommon. Subperiosteal hemorrhage along the femur, tibia, and fibula can cause significant pain and tenderness in the lower extremities.

Adults with scurvy develop a coarsening and keratosis of the hair follicles primarily on the upper arms. Within a few weeks this condition leads to

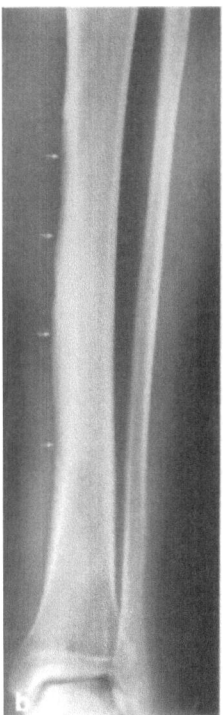
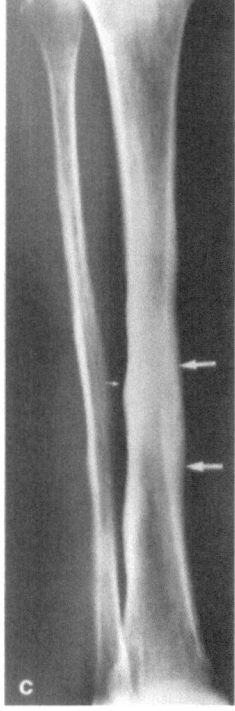

a *rasp-like transformation of the skin* also involving the anterior tibial and gluteal skin areas. Localized bleeding leads to a hemorrhagic zone around the keratotic follicles, promoting the development of *hemorrhagic papules with hyperkeratosis*. Impaired collagen synthesis resulting from the vitamin deficiency leads to poor wound healing. Fresh wounds typically show a reddish or livid discoloration.

When the deficiency state has been present for about 6 months, the oral mucosa becomes red and swollen and bleeds easily. This *gingivitis* gradually becomes spongy, and teeth become loosened and lost. *Necrotic ulcerations* may finally develop.

Radiology

Vitamin C is essential for normal osteoid formation (type I collagen). A deficiency leads to osteoporosis in adults and also to growth disturbances in children. Deficient osteoid formation in the metaphyses and at the periphery of ossification centers tends to retard bone growth while calcium phosphate deposition in the deficient osteoid matrix continues, resulting in a net increase in bone density. This produces the characteristic *"white line"* of scurvy directly adjacent to the epiphyseal plate. A ring of increased density may form around the epiphysis itself (Wimberger's sign).

The zone of provisional calcification on the diaphyseal side of the white line is soft and fragile and appears radiographically as a lucent band, the *Truemmerfeld zone*. This osteoporotic zone is easily fractured by minor trauma, causing the appearance of *metaphyseal beaks* due to corner fracturing (Pelken's spurs, corner sign). A *pseudo-double epiphysis* may appear during the healing stage. Another important radiographic sign of scurvy in children is *periosteal new bone formation*, at times extensive, as a result of subperiosteal hemorrhage. The underlying cortex is usually atrophic and is easily fractured. *Differentiation* is mainly required from battered child syndrome.

References

Arlart I, Bargon G (1981) Periostale Knochenneubildungen bei Colitis ulcerosa im jugendlichen Alter. Röfo 135: 577

Bhate DV, Chandrasekhar H, Greenfield GB et al. (1980) Secondary hypertrophic osteoarthropathy associated with excavating pulmonary metastases from squamous cell carcinoma of the cervix. Case report 126. Skeletal Radiol 5: 258

Glickstein M, Neustadter DO, Dalinka M et al. (1986) Periosteal reaction in systemic lupus erythematosus. Skeletal Radiol 15: 610

Joseph B, Chacko V (1985) Acro-osteolysis associated with hypertrophic pulmonary osteoarthropathy and pachydermoperiostosis. Radiology 154: 343

Lubach D, Freyschmidt J (1981) Das EMO-Syndrom. Hautarzt 32: 91

Lubach D, Freyschmidt J, Bolten D (1981) Pachydermoperiostose (Touraine-Solente-Golé). Z Hautkrankh 56: 175

Moule B, Grant MC, Boyle IT, May H (1970) Thyroid acropachy. Clin Radiol 21: 329

Schawarby K, Ibrahim MS (1962) Pachydermoperiostitis. A review of the literature and report of four cases. Br Med J 1: 763

Torres-Reyes E, Staple TW (1970) Roentgenographic appearance of thyroid acropachy. Clin Radiol 21: 95

Uehlinger E (1942) Hyperostosis generalisata mit Pachydermie (Idiopathische familiäre generalisierte Osteophytose Friedreich-Erb-Arnold). Virchows Arch [Pathol Anat] 308: 396

8 Other Diseases

8.1 Nonsystemic Trophic Disorders of the Hands and Feet with Acro-osteolysis

Scarred lesions and strictures involving the acral portions of fingers and toes may cause a deficiency of peripheral blood flow. If the blood supply to the bone is significantly impaired, osteolytic lesions may develop (e.g., in the terminal tufts of the distal phalanges). The precipitating causes are usually chronic and traumatic in nature (see below). Acute traumatization by heat, cold, electric shock, etc. is relatively uncommon. The pathogenesis of acro-osteolysis occurring in systemic diseases with peripheral blood flow disturbances (e.g., progressive scleroderma, hypertrophic osteoarthropathy; Table 8.1) is ultimately the same as in nonsystemic causes: whenever the "principal players" in bone remodeling, the osteoclasts and osteoblasts, are deprived of nutrition, the balance between production and resorption is tipped toward lysis, and bone substance is lost.

This section deals with two disorders that have a nonsystemic cause of acro-osteolysis and present with marked acral changes in the skin and subcutaneous tissues.

Ainhum Syndrome (Spontaneous Dactylolysis)

In this syndrome, hyperkeratotic lesions of the toes cause constriction of the soft-tissue envelope, disrupting the blood supply to the distal portions of the phalanges, which undergo resorption (Fig. 8.1). The disease is most common in persons who frequently go barefoot, such as the dark-skinned inhabitants of western Africa and other warm climatic regions. Ainhum syndrome has an estimated prevalence of 2% in the Nigerian population. It also occurs in the West Indies and in Central and South America.

Table 8.1. Principal causes of acro-osteolysis in *systemic* diseases that may be associated with dermatologic changes

- Trophic (vascular, neurogenic)
  Raynaud's syndrome
  Scleroderma, Sharp's syndrome
  Epidermolysis bullosa
  Congenital ichthyosiform erythroderma
  Mutilating palmoplantar keratoderma
  Hereditary palmoplantar keratosis
  Werner's syndrome
  Fabry's disease
  Chronic acrodermatitis
  Neurosyphilis, syringomyelia, leprosy
  Hyperostosis with pachyderma (Uehlinger's syndrome)
  In hypertrophic osteoarthropathy
- Goltz-Gorlin syndrome
- Sarcoidosis
- Psoriasis
- Gout
- Tumors (metastases)

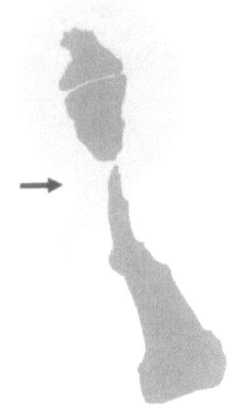

Fig. 8.1. Toe in Ainhum syndrome. *Arrow:* coarse annular constriction similar to that in mutilating palmoplantar keratoderma (see Fig. 1.17). The pathogenic mechanism of resorptive osteolysis with pencil-like tapering of the affected bone is identical in both diseases

The peak incidence is in the fourth and fifth decades, but fully blown cases have been seen in children. The distal portions of the toes are extremely hyperkeratotic and atrophic, usually showing bilateral involvement. Secondary infections of the poorly perfused acral parts are not uncommon and promote the acro-osteolytic changes. Approximately 80% of patients have pain in the affected toes.

Acro-osteolysis in Guitar Players and Violinists

Chronic fingertip trauma from instrument strings in professional guitarists and violinists initially causes small, poorly healing ulcerations on the affected fingers, with the gradual development of cicatricial and hyperkeratotic changes. With repeated trauma the ulcerations recur, perpetuating the process and leading to a severe, stricture-producing atrophy of the distal fingers. One of our patients was a zither player who developed extremely severe cicatricial, ulcerative, and hyperkeratotic changes in the fingertips, which were transformed into bony hard plates. Radiographs demonstrated resorption of the terminal tufts.

References

Bertoli CL, Stassi J, Rifkin MD (1984) Ainhum – an unusual presentation involving the second toe in a white male. Skeletal Radiol 11: 133

Destouet JM, Murphy WA (1981) Guitar player acroosteolysis. Skeletal Radiol 6: 275

8.2 Sudeck's Syndrome

Synonyms: reflex sympathetic dystrophy syndrome, Sudeck's atrophy of bone

> Swelling of the affected extremities; livid, shiny skin; hyperhidrosis, pain.
> **Roentgen signs:** patchy periarticular osteoporosis.

This syndrome will be discussed only briefly, as its dermatologic manifestations are not specific for this medical specialty and actually are within the scope of general medical knowledge. Nevertheless, it is not unusual for patients with an affected hand or foot to be referred to a dermatologist.

The disease is based on a multifactorial trophic disturbance involving the bone and soft-tissue envelope of an extremity or one of its segments. The precipitating factor in reflex sympathetic dystrophy syndrome is severe pain, which need not be localized to an affected extremity. Cases are known in which a very severe toothache, the excruciating pain of myocardial infarction, or severe regional pain in herpes zoster has precipitated the syndrome. But the most frequent causes are traumatic fractures of the affected skeletal segments and painful immobilization (e.g., by a tight-fitting cast). Blumberg (1988) believes that the symptoms are caused by microcirculatory disturbances based on a dysfunction of sympathetic vasoconstrictor neurons. This concept has formed the basis for promising sympatholytic treatment modalities (e.g., sympathetic blockade, prevention of norepinephrine release from vasoconstrictor neurons by the i.v. administration of guanethidine in an exsanguinated field). Six criteria must be met in order for reflex sympathetic dystrophy syndrome to be diagnosed:

1. Pain and hypersensitivity affecting all or part of an extremity.
2. Soft-tissue swelling.
3. Vasomotor instability (hyperhidrosis).
4. Patchy osteoporosis on radiographs.
5. Partial loss of motor function.
6. Trophic skin changes, including shiny skin with livid discoloration (Fig. 8.2 a).

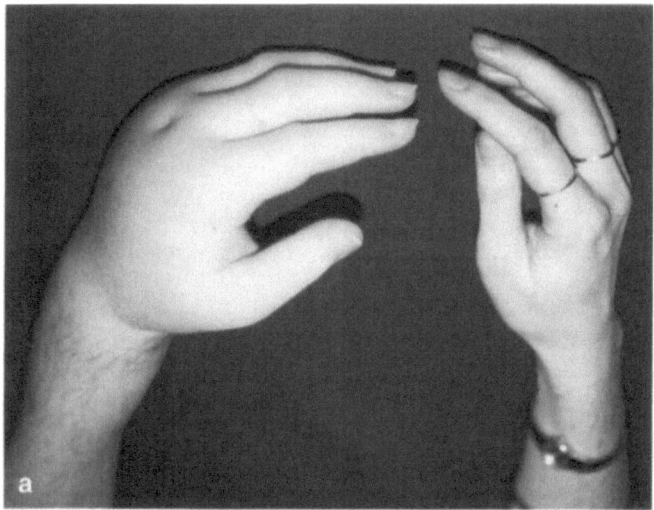

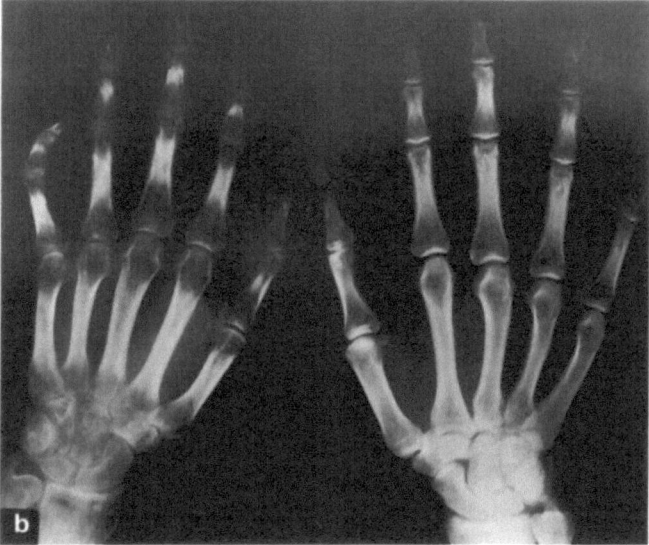

Fig. 8.2 a, b. Sudeck's syndrome. Massive soft-tissue swelling with tense, shiny skin showing livid discoloration (**a**). Severe pain, hypersensitivity, and hyperhidrosis were present in the affected hand. Radiograph (**b**) shows coarse, patchy areas of periarticular osteoporosis in the left hand

The *clinical symptoms* can be very dramatic and may include a severe aching pain that responds poorly to analgesic medication.

Radiographs in the early stage of the disease (usually 3–4 weeks after the clinical onset) show a patchy periarticular osteoporosis (Fig. 8.2 b) that is generally accompanied by marked soft-tissue swelling. This is followed by the development of a uniform cortical and cancellous bone atrophy that progresses in weeks or months to an "end stage" marked clinically by extensive skin and muscle atrophy with painless limitation of joint motion and deformities.

References

Blumberg H (1988) Zur Entstehung und Therapie des Schmerzsyndroms bei der sympathischen Reflexdystrophie. Schmerz 2: 125

Genant HK, Kozin F, Bekerman C et al. (1975) The reflex sympathic dystrophy syndrome. Radiology 117: 21

8.3 Lipoatrophic Diabetes Mellitus

Synonym: generalized lipodystrophy

Congenital: gigantism, diabetes mellitus, hirsutism, skull-like facial appearance, acanthosis nigricans.

Roentgen signs: premature closure of epiphyseal plates, epimetaphyseal sclerosis; focal osteoporosis of tubular bones.

Acquired: absence of subcutaneous fat, hypersensitivity to cold, increased bone density, cortical thickening, prominent metaphyseal sclerosis.

Definition

Lipoatrophic diabetes mellitus is a rare disorder characterized by the absence of body fat. It may be associated with various skeletal and cutaneous abnormalities. The congenital form of generalized lipodystrophy is distinguished from the acquired form.

General Clinical, Dermatologic, and Radiologic Features

The term "lipoatrophic changes" has various meanings in dermatology and radiology, perhaps due partly to the fact that very few cases have been described to date and it has not been possible to establish a clear classification. The most useful classification at present is to differentiate the disease into its congenital and acquired forms. Insulin deficiency is common to both forms and may well be the initiating pathogenic factor.

Congenital Form

Congenital generalized lipodystrophy is an autosomal recessive disorder characterized by an absence of body fat combined with gigantism and an insulin-resistant diabetes mellitus and hypertriglyceridemia that develop between 10 and 20 years of age. Other features are prominence of the skeletal muscles, organomegaly, and hirsutism in women. A striking external feature is the *skull-like facial appearance* caused by the absence of subcutaneous fat (Fig. 8.3 a). *Pigment-*

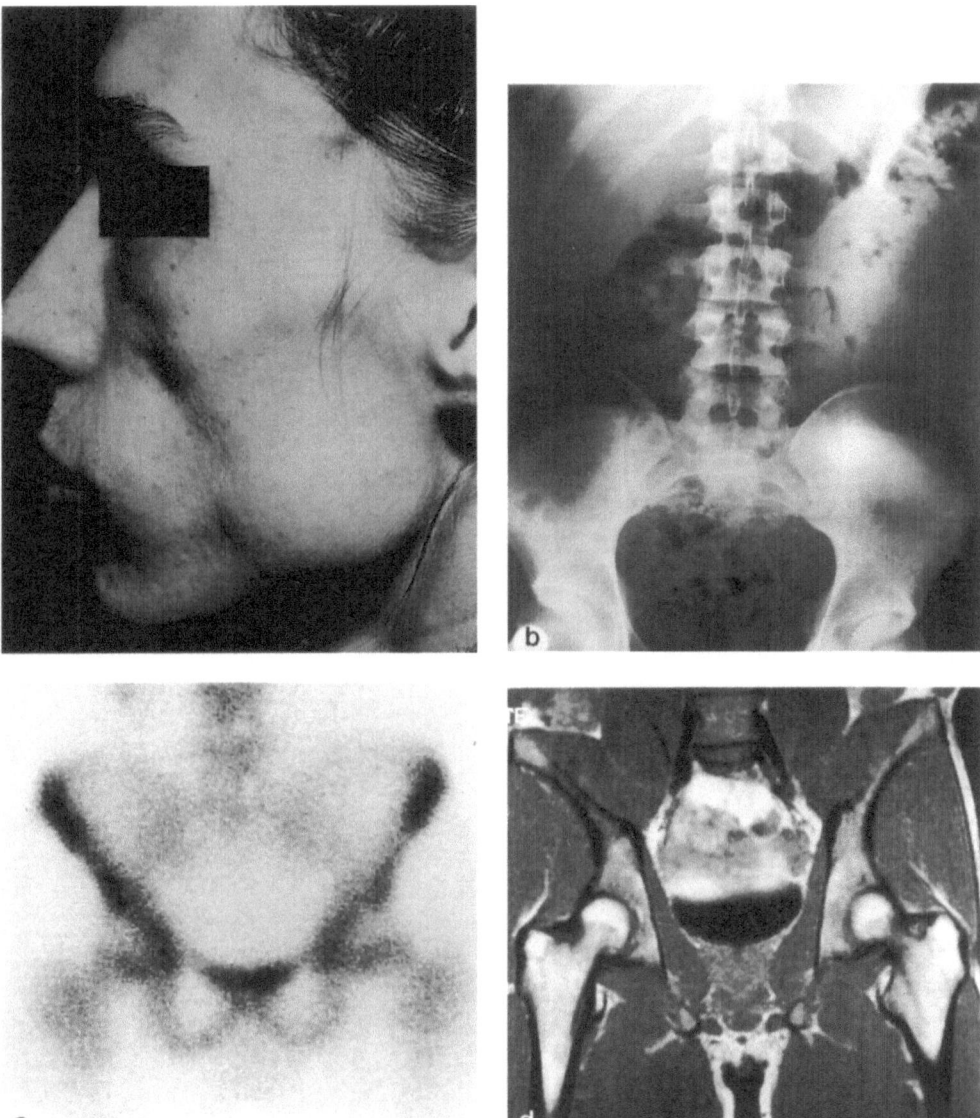

Fig. 8.3 a–i. Lipoatrophic diabetes mellitus. **a** Typical skull-like facial contours. **b–i** Acquired form. This is a 19-year-old man with insulin-dependent diabetes mellitus (type I) and a 6-month history of pain in the right buttock and hip region. Scintigraphic bone scan revealed increased tracer uptake in the right anterior iliac bone. X-rays of the abdomen and pelvis demonstrated reduction of retroperitoneal and pelvic fat planes (**b, c**). MR images confirm the reduced fat content in the pelvic soft tissues and in the bone, especially on T1-weighted images (**d, e**). T2-weighted images (**f, g**) show increased signal intensities in the right iliac bone, upper acetabulum, and upper diaphysis of the femoral bones. The higher single intensities may be explained by liquid formations. The CT scans in **h** and **i** show diffuse sclerosis in the iliac bones and an osteolytic lesion in the right iliac wing (**i**), corresponding to one of the hyperintense lesions in the MR images. CT-guided bone biopsy of the osteolytic lesion in the right iliac wing revealed bone necrosis with saponification of fatty tissue. Given the outer aspect of the patient with severe loss of facial subcutaneous fat, it was possible to interpret the bony changes as associated with lipoarthrophic diabetes mellitus

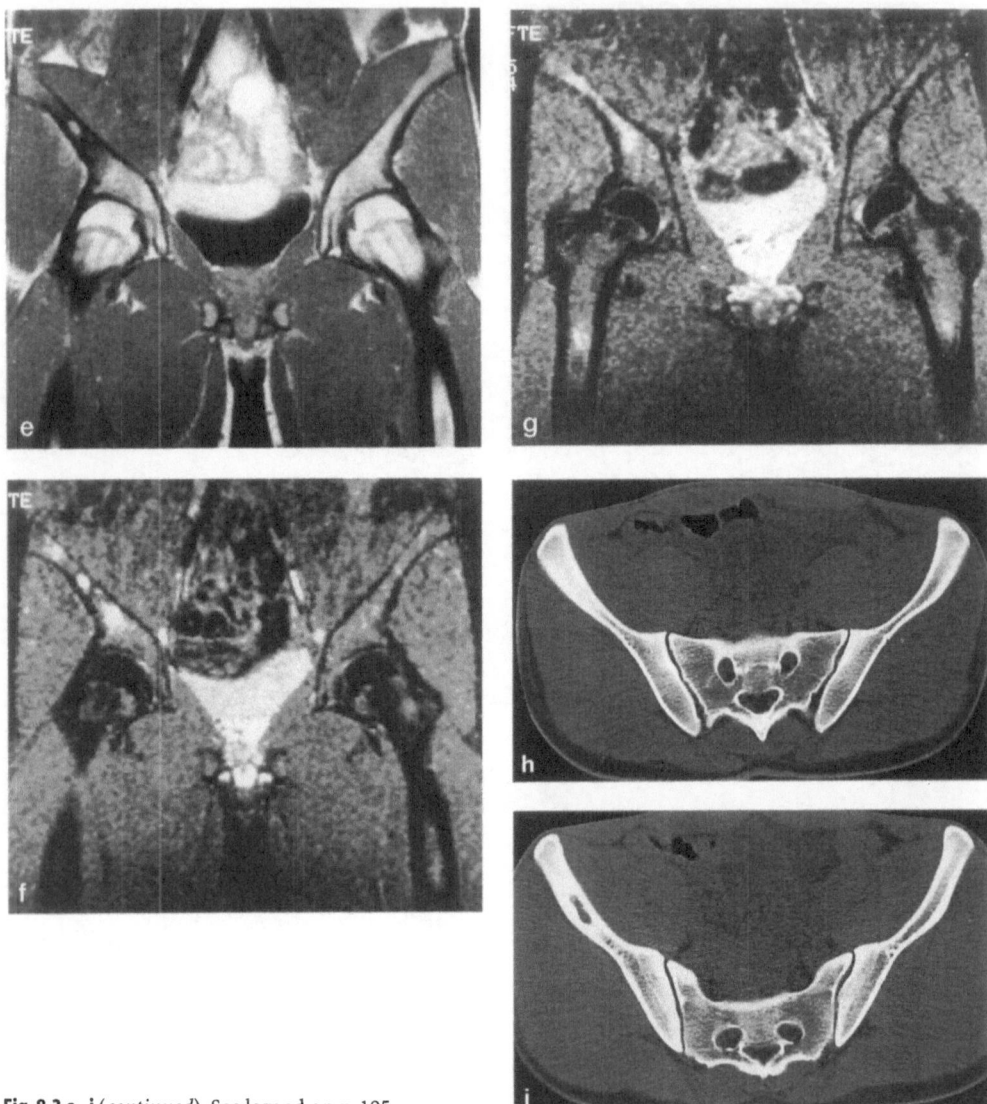

Fig. 8.3 e–i (*continued*). See legend on p. 195

ed skin lesions resembling acanthosis nigricans develop early in the course of the disease and may progress to true acanthosis nigricans. The skin changes appear as dirty-brown to grayish, papillomatous, keratotic lesions that may be pruritic and most commonly involve the neck, axillae, inguinal region, and feet, generally sparing the extremities. Radiographs show *pathologic sclerosis about the prematurely closed epiphyseal plates*. Focal osteolytic lesions may occur in the large and small tubular bones and, when extensive, resemble lytic foci of fibrous dysplasia (Fleckenstein et al. 1992). MRI of the lytic areas may demonstrate fluid levels (replacing marrow fat?) (Fleckenstein et al. 1992).

Acquired Form

Acquired generalized lipodystrophy occurs predominantly in women and initially may be associated with infections (e.g., mumps or whooping cough). Patients suffer from diabetes mellitus. The complete absence of subcutaneous fat is an early symptom primarily affecting the face, upper body, and retroperitoneal and pelvic regions. An increase of subcutaneous fat may be observed in the lower body. Female patients occasionally have menstrual abnormalities. Intellectual deficits are present. Cold sensitivity is markedly increased due to the lack of subcutaneous fat.

Radiographs of the abdomen show a complete absence of fat stripes, resulting in nondelineation of the retroperitoneal and pelvic organs (Fig. 8.3 b). Skeletal investigations (Fig. 8.3 c–i) show an *increase in bone density, cortical thickening*, and *prominent metaphyseal sclerosis*. These changes probably represent the response of the osteoblasts to a reduction of fat in the bone marrow. Radiographs also show small cysts in the trabecular bone that may be caused by circumscribed zones of hypervascularity or bone necrosis with saponification of fatty tissue.

References

Fleckenstein JL, Garg A, Bonte FJ et al. (1992) The skeleton in congenital, generalized lipodystrophy: evaluation using whole body radiographic surveys, magnetic resonance imaging and technetium-99m bone scintigraphy. Skeletal Radiol 21: 381

Gold RH, Steinbach HL (1967) Lipoatrophic diabetes mellitus (generalized lipodystrophy); roentgen findings in two brothers with congenital disease. AJR 101: 884

Guell-Gonzalez JR, De Acosta OM, Alavez-Martin E et al. (1971) Bone lesions in congenital generalized lipodystrophy. Lancet 2: 104

Reed WB, Dexter R, Corley C, Fish C (1965) Congenital lipodystrophic diabetes with acanthosis nigricans: Seip-Lawrence syndrome. AMA Arch Dermatol 91: 326

Sebrechts CH, Garvey WT, Sartoris DJ et al. (1987) Lipoatrophic diabetes mellitus (generalized lipodystrophy). Case report 417. Skeletal Radiol 16: 320

Wesenberg RL, Gwinn JL, Barnes GR Jr (1968) The roentgenographic findings in total lipodystrophy. AJR 103: 154

8.4 Pancreatitic Bone Lesions

> Soft, erythematous subcutaneous nodules resembling erythema nodosum but ubiquitous; arthritis-like joint symptoms.
> **Roentgen signs:** small osteolytic lesions in the cancellous and cortical bone with periosteal reactions (simulating osteomyelitis); bone marrow infarcts, bone necrosis.

Excessive serum levels of lipase can lead to the hydrolysis of neutral fat in adipose cells and to secondary inflammation, resulting in a fat necrosis that affects not only the fat in bone marrow but also the subcutaneous fat. The process may be triggered by acute and relapsing pancreatitis or by an acinar cell carcinoma of the pancreas that affects the exocrine function of the gland (Radin et al. 1986). The latter condition shows a

marked predilection for older males and presents clinically with fever, leukocytosis, and eosinophilia. In pancreatitis, subcutaneous fat necrosis and skeletal changes occur approximately 2–3 weeks after an active episode of the disease.

The *dermatologic* changes consist of soft, erythematous subcutaneous nodules (panniculitis, Fig. 8.4f) that are easily mistaken for erythema nodosum (see Fig. 3.6.4 a). But the latter disease chiefly affects the lower legs and forearms, while the subcutaneous fat necrosis shows a generalized, ubiquitous distribution. If the nodular lesions undergo significant liquefaction, they may break through the skin and discharge a sterile, creamy material that contains fat globules (Fig. 8.4 g).

Fat necrosis near joints can produce arthritis-like symptoms most commonly involving the ankles, knees, elbows, wrists, and the small joints

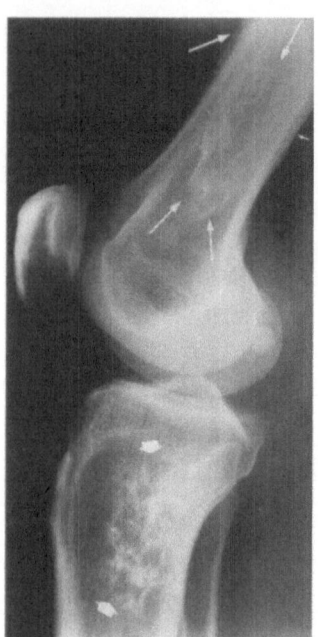

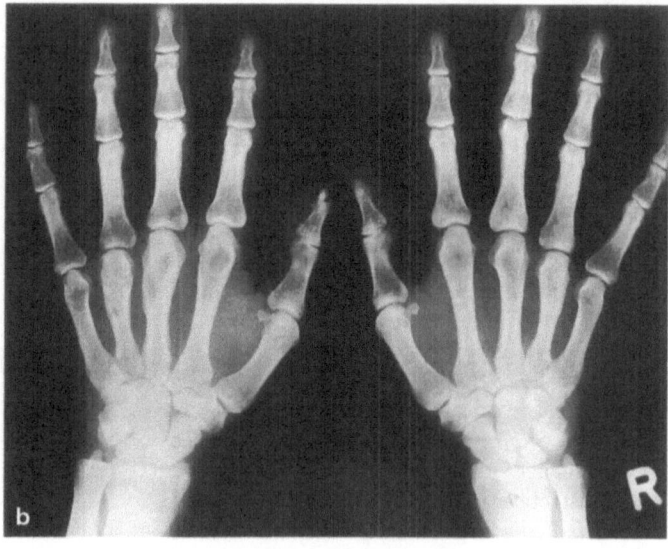

Fig. 8.4. a Areas of bone marrow infarction in the distal femur and proximal tibia (bilaterally symmetric) are manifested by irregular dystrophic calcifications (*arrows in the bones*). The *arrows* pointing to the distal femoral cortex indicate faint areas of periosteal new bone formation. Clinically, the patient had chronic recurrent pancreatitis. **b–g** 40-year-old patient with chronic relapsing pancreatitis. Remittant "rheumatic" pain in the hands, legs and feet. In **b** osteolytic lesions in the shafts of the metacarpal bones III, IV of the left

and – more discrete – on the contralateral side. Increased volume of the involved bones, resulting from resorption of the original cortices and formation of a neocortex. Mixed osteolytic and osteosclerotic changes in the distal tibia and the carpal bones, corresponding with fresh and older bone infarctions, demonstrated in the MR-images in **d** (T1) and **e** (T2). **f, g** Typical pictures of panniculitis with an erythema nodosum-like aspect in **f**. At the right buttock a perforated subcutaneous nodule of fat necrosis. **c–g** see p. 199

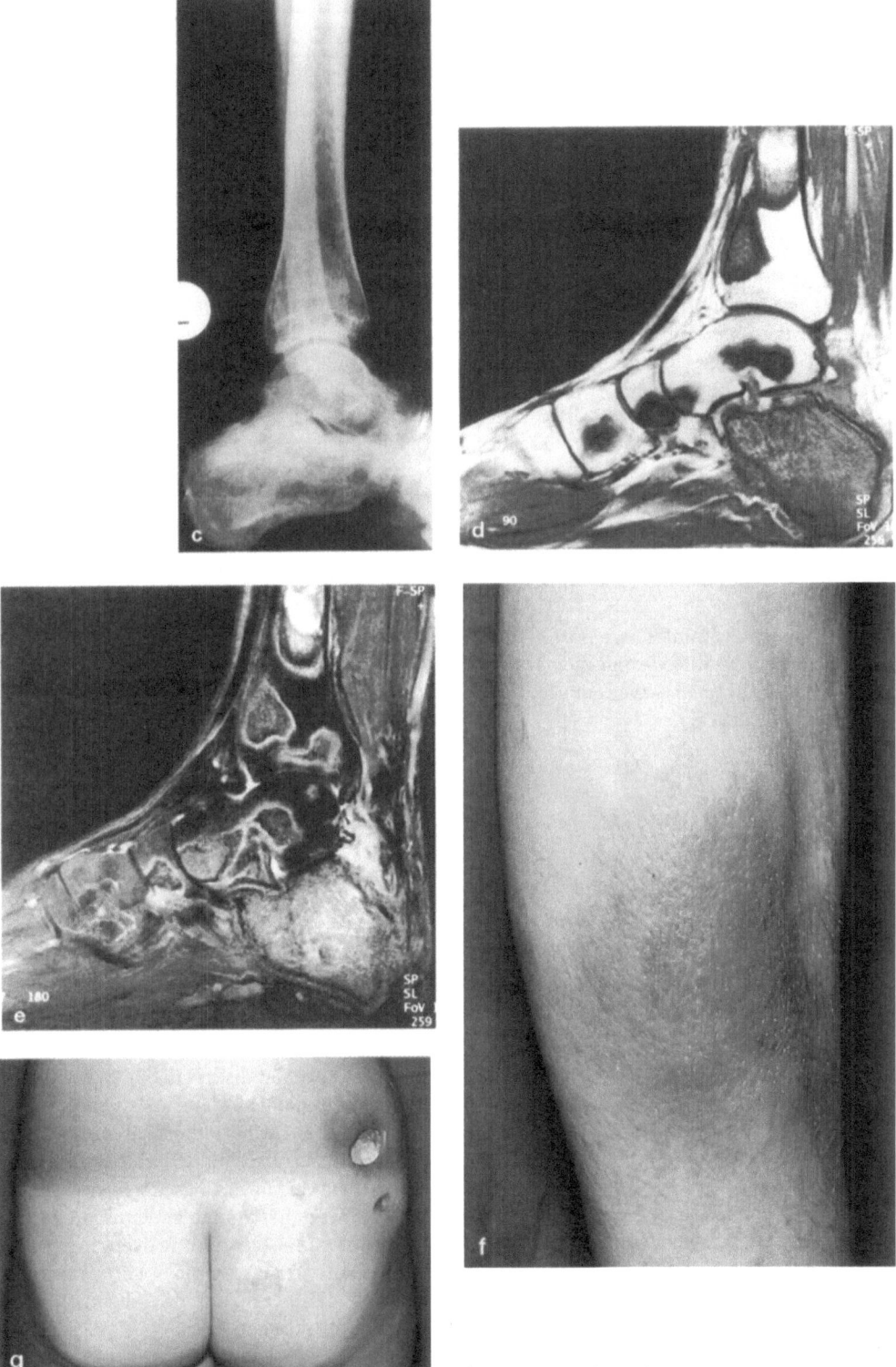

Fig. 8.4 c–g. See legend on p. 198

of the hands and feet. The symptoms are due less to synovitis than to the painful necrosis of juxta-articular fat.

The *radiographic features* of pancreatitic skeletal changes are very diverse (Fig. 8.4 a–e). *Small osteolytic lesions* may appear in the cancellous and cortical bone and may be mistaken for foci of plasmacytoma. Lytic lesions are most common at sites distal to the knee and elbow. Interestingly, these lesions are often located below areas of subcutaneous fat necrosis. Occasionally they are accompanied by *periosteal new bone formation*, simulating the appearance of osteomyelitis.

Other necrotic changes in the bone marrow consist of multiple *bone marrow infarcts*, appearing as a garland-like series of sclerotic islands in the bone marrow, usually centrally located and favoring the distal femoral and proximal tibial metaphyses. The infarcts are distinguished from calcifying enchondromas by their sclerotic margins (dystrophic calcification) and by the absence of lacunar erosions (scalloping) in the overlying cortex.

Besides bone marrow infarcts, a potential complication in patients with chronic recurring pancreatitis (especially when alcohol-induced) is *femoral head necrosis*.

References

Bennett R, Petrozzi J (1975) Nodular subcutaneous fat necrosis. Arch Dermatol 111: 896

Gibson TJ, Schumacher HR, Pascual E, Brighton C (1975) Arthropathy, skin and bone lesions in pancreatic disease. J Rheumatol 2: 7

Haller J, Greenway G, Resnick D et al. (1989) Intraosseous fat necrosis associated with acute pancreatitis: MR imaging. Radiology 173: 193

Radin DR, Colletti PM, Forrester DM et al. (1986) Pancreatic acinar cell carcinoma with subcutaneous and intraosseous fat necrosis. Radiology 158: 67

Simkin P, Brunzell J, Wisner D et al. (1983) Free fatty acids in the pancreatic arthritis syndrome. Arthritis Rheum 26: 127

Smukler N, Schumacher H, Pascual E et al. (1979) Synovial fat necrosis associated with ischemic pancreatic disease. Arthritis Rheum 22: 547

Tannenbaum H, Anderson L, Schur (1975) Association of polyarthritis, subcutaneous nodules, and pancreatic disease. J Rheumatol 2: 14

Wilson H, Askari A, Neiderhiser D et al. (1983) Pancreatitis with arthropathy and subcutaneous fat necrosis. Arthritis Rheum 26: 121

8.5 Interstitial Calcinosis

Interstitial calcium deposits may form in the setting of necrotic tissue changes, because necrotic soft tissue with an altered pH creates a potential "calcium sink." Cutaneous and subcutaneous necrosis can have many causes ranging from trivial trauma to vasculitis, especially in patients with collagen diseases. Cutaneous and subcutaneous calcium deposition can also have a biochemical cause: if the calcium – phosphate product is greater than 70, calcium phosphate will precipitate in the soft tissues, especially around vessels and joints and in the skin and subcutaneous tissues. This may occur in generalized osteopathies, primary and secondary hyperparathyroidism, or hypervitaminosis D. Conditions that promote the precipitation of other calcium compounds such as calcium carbonate or calcium oxalate can produce the same result.

The nomenclature of interstitial calcinosis is far from standard, especially in the fields of dermatology and osteology. Here we shall follow the international nomenclature and discuss several primary forms of calcinosis that generally are less well known than, say, secondary (symptomatic) interstitial calcinosis like that occurring in hypercalcemic states (metastatic calcinosis). It should be added that the morphologic manifestations of interstitial calcinosis in the skin and subcutaneous tissue are relatively uniform and are virtually the same for both the primary and secondary forms.

Circumscribed Calcinosis

The cause of this localized calcium deposition is unknown in about 60% of cases. The remaining 40% are referable to scleroderma, dermatomyositis, or a Raynaud disease (Thibièrge-Weissenbach syndrome). Laboratory tests show no abnormalities of calcium phosphate metabolism. Older women apparently are predisposed to circumscribed calcinosis (Fig. 8.5). Physical examination reveals hard granular deposits, visible as whitish areas beneath the thin overlying skin, located on one or more of the fingertips (acrocalcinosis). These calcium deposits may break through the skin and discharge a grayish-white "mushy" material.

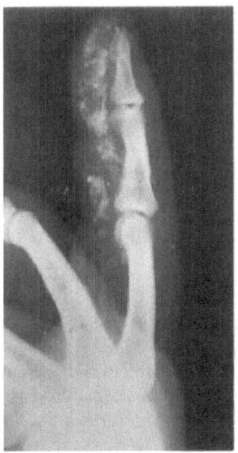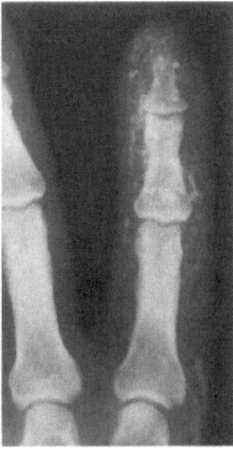

Fig. 8.5. Circumscribed calcinosis in the left index finger of a 48-year-old woman who was otherwise healthy. Pressure occasionally yielded a grayish-white "mushy" material

Universal Calcinosis

As with the localized form, the cause remains unknown in a large percentage of cases. Children and young adults are predominantly affected. From 30% to 40% of cases have a recognized association with a collagen disease (Thibièrge-Weissenbach syndrome, see Fig. 2.1 e, f). Laboratory findings are normal. The calcium deposits are widespread and consist of thin plaques of varying size and thickness in the skin and subcutaneous tissue (especially in pressure areas such as the fingertips, the soles of the feet, etc.). Calcifications are also found between deep muscle planes and in periarticular tissues. Secondary muscular atrophy and contractures with limb deformities may develop in severe cases. The dermatologic lesions consist of multiple calcium deposits in the form of hard white papules that frequently are surrounded by an inflammatory skin reaction. Plaquelike lesions also occur. The lesions may rupture and ulcerate much as in circumscribed calcinosis. Radiographically, the dermatologic lesions correlate with amorphous calcifications that may reach considerable size, especially in the subcutaneous tissue.

Tumoral Calcinosis

Tumoral calcinosis is a rare, often familial disorder that is associated with the formation of calcific masses, usually in periarticular soft tissues. Teutschländer described this entity in 1935, referring to it as "progressive lipogranulomatosis of muscle."

Pathologically, the early stage of the disease is marked by the formation of an initially soft and later firm soft-tissue mass that may attain a weight of 3–4 kg. Generally the mass is enclosed within a dense capsule, and it rarely infiltrates adjacent muscle or skin. The cut surface is yellowish or grayish-white and has a honeycomb appearance because of its multicystic structure. Some of the cysts are separated from one another by firm septa up to 2.5 cm thick. The cysts are filled with a white to grayish-white liquid or pasty material identified chemically as calcium phosphate and/or calcium carbonate. The term "lipogranulomatosis" is derived from the gross lipid deposits that are found in the cyst walls. Metaplastic ossification of the soft-tissue masses may occur.

The etiology and pathogenesis of tumoral calcinosis are not fully understood, but a familial aggregation has been confirmed. It is very common to find hyperphosphatemia in patients with normocalcemia and decreased renal phosphate excretion (Lufkien et al. 1980). But the hyperphosphatemia alone cannot explain why the calcific masses in tumoral calcinosis occur almost exclusively near large joints, especially the shoulder, hip, and elbow, and why calcium deposits do not occur in visceral organs or other soft-tissue structures.

Like universal calcinosis, the disease is most common in children and young adults (first and second decades), though any age group may be affected. Tumoral calcinosis differs from universal calcinosis in that calcium deposits do not often occur in the skin and subcutaneous tissue. When they do occur, the diseases are indistinguishable. The calcific masses cause little discomfort or disability. They rarely cause nerve compression and very rarely cause erosion of the underlying bone, but they do limit the mobility of the associated joint. Masses that break through the overlying skin create sinus tracts that may become infected. The overall rate of progression of the disease is very slow.

Classic tumoral calcinosis appears *radiographically* as a well-defined, multinodular calcified mass that most commonly occurs on the extensor side of large joints such as the hip, elbow, and shoulder. Other possible sites of occurrence are the gluteal region and thigh. Tumoral calcinosis apparently does not occur in the hand or about the knee. Bilateral occurrence is common. If the calcifications are still in a liquid state, fluid levels may be seen.

Martinez et al. (1990) described five cases in which tumoral calcinosis was combined with a *pseudoxanthoma elasticum-like syndrome* (degeneration of elastic connective-tissue fibers with calcium deposition in the skin, vascular calcifications and angioid streaks in the retina) and with patchy areas of bone marrow calcification in the long tubular bones and calvarium accompanied by periosteal new bone formation. Three of the patients were related to one another (all male, ages 10, 53, and 58). The other two patients, not related, were 30 and 77 years of age. In three patients the combinations were present in varying degrees, and two patients additionally had chondrocalcinosis or pseudogout. The bone marrow calcifications, which were clearly visible on CT scans and showed intense uptake on radionuclide scans, are also known as *diaphysitis*. Clarke et al. (1984) described diaphysitis based on the criterion of calcium deposits in large tubular bones in three hyperphosphatemic children. These patients also had pronounced periosteal changes simulating the appearance of osteomyelitis.

References

Bishop AF, Destouet JM, Murphy WA et al. (1982) Tumoral calcinosis: case report and review. Skeletal Radiol 8: 269

Clarke E, Swischuk LE, Hayden CK (1984) Tumoral calcinosis, diaphysitis, and hyperphosphatemia. Radiology 151: 643

Feldman ES, Dalinka MK, Schumacher HR (1981) Diffuse soft tissue calcification in tumoral calcinosis. Skeletal Radiol 7: 33

Harkess JW, Peters HJ (1967) Tumoral calcinosis. A report of six cases. J Bone Joint Surg Am 49: 721

Lufkin EG, Wilson DM, Smith LH et al. (1980) Phosphorus excretion in tumoral calcinosis: Response to parathyroid hormone and acetazolamide. J Clin Endocrinol Metab 50: 648

Manaster BJ, Anderson TD (1982) Tumoral calcinosis: serial images to monitor successful dietary therapy. Skeletal Radiol 8: 123

Martinez S, Vogler JB, Harrelson JM et al. (1990) Imaging of tumoral calcinosis: new observations. Radiology 174: 215

Sissons HA, Steiner GC, Bonar F et al. (1989) Tumoral calcium pyrophosphate deposition disease. Skeletal Radiol 18: 79

Teutschländer O (1935) Über progressive Lipogranulomatose der Muskulatur. Zugleich ein Beitrag zur Pathogenese der Myopathia osteoplastica progressiva. Klin Wochenschr 14: 541

8.6 Chromium and Nickel Allergy Due to Internal Fixation Material

The chromium-nickel-steel alloys that are used in internal fixation devices are subject to eventual corrosion in the physiologic milieu, causing chromium and nickel to be released into the tissues. When infection is present, this process is intensified. The incidence of allergic reactivity to these elements is approximately 2% in the absence of infection and slightly more than 10% in the presence of infection.

The skin may manifest typical chromium-nickel allergic reactions, which are ubiquitous and not localized to the skin over the internal fixation material. The dermatologic correlate is a more or less circumscribed eczema with disseminated foci.

References

Hierholzer S, Hierholzer G (1984) Metallallergie als pathogenetischer Faktor für die Knocheninfektion nach Osteosynthesen. Unfallheilkd 87: 1

Subject Index

Basic descriptive terms and their possible differential diagnostic relationships in dermatology and radiology are listed in the 'Tables of Differential Diagnoses', pp 4–12

---

[1] The page numbers printed in **bold italic** type refer to those pages dealing with the corresponding subject in depth.

Springer
and the
environment

At Springer we firmly believe that an
international science publisher has a
special obligation to the environment,
and our corporate policies consistently
reflect this conviction.
We also expect our business partners –
paper mills, printers, packaging
manufacturers, etc. – to commit
themselves to using materials and
production processes that do not harm
the environment. The paper in this
book is made from low- or no-chlorine
pulp and is acid free, in conformance
with international standards for paper
permanency.

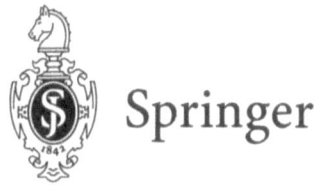 Springer